ADVANCES IN
DISEASE PREVENTION

Volume 1

ADVISORY BOARD

ADVANCES IN DISEASE PREVENTION

Volume 1

Charles B. Arnold, M.D., M.P.H.
Editor-in-Chief

Lewis H. Kuller, M.D., Ph.D.
Merwyn R. Greenlick, Ph.D.
Co-Editors

SPRINGER PUBLISHING COMPANY
NEW YORK

Springer Publishing Company, Inc.
200 Park Avenue South
New York, New York 10003

81 82 83 84 85 86 / 10 9 8 7 6 5 4 3 2 1

ISBN 0–8261–2830–0

ISSN 0277–0687

Printed in the United States of America

Contents

Contents

Contributors

Charles B. Arnold, M.D., M.P.H.
Mahoney Institute for Health Maintenance
American Health Foundation
New York, New York

Henry Blackburn, M.S., M.D., F.A.C.C.
Laboratory of Physiological Hygiene, School of Public Health;
Department of Medicine, School of Medicine
University of Minnesota

Nemat O. Borhani, M.D., F.A.C.C.
Department of Community Health
School of Medicine
University of California
Davis, California

Gilbert Botvin, Ph.D.
Department of Public Health
Cornell University Medical College
New York, New York

Allan L. Drash, M.D.
Division of Pediatric Endocrinology, Metabolism and Diabetes Mellitus
Children's Hospital of Pittsburgh

Howard A. Fishbein, Dr.PH
Diabetes Program
Rhode Island Department of Health
Providence, Rhode Island

Merwyn R. Greenlick, Ph.D.
Health Services Research Center
Portland, Oregon

Lewis H. Kuller, M.D., Ph.D.
Department of Epidemiology
Graduate School of Public Health
University of Pittsburgh

Norman L. Lasser, M.D., Ph.D.
College of Medicine and Dentistry of New Jersey
New Jersey Medical School
Newark, New Jersey

Arthur S. Leon, M.S., M.D., F.A.C.C., F.A.C.S.M.
Laboratory of Physiological Hygiene, School of Public Health;
Department of Medicine, School of Medicine
University of Minnesota

Alfred McAlister, Ph.D.
School of Public Health
Harvard University

Walter Rogan, M.D.
Department of Health and
Human Services
Public Health Service
National Institutes of Health;
National Institute of Environ-
mental Health Sciences
Research Triangle Park,
North Carolina

Introduction

The knowledge that is derived from science will always be the key to good preventive care. However, knowledge is time limited. In view of its changing character, it is essential that clinicians have available to them up-to-date scientific knowledge applicable to disease prevention. Progress in prevention at the population level will result, in large measure, from health care practitioners' greater familiarity with new findings about cause and prevention.

Because chronic disease prevention has become a popular topic in the United States in recent years, the public pressures for prevention services relative to chronic disease prevention have grown tremendously. Despite prevention's public popularity, the insurance industry as well as federal administrators and practitioners have often found chronic disease prevention a slippery concept, especially when the diseases are unspecified. Since the authors of this volume are practitioners as well as researchers, they are familiar with the dual problems of intellectually assessing new developments and putting them into clinical practice.

Advances in Disease Prevention highlights recent developments in science and clinical practice in chronic disease. In doing so, emphasis is placed in three main areas:

1. strategies and methods for the improvement of clinical disease prevention;
2. analyses of detailed knowledge regarding specific risk factors; the diseases for which they are applicable; and their most appropriate treatment;
3. reviews of developments in health protection, i.e., acceptable alteration of the physical environment to reduce populations' risks.

Clinical Methods

In this volume two chapters are concerned with clinical methodologies in disease prevention. The first, by Charles B. Arnold (Chapter 1,

Clinical Strategies for Chronic Disease Prevention: 1981) examines a number of fundamental precepts underlining the development of chronic disease preventive care. Historical aspects of disease prevention and the roles of epidemiology and causal reasoning are highlighted. The changing nature of patient/practitioner relationships with respect to chronic disease prevention strategies are analyzed from the perspective of the clinician's role in prevention. Chapter 1 sets forth issues, their background, and various methods that will shape the future of clinical practice in this area.

Merwyn R. Greenlick (Chapter 2, Helping Patients Achieve Risk-Reducing Behavior) has reviewed specific recent clinical methods in health behavior change that can assist clinicians to change unhealthy habit patterns in patients. In this chapter, Greenlick, who does research and practice in this problem area, discusses a number of important assumptions behind current methods that have significance for other practitioners. These assumptions include: (1) the need to gain patient adherence to behavior change methods; (2) techniques to gain their commitment to the adoption of new health practices; (3) implementing specific behavioral changes with patients; and (4) means by which changes can be maintained in the future.

Adult Risk Reduction

Nemat Borhani, (Chapter 3, Hypertension) observes that despite the impressive decline in mortality since 1968, the death rate associated with hypertensive disease remains high. Problems such as coronary heart disease, stroke, and congestive failure constitute major threats to community health. Borhani reviews the epidemiology of hypertension including its trends within different risk groups in American society. His discussion of etiologic factors in hypertension has an important relationship to treatment rationale. His authoritative review will be found useful for virtually all clinicians with responsibilities for hypertensive individuals. By providing an analysis of the results from the major clinical trials, including the recently concluded Hypertension Detection Follow-up Program, Borhani enables the reader to become thoroughly familiar with the most recent therapeutic concepts, including some methodological problems in the diagnosis, treatment, and maintenance of goal blood pressure values.

Perhaps, no subject has aroused more widespread public discussion concerning prevention than the role that physical activity may take in reducing the risk of coronary heart disease. In Chapter 4, Arthur Leon and Henry Blackburn carefully review the results of clinical and population research that can provide guidance to clinicians wishing to incorporate physical activity regimens into their practices. The authors discuss the limitations of exercise studies as well as the nature of cardiovascular, metabolic, and muscular adaptations to exercise. Their review of the metabolic effects of exercise on obesity, as well as the lipid and glucose metabolism, have inherent interest for all concerned with clinical care of physically active populations. The reader will discover that a number of Leon and Blackburn's recommendations can be relatively easily incorporated into current medical practice.

In Chapter 5, (Nutrition and Prevention of Coronary Heart Disease), Norman Lasser reviews the omnibus literature relating nutritional factors to the etiology and preventive therapy of atherosclerosis. The chapter proceeds from the epidemiologic evidence linking dietary fat, blood cholesterol levels, and transportation with the abundant epidemiological, clinical, and experimental evidence in this disease complex. In addition to reviewing the interstices of this important problem area, Lasser provides guidelines for the practitioner to modify food patterns for the purpose of achieving reduced serum cholesterol levels. An issue that has received much controversial attention in recent years is the relationship between dietary fat, cholesterol, and heart disease. In a thorough analysis, Lasser reviews the literature, its conclusions, and its practical implications for patient populations.

Childhood Cause and Prevention

The causes and prevention of cigarette smoking among children and adolescents is the subject of Chapter 6 by Gilbert Botvin and Alfred McAlister. This subject is of great importance and urgency with respect to the future of the nation's health. Of particular interest is the discussion of the factors contributing to the onset of cigarette smoking—familial, peer, and general societal pressures. Personality attributes and behavioral correlates that affect smoking behavior complete the review of causal considerations and lead to a detailed review of smoking prevention strategies for children. In this section of Chapter 6, clinicians can find considerable guidance for specific counseling and programming strategies to reduce the smoking rate among children. Recommendations are given for specific activities that can be undertaken by clinicians in schools, communities, and in research.

Research on the causes of childhood diabetes—an important but poorly understood disease of children—is the subject of Chapter 7 by

Howard Fishbein, Allen Drash, and Lewis Kuller. Because causal mechanisms for the metabolic disorders called juvenile diabetes have been illusive, the authors review the epidemiology, genetics, and the newest research on such markers as histocompatibility systems and the human leukocyte antigen (HLA). They also review several recent findings that link some juvenile diabetes to viral infections. While answers to this troublesome disease are not easily forthcoming, the authors conclude with possible pathophysiologic explanations for causal mechanisms.

Environmental Issues

Environmental and occupational health topics have received much attention in the nation's press as well as in the professional literature. Walter Rogan (Chapter 8) addresses the risks of disease caused by exposure to the toxic substances asbestos, lead, and halogenated hydrocarbons. For each substance, Rogan has reviewed the etiology, clinical diagnosis and management, and prevention aspects. Clinicians are told how to identify potential hazards as well as how to prompt earlier diagnosis and administer more effective treatment.

CHARLES B. ARNOLD, M.D., M.P.H.
MERWYN R. GREENLICK, PH.D.
LEWIS H. KULLER, PH.D.

CHAPTER 1

Clinical Strategies for Chronic Disease Prevention: 1981

CHARLES B. ARNOLD, M.D., M.P.H.

Over the past century American medicine and public health have gained remarkable control over communicable and deficiency diseases. Despite recent reductions in mortality rates for cardiovascular diseases, however, prevention strategies for the major chronic conditions have often seemed elusive. Nevertheless, recent optimism has been expressed about clinical strategies for prevention of cancer, heart disease, and other chronic illnesses (USDHEW, 1979b; Sheps, 1979; Stokes, 1979), which is based primarily on the growth of recent biological and behavioral scientific research that is applicable (International Agency for Research on cancer, 1979; Blackburn, 1979).

We are clearly in a state of transition concerning prevention of many chronic diseases. Not surprisingly, it is difficult to know the best measures to take. In this setting this chapter examines some origins of the current strategies for chronic disease prevention as they may apply to conventional clinical practice.

Disease prevention is probably best defined as a reduction in the number of new illnesses arising in a population during a specific time period. Decreases in new chronic illness rates are generally first recognized statistically, such as in the case of cardiovascular deaths, where a clear downward trend has been established since 1968 (USDHEW, 1977). Without understanding the precise mechanisms that have caused the reduction in cardiovascular disease deaths, it is likely that population changes in risk factors for this disease have produced this improvement (Beaglehole et al., 1979). Though it may be possible that improved survival of heart attacks has accounted for the lower death rates, a strong statistical case can be made for primary prevention practices of the American public as the basic cause. For example, butter consumption in the period 1963–1975 decreased by 32 percent, with animal fats and oils down by 57 percent and cigarette consump-

1

tion 22 percent (Levy, 1979; USDHEW, 1979a). These striking preventive practices have resulted from greater public awareness of cause and effect factors in heart disease. Further, it indicates enormous latent interest in millions to make and sustain lifestyle changes. Interestingly, no other Western industrialized country has experienced such a decrease in heart disease death rates, or a change in public consumption patterns of foods shown to be associated with hypercholesterolemia and heart disease risk (Stamler, 1979).

EVALUATION OF PREVENTION STRATEGIES

As the reduction in heart attack death rates illustrates, though the public's health may be improved by personal prevention practices, the biological mechanisms underlying the improvement may not be well understood. The example of the reduction in coronary heart disease death rate is not an isolated one, however. For nearly 30 years there has been a steady decrease in deaths from stomach cancer in the United States. There has been a decline, though smaller, in Japan. Dietary factors are hypothesized to be involved in these changes (Wynder and Hirayama, 1977). Typically, a disease like stomach cancer has multiple factors contributing to its causation, so that prevention strategies by necessity are often complicated to formulate. Epidemiological studies, however, have enabled us to grasp many of the fundamental interactions among the factors causing these diseases.

Classically, it is recognized that a combination of disease agents, susceptible populations, and appropriate environmental factors are necessary to produce changes in the health status of human groups. Because of the complex nature of epidemiological interactions, frequently prevention strategies derived from epidemiology may not fit intuitive formulations. For example, in 1855 when John Snow discovered that one of London's water supplies was contaminated with cholera, modern microbiology had not come into existence. Despite the lack of knowledge of the transmissibility of cholera through water supplies, Snow was, however, able to prevail on London's government at the time to close the affected water system (Snow, 1964).

Similarly, Goldberger's 1920 findings that pellagra was caused by deficiency in niacin-rich foods was a counterintuitive formulation at that time because most medical reasoning held that epidemic conditions resulted from communicable diseases (Terris, 1964). Deficiencies in micronutrients were not unknown in 1920 (e.g., scurvy and beri-beri were recognized deficiency conditions), but in the case of pellagra, relationship to a deficiency condition was unsuspected. When dramatic proof can be offered, such as the abrupt decrease in cholera incidence in London, or the recovery of pellagra cases, acceptance of counterintuitive prevention strategies usually occurs. In chronic diseases, however, the proof is expected to emerge more slowly.

With additional biological research, improvements in preventive methods can be expected, if the results can be applied clinically. For example, in the case of poliomyelitis immunization there was initial dependence on a heat-killed virus strain (Salk), but with subsequent development by Sabin of attenuated live virus, the former was clearly surpassed in preventive value. Occasionally, the transition from earlier methods to later, more specific ones may be slowed by controversy and lack of scientific consensus. Attempts to determine appropriate environmental standards for air and water pollution seem to exemplify such transition problems for chronic disease prevention in 1980.

In general, prevention is the most prudent approach to improving the public's health. In the case of the diet–heart hypothesis, stated acceptance of the scientific evidence seems to have proceeded more slowly among the researchers than it has among the public at large. Despite this apparent ambiguity, it appears that food product modification is well underway. Together with changes in food patterns, smoking habits, and hypertension control, risk reduction should continue for the foreseeable future. For these reasons, it seems that clinical disease prevention may have as marked an impact on the practice of medicine as Snow's and Goldberger's findings had on practitioners after 1855 and 1920. As noted earlier, emerging changes in prevention practice have often been initiated by epidemiological studies. Furthermore, these therapies have been evaluated using epidemiological methods. It seems useful to consider next the elements of epidemiology that have made possible the development of contemporary cause and prevention clinical practices.

EPIDEMIOLOGICAL STRATEGIES AND
DISEASE PREVENTION

Heart disease and cancer prevention was given valuable impetus from several epidemiologic studies begun between 1945 and 1955. Important among them were the coronary disease epidemiological surveillance projects begun in Framingham, Massachusetts, but later joined by comparable studies in Tecumseh, Michigan; Albany, New York; Chicago, San Francisco, and Los Angeles. Much of our understanding about heart disease risk came from them (Stamler, 1978). Ancel Keys' seven-country study of cardiovascular disease risk added a comparative international perspective that confirmed the American results (Keys, 1980). These studies eventually described the powerful independent statistical associations of cigarette smoking, elevated serum cholesterol, and hypertension on the development of heart disease. Subsequent clinical and experimental investigations have confirmed and extended these initial epidemiologic findings, and provided concepts for understanding the interaction of these three in the basic disease mechanisms (Lewis, 1979; Whissler, 1979).

More recently, epidemiological methods have been used to evaluate large clinical trials designed to extend the prevention hypothesis to applications at the clinical and population level. These contributions from epidemiology as illustrated by the causal research on atherosclerosis have been both conceptual and methodological.

Methodological Contributions

John Galbraith, the economist, is reported to have said that only through measurement of social problems can their existence and magnitude become recognized (Moynihan, 1968). Epidemiology has such a measurement role in public health and program evaluation. It tends to be diverse, ranging from statistical definitions of population at risk to complex multivariate analytical procedures designed to sort out confounding variables in causal research (Susser, 1973). Recent epidemiological studies of the potential impact of the food additive saccharine have illustrated this. Wynder, for example, has shown that to avoid confounding saccharine use among research subjects one must partial out the effect of certain personal consumption characteristics (Wynder and Stellman, 1980). For example, obese people, better educated persons, and Jews tended to use saccharine more frequently than other individuals. By using these variables in the analysis of the bladder cancer risk–saccharine use problem, it was found that a previous weak, statistical association between saccharine and bladder cancer virtually disappeared.

The integration of various epidemiological methods with metabolic studies enables scientists to infer causality. These relationships are further discussed later in this chapter in analyzing colon cancer risk and its research. The term *risk factor* from epidemiology has achieved veritable cornerstone status in designating the relationship between risk and disease causation. The term was coined by Stamler (1980) in 1958 and has been in common usage ever since.

Conceptual Epidemiological Contributions

Conceptually, epidemiology has enabled the health field to develop a clearer understanding of host-agent-environment interactions in chronic disease and injury causation. An example of this conceptual application was Haddon's finding that alcohol exposure, driver intoxication, and speeding interact in auto crash injury and death (Haddon, Suchman, and Klein, 1964). As derivatives of the agent-host-environment triad, four basic disease prevention strategies have emerged from epidemiology which indicate that risks can be reduced when one:

Increases individual resistance to the agent
Protects susceptible individuals from contact with the agent
Isolates the agent so that it cannot reach susceptible persons
Modifies the agent to reduce its injurious effects

Increase Personal Resistance to Disease

Immunizations and micronutrient supplements (e.g., addition of iron or thiamin to the diet) have long represented the prototype for strengthening individual resistance to disease. Most chronic diseases have causes that are too complex biologically to yield to a single clinical intervention, yet there are examples of important chronic conditions for which single factors have been used effectively. Dean (1949) showed the addition of one part per million fluoride to water supples markedly reduced tooth decay in treated populations. Another example was in Sweden, where the addition of micro-amounts of dietary iron to food suplies (particularly bread) resulted in the virtual eradication of Plummer-Vinson syndrome, a condition associated with a high incidence of oral cavity and upper gastrointestinal cancer (Waldenstrom, 1946). By way of contrast, in prevention of atherosclerosis and certain cancers, it is not deficiency per se, but moderation of dietary excess or substance abuse which may have the principal preventive effect—for example, obesity (overeating); smoking cessation for lung cancer, obstructive lung disease and peptic ulcer prevention; and moderation of alcohol intake for prevention of liver cirrhosis, acute pancreatitis, and various peripheral and central neurological diseases.

Protect Susceptible Persons from Agent

Prevention is not often considered a clinical management function, though protection of susceptible persons by physical measures is conventionally regarded as a prevention strategy. For example, in burn units, patients are routinely isolated to prevent infections. Comparably, renal dialysis units observe special hygienic procedures to limit infections. Control of hospital-type (nosocomial) infections have used special epidemiological methods to assist in their control. In injury prevention, auto seat belt restraints may also be regarded as a form of passive protection of drivers and passengers from risks of high-velocity impact-type auto crashes. In occupational health it is known that virtually everyone is susceptible to the pathological effects of certain toxic substances such as asbestos, benzidine, coke oven emissions, and uranium dust. Not only are specific industrial processes modified to reduce exposure to these agents, but industrial environments are now monitored to insure that when exposures do occur, concentrations are so low that disease risk is greatly minimized.

Isolate the Agent from Susceptibles

Toxic substances need to be kept away from workers and the public, particularly those work groups in which high exposure levels may occur. Potts (1975) first stated the principle in his paper identifying scrotal cancer risks in chimney sweeps, thus initiating industrial preventive carcinogenesis. Today's industrial processes with potential harmful emissions are isolated with special equipment to protect workers; e.g., machines admitting gamma or other ionizing radiation are specially covered, together with the provision of protective personal shields and certain technical procedures for radiologists and their technicians. In the plastics industries, vinyl chloride processes are now contained so that exposures have been limited to less than 30 ptm (time-weighted exposure), an 80 percent reduction since 1950 (Cralley and Atkins, 1975). Asbestos dust has been reported as decreased following improved industrial engineering (Gibbs and du Toit, 1979).

Modify the Agent to Reduce Risk

Few recent environmental challenges seem greater than those derived from risks associated with public exposure to products or services with potential pathological significance. The possible carcinogenicity of saccharine (bladder cancer) (Wynder and Weisburger, 1977), or low dosage radiation in mammography (breast cancer) (Jablon and Bailar, 1980) has received much recent public and scientific attention. There appears to be sizable public demand for safe artificial sweeteners, and a public health need for safer breast cancer detection means. The attempts to develop less harmful cigarettes in the past 20 years may be an example of a successfully modified product (Wynder and Stellman, 1977; Wynder and Hoffman, 1979). A recent paper by Auerbach reports a marked reduction in histopathological changes in the lungs of smokers since 1959 (Auerbach, Hammond, and Garfunkel, 1979). This report provides some optimism that product modification can be achieved when the scientific case is strong and public awareness is at a high level. Environmental manipulation, such as that described for cigarettes, often requires sophisticated engineering collaboration. The changes made in automobile design to protect passengers from crash injury, for example, padded dash boards, seat belts, and shatter-proof glass, are also illustrations of this principle.

The impact of scientific studies on diet and disease may also prove instructive concerning product modification. Changes in consumer preference patterns for foods low in fat and high in fiber are clearly illustrated in supermarkets as well as in the consumption patterns mentioned earlier. These changes represent substantial product modifications and altered public tastes, resulting in the eventual lower risk. Examples of these modifications include corn and sunflower oil margarines, egg substitutes, partial skim milk cheeses, and skim milk yogurts.

The choice of an appropriate prevention strategy often depends on practical contingencies. Some risk factors can be more easily managed clinically than others. For example, with existing methods, hypertension is more easily controlled than obesity. When the proven benefits seem to outweigh the cost, it is also easier to proceed with therapy. Where the general social desirability of risk reduction is preceived as high by the public, the development of programs is easier, too. Drug abuse education for children in schools has proceeded far more rapidly than other newer forms of health education because of the public's fears about drugs. In addition, the technology required to reduce risk must be widely available. For example, stroke prevention through hypertension control will undoubtedly enable it to continue to outpace other chronic disease prevention control efforts because of the widespread availability of hypertension services. Contingencies such as easy manageability, high social desirability, and availability of technology greatly constrain the structure of preventive medical services.

For public health reasons, prevention strategies are often initiated when it is easy to apply the recommended procedures. Fluoridating water for dental care prevention or mass immunizations for health care personnel under epidemic conditions are examples of relatively easy applicability. As time and technology change, preventive strategy previously held more difficult (e.g., smoking cessation) can gradually become more widely available. The rate at which constraints drop away cannot be easily predicted. Which of the four basic epidemiological strategies will prove most applicable in a specific occupational health problem may not always be clear. Often a combination of strategies is required. For example, in India the smallpox control program found that eradication could probably be achieved by systematic isolation of individual cases over the country with immunization of all village residents, when cases occurred (Henderson, 1976). These two steps (isolation, increasing resistance) have the effect of invoking a third: susceptible persons outside the involved village would be thereby protected from future potential smallpox contacts. The worldwide eradication of smallpox has been a remarkable public health achievement. It is interesting that the success of the smallpox prevention program was primarily based on the effectiveness of risk reduction strategies with epidemiological origins.

THE ROLE OF CAUSAL RESEARCH

Primary prevention requires the interruption of at least one part of a disease pathway starting from the earliest known biological stage. Once a disease is clinically detectable, interventions are referred to a secondary or tertiary prevention. In coronary artery disease, for example, the preclinical stage includes arterial plaque formation with repeated intimal injury stemming from proliferation of smooth muscle cells with lipid deposition. Eventual distortions in blood flow begin to occur with resulting disease symptomatology. Complications of plaque formation, such as erosion or hemorrhage, further alter the process and, together with thrombosis, are responsible for many of the acute syndromes attributable to coronary disease.

Interruption of these processes of frank reversal may well occur even in advanced stages, through dietary modification, blood pressure control, or smoking cessation. Regression of coronary lesions has been clearly shown in nonhuman primates. If these primary prevention efforts begin early in life, it may permanently prevent the occurrence of coronary heart disease. One program to promote prevention behavior in children is a research program at the American Health Foundation, entitled "Know Your Body." It is testing the effectiveness of a risk factor-oriented health education program designed to prevent coronary heart disease and tobacco-related cancers (Williams, Arnold, and Wynder, 1977). Preliminary results have been encouraging concerning the program's acceptance by children, teachers, and parents (Williams et al., 1979).

In all diseases, as scientific research progresses, consensus about disease causation emerges. In coronary heart disease, for example, general agreement about causation has occurred as scientific communication between relevant disciplines has demonstrated comparability in their investigative findings. Research in cancer also exemplifies this principle. Colon cancer research can be used to illustrate recent evolution of consensus on disease etiology. In the balance of this section we will examine the framework of scientific findings about environmental factors in colon cancer. The major sources of colon cancer research have been derived from:

Epidemiological investigations
Clinical studies
Animal experimentation

Epidemiologically, colon cancer is an important public health problem. Over 100,000 new cases have occurred in the United States recently with an overall mortality rate placing it second highest among all cancer sites in American men and women. Its incidence is low among populations consuming low-fat diets (Armstrong and Doll, 1975), primarily those peoples live in non-Western, non-industrialized societies.

Clinical studies of colon cancer patients have shown higher concentrations of bile acid metabolites and free cholesterol in the feces than in controls free of intestinal disease; colonic polyp cases have bile metabolite concentrations intermediate to cancer and normal controls. Further, it has been shown in clinical studies that concentrations can be modified in two ways: either by decreasing the fat content of the diet, or by increasing the fiber content (Watanabe et al., 1979).

Experimental animal studies have shown that rodents on high-fat diets are more susceptible to carcinogens acting primarily on the colon compared to rodents on normal animal chow; evidence from all three areas strongly suggests total fat in the diet as a promoting factor, with certain types of vegetable fiber having an apparent protective effect (Reddy et al., 1980).

To decide whether the extant research on a disease's etiology justifies causal inference (Susser, 1973) necessitates a careful examination of substantiating and refuting evidence. There are several criteria classically used to judge the extent to which causal mechanisms are understood:

> Biological plausibility of risk concepts
> Specificity of the findings for the given disease
> Significance level of the statistical results
> Consistency of findings among similar studies and between different fields
> . Temporal associations shown between exposure and disease onset
> Dose response relationships which correlate with disease severity

Let us use the example of colon cancer etiology to illustrate the formulation of a causation mechanism in anticipation of a primary prevention strategy. To do this we will examine epidemiological, clinical, and animal research findings within these six categories to demonstrate the scientific process in unraveling cause and prevention strategy in a complex disease.

Biological Plausibility

Since the colonic mucosa is in constant contact with fecal contents, it seemed reasonable that any putative carcinogens consistently present in the feces should be suspect. Since over 95 percent of fat is absorbed in the small intestine, it is likely that fat contributes indirectly to risk through a metabolic pathway.

Fecal bile, however, contains sterols whose biosynthesis is associated with dietary fat metabolism. Biochemically it has been shown that certain stool substances (presumably sterols) can be converted into reactive carcinogens in the gut.

Specificity

Animal models for colon cancer have been developed. Certain rodent strains when treated with a chemical carcinogen consistently develop colonic tumors. Increasing the total fat content of the animals' diet has significantly increased these tumor yields, thus confirming the epidemiological findings. In clinical studies it was further shown that colon cancer cases had higher levels of bile metabolites in their feces than normal controls. Fecal bile metabolite levels in persons with precancerous polyps were found to be intermediate between persons with cancers and healthy controls. Dietary fiber increases the water content of feces, which may dilute the concentrations of the suspected reactive carcinogens to relatively harmless levels. Further, there seemed to be no other colonic condition which might be caused by fat in the diet which in turn might confound the noted relationships.

Consistency

The findings to date appear consistent among all the major studies, including additionally Japanese migrants and Seventh Day Adventists. The close agreement among animal, clinical, and population studies also strengthens the fat–cancer hypothesis.

Significance

The level of statistical significance in the various studies strongly confirms the hypothesis as well.

Temporal Associations

The timing of onset of cancers in experimental animals is also consistent with the hypothesis. The trend toward increased colon cancer in Japanese immigrants to the United States over two to three generations is consistent with current concepts of environmental carcinogenesis; e.g., a gradual Westernization of the migrants' diet with its higher fat content.

Dose Response Relationship

The proportion or quality of dietary fat calories is not known to increase the risk of colon cancer. Whether, for example, a threshold for fat intake exists beyond which cancer is promoted remains unknown in 1980. Clearly, native Japanese whose diet contains about 8–10 percent fat calories have dramatically lower colon cancer death rates than their American relatives on a higher fat diet.

Summary

There is a strong association between dietary fat and colon cancer, derived from animal, clinical, and epidemiological studies. While a causal relationship is apparent, the biological mechanism by which dietary fat contributes to risk is not yet well understood, though it apparently involves bile metabolites. The proportion and kind of dietary fat calories responsible for increased risk is unclear; however, epidemiological migration studies suggest it is lower than the current American level (38 percent). Accordingly, it seems reasonable to encourage all individuals, particularly those in families with colon cancer histories, to reduce their dietary fat intake through consultation with a nutritionist. The causal reasoning from the scientific evidence warrants this recommendation.

PRIMARY PREVENTION STRATEGY

For primary prevention of chronic disease to succeed, high-risk persons must become known to themselves and to a therapist. Screening of asymptomatic persons for risk factors is the only feasible means to make such identification. From a cost-effective standpoint, it needs items with likelihood of clinical results (Kristein, 1977). These should include most of the following: personal history (demographics, occupational exposures, medical and familial health), health-related behaviors (eating pattern, smoking, alcohol, licit and illicit drugs, physical activity), and a mini-exam (height, weight, blood pressure, and total serum cholesterol). Many clinicians become discouraged because a seemingly sizable percentage of persons may not be ready to participate. Moreover, high-risk persons may not want to reduce their risk, and dropouts in treatment occur. It becomes important to anticipate and plan for varying levels of motivation.

One rule of thumb developed at the American Health Foundation can be used to estimate the proportion of any group that would participate in a prevention program. Called the "rule of halves," it states: half a population will participate in a screening when offered; half the high-risk persons identified will want to start in an intervention program; about half those starting intervention programs will reach a predetermined goal. Through repeated application, the rule has been found applicable during 1976–1980. The rule of halves is based on several assumptions; for example, the initial motivation of the population is not extremely positive or negative; any advance educational program used before the program starts has a positive effect, but lasts only one to two weeks; the experience and skill of the professional staff is good, but not exceptional; and the cost structure (fees or payments) is appropriate to the specific situation.

This rule has been found to apply rather well to observed averages in screening, starting, and maintaining risk reduction therapy, such as cigarette smoking cessation and weight and cholesterol reduction. Hypertension control, however, tends to get better continuous participation than 50 percent, whereas physical activity programs have had a much higher dropout rate. Moral: at a given time only part of a population is usually ready for change. Of the remainder, it is probable that some may never change. Beyond initial participants, the more important other group, though, consists of those who may want to wait until "a better time" to initiate change.

To start primary prevention programs in a clinical setting, it is essential to accept the inevitability of this differential participation behavior. With this perspective, developing a clinical strategy for disease prevention can be made simpler from screening to follow-up.

An algorithm for a clinical prevention strategy which incorporates the rule of halves is shown in Figure 1-1. In this schema, a population can be subdivided into several groups depending on their response to the specific phase of the program: risk identification, risk reduction, or follow-up. Particular importance is attached to the four nonparticipation branches that derive from the individuals' initial motivation level. This is intended as a positive approach. That is, one's first tendency may be to count the dropouts and decry prevention. This strategy urges maximum attention be given the ongoing participants. Nonparticipants, however, would not be ignored, but rather systematically recontacted after an appropriate time interval to determine their readiness for screening at a later date. In this way those who have the most readiness for primary prevention assistance are served first.

Experience at the American Health Foundation has shown this strategy to bring results. Participant involvement tends to have a "ripple effect." That is, though the risk reduction services may begin with a few individuals, others will soon learn of the services through "innovators," participants whose behavior sets trends for other members. Cigarette smoking cessation provides a good example. The current 30 percent reduction in adult smoking in the United States has not occurred evenly across educational and sex groups. Well-educated men, for example, have a decidedly higher quit rate than men who are high school drop-

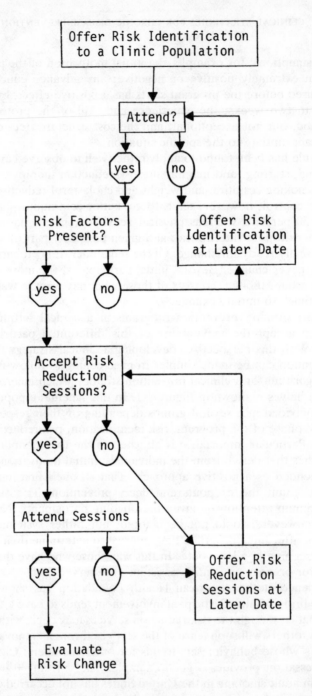

Figure 1-1. Algorithim for risk identification, treatment, follow-up of a clinic population with options for nonparticipants.

outs, a change that has occurred in the past 15 years. Though men's reported reasons for quitting vary, these college educated men have been the most responsive group thus far among Americans. No educational trend yet exists among women, however. According to sociological concepts, one can expect the personal influence of early primary prevention adopters (e.g., educated men) to affect others (i.e., other men, and women). In this volume, Merlyn Greenlick extensively discusses these concepts and their application to risk reduction.

Systematic screening of large numbers of healthy persons is not within the realm of most clinical practices, although specialized centers for screening have existed for several years. Furthermore, periodic executive examinations have become an established part of corporate health programs, though these services have not included follow-up care when risk factors are identified. These screening efforts have tended to remain separate from most community clinical care and have rather narrowly defined corporate persons eligible for them. Office-based prevention presents certain organizational problems too. For example, periodic screening requires special efforts to organize clinical records so that clerical staff can follow up the various groups delineated in Figure 1-1. It is beyond the intended scope of this chapter to discuss organizational systems for prevention because of their scope and complexity. Regrettably, there are virtually no references on this subject in the literature at this time.

When focused screening occurs in conjunction with planned interventions, an unparalleled opportunity arises for a clinical program to improve the health of a patient population. Through the development of practice-based prevention programs, clinicians can play a direct role in reducing risk factors for several major causes of death for which risks are well established, e.g., myocardial infarction and hemorrhagic stroke (hypertension control); lung cancer, sudden death, and chronic obstructive lung disease (cigarette smoking cessation); auto crash injury; cirrhosis of the liver, central and peripheral neuropathic diseases (alcohol abuse).

CLINICAL MANAGEMENT STRATEGIES
FOR PREVENTION

The contrasts between clinical management of asymptomatic high risk persons and symptomatic patients are substantial, when fully considered. The two key initial issues for practice-based prevention programs—health education and personal motivation for change—are different for well people than for the sick. Though these differences appear obvious, they are worth reviewing briefly. Previous clinical training and experience may create difficulties in preventive care for the unsuspecting clinician. Because of the sick person's symptoms (e.g., pain), therapeutic compliance can be assumed to be virtually complete, at least until the acute phase has subsided. No such easy assumption can be made with the well person. If one contrasts four fundamental clinical strategies, these issues may become clearer: (1) role of pharmacological agents; (2) compliance with a standardized regimen; (3) therapeutic latitude permitted patients; and (4) patient–therapist relationship (see Table 1-1).

Pharmacologic methods are an indispensable part of sickness care, but play a minor role in disease prevention, except for hypertension therapy. In general, however, new behaviors rather than drugs are used in preventive care. This difference necessitates a less standardized form of treatment and certain changes in therapeutic style which become clearer when compliance is considered.

Compliance and adherence in standardized treatment regimens. The

Table 1-1
Comparison of Selected Basic Elements of Medical and Behavioral Change Models in Prevention

	Medical-Therapeutic	Behavioral Change
Involves pharmacological methods	usually	rarely, except hypertension control
Strict adherence to clinical protocol, a key factor in therapy	yes	no
Patient can help determine best therapeutic approach	rarely	often
Patient-therapist relationship		
• length of time	usually short term	often lengthy
• degree of patient dependence	high degree	independence encouraged early
• who solves most problems	therapist	patient, with assistance from therapist
• symptoms present	often	rarely

greater the extent that disease processes are scientifically understood, the more specific therapies usually become. This is true for prevention as well as treatment. While there may be controversy over the precise individual benefits of habit modifications, e.g., smoking or overeating, it is generally agreed that the public health would be greater without either habit. This assumption would be equally true for well or sick individuals. The problem exists at the next level: prescribing a specific individual management for such habits.

Standardization of preventive care (e.g., for treatment of overeating disorders) does not exist. In all likelihood it may never be present in the form associated with most disease care therapies (e.g., management of peptic ulcer, or surgical approaches to inguinal hernias). In most instances, despite the range of choices available to the clinician, the treatment decisions in acute care are made exclusively by the therapist. While a partnership exists, the active part is taken by the clinician in initiating care for an acute pathological process. The information needed to manage disease treatment is complex, not easily comprehended by the patient, especially under the anxiety often accompanying acute illness, and is usually coupled with the problems in understanding medical care organizations.

In long-term therapies like habit modification, the underlying organic pathology is also complex, but the individual's capacity to participate may be enhanced if there are lower anxiety levels and a relative ease with which the therapy can be understood by the patient (e.g., modifying an eating pattern, the need to take medication, or smoking cessation). While these conditions may be favorable to the participant, this is offset by uncertainties associated with clinical management of behavioral change. Regrettably, simple formulas cannot be readily applied. Human behavior is simply too varied. As a result, so-called multi-component therapies have been developed. Cafeteria-like in style, participants can select the habit change method(s) that suit them. Intellectually this situation is interesting because the patients may be more active than the clinician, selecting methods through trial and error or by personal preference. Once committed to changing, participants' involvement can be intense. Though in a different role than for disease care, the therapist remains a key figure by offering guidance toward those methods most likely to be suitable. Because persons differ in intellectual style and behavior, patience may be required while participants experiment with methods. In all, latitude is increasingly given to the participants. Adherence to therapy gradually becomes relative to the individual's stated goals.

Therapeutic Autonomy

In most disease care situations, therapists unilaterally determine the best clinical management, and patients are given limited latitude, if any, to individualize the treatment. There are some exceptions. It is widely recognized among physicians, for example, that patients with certain chronic diseases, (e.g., bronchial asthma, gout, psoriasis, peptic ulcer, and arthritis) often become very skillful in making periodic modifications in their drug therapy in order to control exacerbation. In general, however, the therapist's management is not questioned.

In disease prevention, participants' therapeutic autonomy, especially in timing and pacing, is essential and not the exception (e.g., control of behaviors such as obesity, tobacco use, alcohol and other substance abuse, or attending prenatal clinics and following immunization schedules). The optimum management of behavior in clinic situations strives for participants gradually to accept control with therapeutic guidance from the clinician. Some clinicians find behavioral counseling for prevention difficult because the independence needed for patient control alters the usual clinical relationships.

Patient–Clinician Relationship

When patients are given greater autonomy in prevention, such as modifying unhealthy behaviors like overeating or tobacco use, a change is necessitated in the accepted patient–therapist interactions. At least four important attributes characterize the relationship difference between most disease treatment and preventive care:

The time span may be lengthy (years)
The condition is usually asymptomatic, thus the patient always feels "well"
The patient may choose the methods to be used
The clinician gradually shifts from therapist to a consultant role

As a result of these changes in the relationship, the patient becomes more adept at assuming responsibility for life-long care. The clinician's role, in turn, increasingly becomes consultative for new problems or for future disease care needs that arise independently.

PREVENTION STRATEGY FOR
CHRONIC DISEASES

Sir George Pickering (1978) has pointed out that it is hard to make an asymptomatic person feel better. This challenge applies to most initial chronic disease prevention efforts, that is, how to motivate people who feel well, but who also have measurable risk (e.g., hypertension or hyperlipidemia). Further, persons who have practiced primary prevention for years cannot be certain whether their health practices were responsible for their good health or whether they were the product of sheer luck, heredity, or other factors. Thus, health gains made by specific individuals are virtually impossible to establish. Often at a population level it is known only by changes in mortality or morbidity rates.

What are the differences between prevention service users and nonusers? Commitment to a healthy lifestyle and motivation are clearly a major (though not exclusive) part of the answer. To the extent that one can promote commitment and enhance motivation, these become the clinician's first prevention responsibility. These tasks may be frustrating, unless one recognizes the process involved. Let us briefly consider it. Interest may have been aroused in the participant before the first clinical encounter. If so, this makes the subsequent work easier. Increasingly, persons first learn of their possible risk from the media, notices at school, work, or through a community center (e.g., immunization bulletins, National High Blood Pressure Education Program). While the numbers of such persons are increasing in frequency, such established commitment probably represents but a small fraction of the total population encountered clinically, perhaps 10 percent. Most often the issue of preventive care must first be raised by the clinician. From population surveys it is reported that most people want their clinicians to broach the subject of prevention. For example, approximately 70 percent of smokers report that though they wanted their physicians to mention smoking cessation to them, it had not occurred.

In reviewing an individual's history, the familial disease pattern may also provide a motivational opportunity (e.g., relatives with early coronary heart disease, certain cancers, stroke, and chronic obstructive lung disease). Adults in such families have probably witnessed these conditions. If so, they may not require detailed explanations of the health consequences, when preventive care is indicated. Of particular interest are younger children in these high-risk families, for whom antismoking and nutrition education may have major disease-sparing effects later in life.

As useful as identifying high-risk families may be, most estimates place the total of such persons in the United States with familially associated disorders at less than 5 percent of the population, compared to 65 percent of the population that die from coronary heart disease, cancer, and stroke mainly due to environmental factors. The specificity of the long-term beneficial effects of lifestyle change are not yet known. It is presumed that many future coronary heart disease, lung cancer, and stroke deaths can be prevented (e.g., through smoking cessation, blood pressure control, and dietary modification), if persons make appropriate modifications early in life. As risk reduction technology improves, the behavioral change results will improve. It is important to help patients select reasonable personal goals, reflecting the state of the art. Table 1-2 summarizes five selected behavioral change goals, and reasonable targets of each, based on current chronic disease prevention technology. Indicative of the rate of change in this field, it is noteworthy that the key work in behavioral medicine has occurred recently (Pomerlau, 1979). This acceleration of interest in this field augurs well for the future.

Setting Individual Goals

Inevitably one is asked by patients how much weight to lose, how much reduction in serum cholesterol or blood pressure must one strive for? Despite the spate of efforts to reduce preventive care into simple formulas such as crash diets, physical activity, holistic medicine, or risk-appraised systems, clinically determined risk continues to be an inexact science. Further, there are only a few diseases that merit the efforts required of patient and clinician for preventive therapy: those conditions with high incidence rates in the population. Here one refers to the major causes of morbidity and mortality in America:

Coronary heart disease (angina pectoris, myocardial infarction, sudden death)
Stroke
Lung cancer
Colon cancer
Breast cancer
Automobile crashes
Cirrhosis of the liver

Table 1-2
Chronic Disease Risk Reduction Goals for Clinical Prevention

Risk Factor	Target Level	Estimated Proportion of Individuals Who Can Achieve Target	Comments
Cigarette Smoking Cessation	Zero Cigarettes Per Day	35-70%	Technology is improving rapidly
Smoking Prevention	Zero Cigarettes Per Day	90-95%	Methods are still developing, early results are promising (see Botvin and McAlister in this volume).
Hypertension Medication Adherence	Goal Blood Pressure (<90mm Hg)	80%+	Stepped care approach best published results (see Borhani, this volume).
Weight Control	<110% Ideal Body Weight	—	A frustrating area, but good results have been increasingly reported
Low-Fat Food Pattern	10-20% Reduction in Low Density Lipoprotein Cholesterol (<140mg%)	35%	A complex nutritional counseling problem, but knowledge/methodology greatly improved.

In addition to their high incidence and death rates, those conditions have in common a set of preventive measures which, regardless of present limitations, are undoubtedly cost-effective (Kristein, 1977). Table 1-3 summarizes the risk factors for these eight diseases. it is noteworthy that the five risk reduction measures mentioned earlier are so prominent in their association with these leading causes of death:

Smoking cessation
Blood pressure control
Dietary change
Seat and shoulder (auto) restraints
Alcohol abuse control

For complex reasons (e.g., long disease latent periods, inadequate noninvasive diagnostic techniques, fallibility of current behavioral methods, and insufficient number of prevention therapists) the complete prevention of these diseases may never occur; however, reduction in their age-adjusted incidence is highly likely. Scientifically speaking, the causal evidence for those risk factors meets almost all the conditions for causal reasoning.

In the United States a major gap in clinical prevention programs stems from deficiencies in health profession's education and training. It is hoped that resolution can occur through a combination of undergraduate, residency, and continued professional education. While it is clear that clinical prevention goals are generally accepted (i.e., reduction in risk and in disease incidence), what remains is the development of better methods, trained personnel, and the supporting resources to accomplish the task.

Behavioral Contracting

It is widely recognized that patients frequently fail to follow treatment management schedules. There have been various explanations offered for this seeming paradox, none wholly satisfactory. Among the better accepted is that patients may not have been given an explanation of their care which fitted their frame of reference. As a result, though they may have behaved rationally according to their beliefs, they erred with respect to current treatment precepts.

One way to counteract this problem has been the advent of the behavioral contract as a clinical management tool (Mahoney and Thoresen, 1974; Thoresen and Mahoney, 1974). The contract represents an

Table 1-3
Risk Reduction Measures, Primary and Secondary Prevention, for Eight Major Diseases

Condition	Primary Prevention		Secondary Prevention	Comments
	Risk Factors	Target Level		
Coronary Heart Disease (CHD)	Decrease dietary fat	Serum cholesterol <220mg%		Saturated fat decrease primary dietary goal. Blood pressure target from clinical trial result.
	Blood pressure	Diastolic <90mmHg		
	Smoking Cessation	Abstinence		
Stroke	Blood pressure control	Diastolic <90mmHg		(see CHD note above)
Lung Cancer	Smoking cessation	Abstinence	—	
Colon Cancer	Decrease dietary fat	Clinical marker not available	Stool occult blood	Total fat decrease is dietary goal. Cost effectiveness limited to persons over 55 years
Breast Cancer	First relative with breast cancer	—	Breast self-examination	
Automobile Crashes	Seat and shoulder restraints	Use	—	Period of abstinence before driving may vary, one hour is minimum
	Alcohol abuse	Abstinence over one hour for drivers		
Cirrosis of Liver	Alcohol abuse	Low intake through-out life	—	Dose-response relationship not quantified.
Cervix Cancer	—		Cervical Smear	

23

agreement stated in the patient's words, making a commitment to a specific regimen. The contract is usually prepared jointly with the therapist. It provides patients an opportunity to state in writing their comprehension of the therapy and their role in it. Past treatment adherence errors by patients have often resulted from overly optimistic assumptions by clinicians about patients' understanding of medication schedules, dosages, food patterns, or other procedures. Contracting appears broadly applicable to clinical therapy. Where behavioral contracts have been used, patient–therapist relationships have been reported enhanced and therapeutic response improved. When a treatment problem involves a habit change, as needed in chronic disease prevention, a contract enables the therapist to educate the patient about their mutual responsibilities in the therapy. Behavioral contracts for medication adherence have been successfully tried in several studies of hypertensive patients to promote better control of blood pressure. Uniformly, the results of such studies have been encouraging.

Six steps in contracting appear necessary to make it work well. Each can be undertaken without prior experience in such contracts and can be managed relatively easily either in groups or individually.

1. Set a Goal. A goal can be any endpoint that the therapist and patient agree upon as desirable. To be effective, a goal needs to be expressed in behavioral terms, i.e., "take medication twice a day," "eat only at mealtime," "don't smoke for 48 hours," and so forth.

2. Self-monitor. Here the patient is instructed to keep a careful record for a period of time (e.g., a week) of the particular behavior. Notes should be kept of the occasions on which it was easy and when difficult to comply. If the person is capable and motivated, the self-monitoring may include a variety of behaviors and their associated social-environmental influences.

3. Assess. It is recommended that self-monitoring data be assessed by clinician and patient together in order to determine which aspects of behavior (e.g., overeating) can be changed. This is a critical stage. The behavioral targets are best set within the person's attainment, or else discouragement ensues. Because clinical indicators are available for most behavioral endpoints (e.g., carbon monoxide in exhalated air; or weight change for obesity), it becomes a simple matter each visit to assess the patient's progress. As a result of this process, goals can be modified periodically, depending on the rate of change made (e.g., the time to reach a goal can be lengthened, if progress has been slower than initially planned).

4. Decide on Appropriate Behavior Change. After assessment, the decision about changing the particular behavior should be completely made by the patient. In practice it is a joint decision because the patient's enthusiasm for change often requires some realistic tempering. To be successful in treatment, some persons, for example, need highly structured activity patterns, while other patients strenuously resist excessive structure. Some gentle questioning often reveals what a given individual's personal style can best accept.

5. Implement Contract. On a regularly scheduled basis the patient should revisit the clinician for feedback and appropriate therapeutic modifications, particularly needed in food pattern management. The strength of the behavioral contract lies in the ease with which a clinical assessment can be made at a revisit. Because the behavioral goals are usually well understood, the consultation can be problem-centered. Consultations clearly focused on the patient's needs build confidence in the clinician and the therapeutic process.

6. Make a Personal Evaluation. Throughout the behavioral contract process, data are provided the patient. Regardless of baseline clinical values in primary prevention, the emphasis is most effectively placed on the self-awareness of risk. Progress toward the goal, as measured by specific results, needs to be interpreted with encouragement and sympathy. Some individuals can seemingly make no progress by external criteria for weeks or months, yet suddenly make major changes. Clinical data must always be judiciously interpreted in behavior change.

FAMILY INVOLVEMENT IN PREVENTION

Even casual examination of the risk factors in Table 1-3 underscores the familial aggregations of risk that occur in many chronic diseases. Put simply, health habits tend to cluster in families; for example, each of the following has such aggregations: cigarette smoking, obesity, high-fat food patterns, elevated serum cholesterol levels, physical inactivity, hypertension, and alcohol abuse. Such lifestyle risk factors are probably transmitted from parents to children through social conditioning, not by genetic mechanisms. From a therapeutic perspective, however, they can seem almost as deeply rooted. To complicate matters, there seem to be interactions between certain habits and phenotypic patterns that may increase risk in certain individuals (e.g., diabetic familial history and obesity, chronic obstructive lung disease history in the family and cigarette smoking).

Behaviorally, smokers seem less likely to quit permanently when their mates smoke and do not quit too. When both parents smoke, their offspring become cigarette smokers four times more often in childhood than children of nonsmoking parents. These relationships also apply to diet. Not only is the trend in obesity a familial one, but it has been shown that weight loss programs are most successful when both spouses participate (Brownell, 1980).

In addition to total calories, fat content of family diets may also contribute to children's subsequent heart disease risk (Williams and Wynder, 1976). Blood cholesterol (Kristein, 1977) and blood pressure (Miall, 1977) have both been shown in twin studies to suggest that environmental as well as genetic factors play a role in their metabolic control, an observation important to recall when families' health status is reviewed clinically. Alcohol abuse has well-known tendencies to family aggregations, although the evidence tends to be somewhat more ambiguous than with obesity, cholesterol, smoking, or blood pressure.

The clinical importance of family history in certain diseases (e.g., see Table 1-3) necessitates a careful review be made with each parent of young children. These adults should probably be given high priority in family health care, when primary precaution is practiced. Young people such as school children should be made the objects of special efforts to reduce future risk through school, community groups, recreation programs, and other institutions with which they affiliate. Health and medical professionals can take important community leadership roles in nonclinical educational activities whose goals are to increase public awareness of risk factors. Several authors in this volume have given children's preventive care special attention.

From a preventive care perspective, these family aggregations of risk create a special responsibility and opportunity for preventists. The family history can become a powerful tool in identifying high-risk persons, thereby promoting health enhancement.

REFERENCES

American Cancer Society: *Cancer Facts*. New York City, 1979.

Armstrong, B., and Doll, R.: Environmental factors and cancer incidence and mortality in different countries with special reference to dietary factors. *Interntl. J. Cancer* 15:617–631, 1975.

Auerbach, Oscar, Hammond, E.C., and Garfunkel, L.: Changes in bronchial epithelium in relation to cigarette smoking, 1955–1964 vs 1970–1977. *N. Engl. J. Med.* 300:381–386, 1979.

Beaglehole et al.: Serum cholesterol, diet, and the decline in coronary heart disease mortality. *Prev. Med.* 8:538–547, 1979.

Blackburn, Henry: Preventive cardiology in practice, in M. Pollock and D. Schmidt, editors, *Heart Disease and Rehabilitation*. Boston: Houghton Mifflin, 1979, pp. 245–275.

Brownell, Kelly: *The Partnership Diet Program*. New York: Rawson Loade, 1980.

Cralley, L.V., and Atkins, P.R.: *Industrial Environmental Health*. New York: Academic Press, 1975, pp. 280–281.

Dean, H.T.: Fluoride: Water-born fluorides and dental, in W.J. Delton and J.M. Wisam, editors, *Dentistry in Public Health*. Philadelphia: W.B. Saunders, 1949.

Gibbs, G.W., and du Toit, R.S.J.: Environmental considerations in surveillance of asbestos miners and millers. *Ann. N.Y. Acad. Sci.* 330:163–178, 1979.

Haddon, William, Suchman, E.A., and Klein, D.: *Accident Research: Methods and Approaches*. New York: Harper and Row, 1964, pp. 172–184.

Henderson, Donald: The eradication of smallpox, *Sci. Am.* 235:25–33, 1976.

International Agency for Research on Cancer: *Carcinogenic Risks: Strategies for Intervention*. Lyon, France, 1979.

Jablon, S., and Bailar, J.C.: The contribution of ionizing radiation to cancer mortality in the United States. *Prev. Med.*, 9:219–226, 1980.

Keys, Ancel: *Seven Countries: Death and Coronary Heart Disease*. Cambridge: Harvard University Press, 1980.

Kristein, Marvin M.: Economic issues in prevention. *Prev. Med.* 6:252–264, 1977.

Levy, Robert I.: Congressional Testimony, May 22, 1979 on Heart Disease: Public Health Enemy No. 1. Subcommittee on Nutrition, U.S. Senate Committee on Agriculture, Nutrition, and Forestry. U.S. Government Printing Office, Washington D.C., p 39, 1979.

Lewis, Barry: Clinical-pathological section, conference on the health effects of blood lipids. *Prev. Med.* 8:679–714, 1979.

Mahoney, M.J., and Thoresen, C.E.: *Self Control: Power to the Person*. Monterey: Brooks/Cole, 1974.

Miall, W.E.: Genetic considerations concerning hypertension, in H.M. Perry and W.McF. Smith: Mild hypertention: to treat or not to treat. *Ann. N. Y. Acad. Sci.* 304:18–25, 1977.

Moynihan, D.P.: Foreword, in Heer, D.M.: *Social Statistics and the City*. Cambridge: Harvard University Press, p. iii, 1968.

Pickering, George, in H.M. Perry and W.McF. Smith: Mild hypertention: to treat or not to treat. *Ann. N. Y. Acad. Sci.* 304:466–471, 1978.

Pomerlau, Ovid: Behavioral medicine: The contributions of experimental analysis of behavior to medical care. *Am. Psychologist* 34:654–663, 1979.

Potts, P.: *Chirurgical Observations Relative to the Cataract, the Polypus of the Nose, the Cancer of the Scrotum, the Different Kinds of Ruptures, and the Mortification of the Toes and Feet*. London: Hawes, Clarke, and Collins, 1975.

Reddy, Bandaru, Cohen, Leonard A., McCoy, David, Hill, Peter, Weisburger, John H., and Wynder, Ernst E.: Nutrition and its relationship to cancer. *Adv. Cancer Res.*, 1980.

Sheps, C.: Preventive medicine. *JAMA*, 241:1384–1385, 1979.

Snow, John: *Snow on Cholera*. New York: Hafner, 1964.

Stamler, Jeremiah: Public health aspects of optimal serum lipid-lipoprotein levels. *Prev. Med.* 8:733–759, 1979.

Stamler, Jeremiah: Lifestyles, major risk factors, proof, and public policy. *Circulation* 58:3–19, 1978.

Stamler, Jeremiah: Personal communication.

Stokes, B.: Self care: A nation's best health insurance. *Science* 205:547, 1979.

Susser, Merwyn. Causal thinking in the health sciences. *Concepts and Strategies in Epidemiology*. New York: Oxford University Press, 1973, p. 75.

Terris, M. (editor): *Goldberger on Pellegra*. Baton Rouge: Louisiana State Press, 1964.

Thorensen, C.E., and Mahoney, M.J.: *Behavioral Self Control*. New York: Holt, Rinehart, Winston, 1974.

USDHEW: *The National Heart, Lung, and Blood Institute's Fact Book for Fiscal Year 1977*. Public Health Service, National Institutes of Health, DHEW Publications No. NIH 78-1419, 1977.

USDHEW: National Center for Health Statistics, Fats, Cholesterol, and Sodium Intake in the Diet of Persons 1–74 years: United States. *Advancedata*, Public Health Service, 54:12/17/79, 1979a.

USDHEW: *Healthy People: The Surgeon General's Report on Health Promotion and Disease Prevention*. U.S. Government Printing Office, 1979b.

USDHEW: *Promoting Health and Preventing Disease*. Office of the Assistant Secretary for Health, Internal Publication, Washington D.C. pp. 155–162, 1980.

Waldenstrom, J.: Incidence of "iron deficiency" (sideropenia) in some rural and urban populations. *Acta Med. Scand.* Suppl. 170:252–279, 1946.

Watanabe, K., Reddy, B.S., Weisburger, J.H., and Dritchevsky, D.: Effect of dietary alfalfa, pectin, and wheat bran on caranogenesis in F344 rats. *J. National Cancer Institute* 63:141–145, 1979.

Whissler, Robert W.: Laboratory experimental section conference on the health effects of blood lipids. *Prev. Med.* 8:715–732, 1979.

Williams, C.L., Arnold, C.B., and Wynder, E.L.: Primary prevention of chronic disease beginning in childhood. *Prev. Med.* 6:344–357, 1977.

Williams, C.L., Carter, B.J., Arnold, C.B., and Wynder, E.L.: Chronic disease risk factors among children. *J. Chron. Dis.* 32:505–513, 1979.

Williams, C.L., and Wynder, E.L.: A blind spot in preventive medicine. *JAMA*, 236:2196–2197, 1976.

Wynder, E.L., Hirayama, Takeshi: Comparative epidemiology of cancers in the United States and Japan. *Prev. Med.* 6:567–594, 1977.

Wynder, E.L., and Hoffmann, Detrich: Tobacco and health: A societal challenge. *N. Engl. J. Med.* 300:894–902, 1979.

Wynder, E.L., and Stellman, S.: Comparative epidemiology of tobacco related cancers. *Cancer Res.* 37:4608–4622, 1977.

Wynder, E.L., and Stellman S.: Artificial sweetner use and bladder cancer: A case control study. *Science* 207:1214–1216, 1980.

Wynder, E.L., and Weisburger, J.H.: Recommendations for modifying federal statutes relating to environmental carcinogens. *Prev. Med.* 6:185–190, 1977.

CHAPTER 2

Helping Patients Achieve Risk-Reducing Behavior Change

MERWYN R. GREENLICK, PH.D.

The purpose of this chapter is to review some of the recent approaches in the field of health behavior change with particular emphasis on those tools which will enable medical care practitioners to enhance their ability to help patients make needed or desired health behavior changes. In reviewing the pages of this book, it will become apparent to medical care providers that an increasing proportion of their practices will revolve around the modification of health behaviors.

Most medical care professionals have had little training in the social and behavioral sciences and have devoted little attention to the science and technology of behavior change. While this science and technology will appear to be relatively diffuse and primitive to people schooled in the traditional biological sciences, it is possible to glean many insights from recent behavioral research advances. A large body of literature has been produced in the past decade and techniques are readily available to busy medical care practitioners to enhance their ability in the practice of behavior change.

This chapter focuses on a clinical rather than public health approach to health behavior change. It is directed toward medical care providers who deal with patients in the traditional medical care setting on a one-to-one basis, rather than toward either public health professionals who design population-based programs or clinical behavioral specialists who deal with patients referred because of motivation or need for specific behavior changes.

There are several implications of this approach. First, it is assumed that patients in providers' offices have not arrived there with the primary intention of making health behavior changes. They are there as a response to a particular disease problem or as a result of a general preventive motivation. Typically, they are not highly motivated or burning to make particular changes or modify their overall lifestyles.

The second implication of a clinical focus is that providers, although motivated to act as behavioral change agents and guides, are not particularly trained or skilled in dealing with health behavior change. Moreover, patients' prior experience with health behavior change will most likely be a series of failures in attempts to change their lifestyles. They may have failed at weight loss, smoking cessation, changes in their physical activity program, and perhaps in a number of other attempts to change their health behavior.

Practitioners probably also have a history of failure in motivating health behavior change and have developed a social and psychological support system to enable "scapegoating" of patients who continue to present them with evidence of the providers' failure. The frustration of practitioners in the face of continuing unsuccessful efforts in treating the medical effects of obesity, alcoholism, and smoking and of the general inability to motivate patients to make changes required for living more healthful lives results in a great deal of resentment of patients by practitioners. Unflattering identification of patients as "crocks," "drunks," "slugs," "blobs," "gorks," and "turkeys" frequently heard in reference to patients by medical care providers is evidence of this frustration and resentment.

This chapter is not intended to provide practitioners a "magic bullet" that can be used easily and with universal success to deal with very difficult behavioral situations. It will, however, review some of the conceptualizations in the field of behavior change and offer some ideas and tools to help practitioners gain a new sense of control and hope in dealing with health behavior changes in their patients. Just as it is important for patients to understand that there is no easy road to success, it is also important for providers to accept that same idea. It is possible, however, for providers as well as patients to learn that by understanding the dynamics of the situation and by applying a few very simple tools, step-by-step improvements can be achieved in the providers' performance and in the ability of patients to achieve desired and important changes in health behavior.

A final general statement is a call for patience on the part of patients and providers. The approaches suggested in this chapter may be new and may seem, in some respects, strange. Since, however, most prior efforts at change have not been successful, it would be wise to refer to an aphorism of Francis Bacon suggested in his classic work, *The New Organon,* produced in the early 17th century. Bacon said, "It would be an unsound fancy and self-contradictory to expect that things which have never yet been done can be done except by means which have never been tried" (Aphorism VI, Book One).

MODELS OF HEALTH BEHAVIOR CHANGE

The function of reviewing models of health behavior and health behavior change is to provide change agents with a comfortable road map for applying common sense and for using a few well-tested techniques and approaches. The models presented for review are basically ones not dependent on such concepts as personality type nor derived from traditional psychoanalytic theory. Since the problem of medical care practitioners is to help their patients make needed or desired risk reducing health behavior changes, it is more useful to focus on models that point the way toward direct behavioral impact than to concentrate on personality types or other such constraints not easily amenable to change.

Achieving Insight into Human Behavior

Some of the material in this chapter is presented to provide background information for practitioners (for example, the perspective of cognitive dissonance theory to be discussed in the next section), and all of it is intended to aid practitioners to achieve the insight into human behavior required to help their patients make behavior changes. It is not the purpose of this chapter to review the total current literature in health behavior and health behavior change. It is, however, necessary to point out and describe briefly the general models upon which the concepts presented in this chapter are based and to review relevant literature.

The Health Belief Model

One such model is known as the "Health Belief Model." (For a review of the literature on this model, see Health Education Monograph 2, 1974, also republished in 1974 in a volume edited by Becker). The health belief model, which derived from the work in the 1940s of Kurt Lewin and others, is predicated on the assumption that good health is generally an important value of people and that, given the correct environment and the correct set of stimuli, individuals are motivated to engage in personal behavior appropriate to increasing their probability of good health.

It has been posited that the health belief model and related psychosocial models of individual health behavior can teach medical care providers that (1) behavior is motivated, (2) certain beliefs seem central to a patient's decision to act, (3) people possess beliefs and motives in varying degrees, and (4) information arrived at through education, while necessary, is often not sufficient to stimulate beliefs needed for making changes in behavior (Becker et al., 1977a).

The literature on the health belief model is varied and rich, and a review might stimulate many new ideas on the part of medical care providers. (See particularly Kasl and Cobb, 1966; Becker, 1974; Rosenstock, 1974; Maiman and Becker, 1974; Kirscht, 1974; Haefner, 1974; Kasl, 1974; Rosenstock and Kirscht, 1974; Maiman et al., 1977; Langlie, 1977; Horn, 1976; Becker et al., 1977a; and Ben-Sira, 1977.) Of particular interest in this review would be Becker and co-workers, 1977a and b, which reviews several psychosocial models and discusses the correlates of individual health-related behavior.

Of particular value because of its specificity is a 1976 paper by Daniel Horn, the former director of the National Clearinghouse for Smoking and Health. Horn's article, "A Model for the Study of Personal Choice Health Behaviour" (Horn, 1976), reports on a project which identified a practical system of measuring a number of factors involved in the development of smoking behavior and produced data from several national studies which characterized the initiation, development, maintenance, and cessation or modification of smoking behavior. Horn's concepts and findings, which follow directly from the early work on health and illness behavior and the health belief model, can be applied to a wide variety of personal choice behaviors that affect health. His findings are used to guide much of the discussion in this chapter.

Other Literature

Practitioners of a psychological bent might refer to a recent review of motivation literature by deCharms and Muir (1978) which discusses the social aspects of human motivation (which the authors refer to as social motivation) and provides some particular insight into the advances of the work originally described in terms of achievement motivation.[1]

1. Some of the work didscussed in deCharms and Muir, particularly the review of Raynor's work on future orientation (which also is an intellectual grandchild of Kurt Lewin's theories) and the discussion of Seligman's "learned helplessness," is particularly useful in the discussions that follow.

Finally, the reader is referred to a review of the field of behavioral medicine by Ovide Pomerleau (1979) which deals particularly with two major intervention techniques in behavioral medicine: biofeedback and behavioral self-management. He discusses how these two techniques are applied to what he perceives as the principal lines of development in clinical behavioral medicine: (1) intervention to modify an overt behavior or physiological response that in itself is a problem; (2) intervention to change the behavior of medical care providers, thereby improving the delivery of medical care services; (3) intervention to improve "adherence" to medical treatment; and (4) intervention to modify behaviors or responses that constitute risk factors for diseases.

Achieving Risk-Reducing Changes

This chapter focuses on achieving changes, especially risk-reducing changes, through encouraging patients to *consider* health behavior change; stimulating them to *attempt* risk reducing change; and helping them *achieve* and *maintain* change. Therefore, those elements of health behavior change theory that are particularly relevant to achieving changes are emphasized. Figure 2-1, adapted from Horn (1976), depicts four sets of factors that Horn argues either enhance or reduce the potential for successful risk-reducing behavior change. The four sets of factors relate to (1) the individual's motivation for changing behavior (values); (2) the perception of the threat of existing behavior; (3) the psychological utility of existing behavior; and (4) the environmental factors facilitating behavior change. These sets of factors will be individually discussed with regard to the particular elements of the change process discussed in the remainder of the chapter.

ENCOURAGING PATIENTS TO *CONSIDER* RISK-REDUCING BEHAVIOR CHANGE

Values Underlying Change

The set of factors Horn identifies as motivation for changing smoking behavior can be generalized to the values underlying change or reasons for changing or not changing any health behavior. Horn points out that motivation for making changes in health-related behavior is certainly

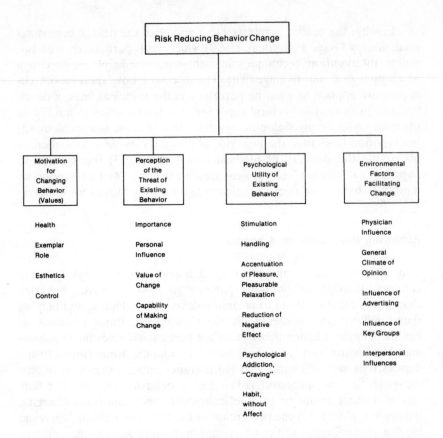

Figure 2-1. Factors affecting the potential for and success of risk-reducing behavior change (adapted with permission from D. Horn, "A model for the study of personal choice health behavior," *International Journal of Health Education,* 1976).

affected by the extent to which the individual perceives that such changes will promote or satisfy personal values.

Horn identifies four specific factors that affect motivation for change and that he asserts are applicable to a variety of personal choice health behaviors as well as smoking behavior. These are the importance of good health, the significance of the exemplar role, the importance of esthetic values, and the importance of mastery or self-control over behavior and its outcomes.

It is clear that these four factors are not necessarily independent; they can be combined in some way to produce interest in thinking about changing health behavior. In assessing patients' values in order to help them find out what the values are and help them better understand the reasons for considering behavior change, practitioners can highlight the value or values that are particularly appropriate to the behavior change under consideration.

For many people health is not necessarily a primary value; health for health's sake may be secondary to the attainment of other goals considered more important to the individual, but whose attainment suffers in the absence of good health. However, general health concepts are becoming very popular in the United States, as illustrated by increasing interest in holistic health and more natural modes of living. It is quite possible that general cultural values for living a more natural and unpolluted life will become a significant motive for behavior change in the future. It seems inconsistent, for example, for a patient with a high commitment to a life close to nature to continue smoking cigarettes.

On the other hand, awareness of their role as exemplar might be the seminal factor producing smoking cessation among parents of young children. Even the most confirmed smokers appear to be concerned that their children not become smokers. Another patient's concern for esthetics may be a particularly potent motive in stimulating him to consider a weight control program. The factor of mastery or self-control over behavior and its outcomes is a tool that providers might find particularly valuable in influencing behavior change efforts among people for whom control is of great value. For example, a busy, harrassed, and stressed business executive might be motivated to consider making health behavior changes when approached through the channel of increased mastery over undesirable health behavior.

The Threat of Existing Behavior

The role of the perception of the threat of existing behavior is very significant in the development of patients' interest in making health behavior changes. The earliest models developed to study health behavior focused upon this area (see particularly Rosenstock, Hochbaum, and Kegeles, 1960; Janis, 1974). Following the health belief model, Horn identifies four aspects of the perception of threat. Patients must be aware not only that a threat exists, but that: (1) it is important, (2) there is direct personal danger inherent in the threat, (3) there is direct value to the patients in making a change, and (4) they perceive themselves as capable of altering their behavior.

In the case of smoking behavior (and presumably in the case of other kinds of health behavior), these different aspects of the perception of threat to health bear quite different kinds of relationships to the various stages of making ultimately permanent and successful behavior change. Horn argues that the effect of the various aspects of the perception of threat is additive when it comes to predicting (or enhancing) the likelihood that an individual will seriously *contemplate* making a change in smoking. In other words, the greater the total strength of the factors, the greater the likelihood that the patient will *consider* undertaking change. Therefore, in order to achieve the patient's contemplation of a health behavior change, it may be necessary only to achieve a relatively large impact in one of the four aspects of threat or medium impact in several aspects.

The Role of Cognitive Dissonance Theory

Given the information available in today's society, it is hard to imagine that all patients are not aware of the threat to their health inherent in some of their current behavior. Few patients do not know about the dangers of cigarette smoking, the potential problems of obesity, the negative effects of excessive alcohol consumption, and the problems of an overly sedentary life. However, in practice, many patients appear to have managed to repress any information they may have ever received concerning the dangers of their negative health behaviors.

Work done in the early 1950s on cognitive dissonance theory provides insight into this behavior (see, for example, Brehm and Cohen, 1962). If an individual engages in behaviors that are known to be dangerous, the result is a very significant amount of dissonant feeling within the individual. The theory argues that since a large degree of dissonance is uncomfortable, individuals seek to achieve equilibrium by reducing the dissonance in one of several ways. One obvious way, of course, is to change the behavior. But when that cannot be or has not been achieved, one or more defense mechanisms may be used to reduce the dissonance.

The most common technique is denial. Many patients continue to be quite willing to deny that there is, in fact, any implied or real threat in their health behavior in the face of increasing evidence or knowledge of the dangers. Every medical care practitioner has heard patients report that some relative or another lived to be 95 years of age in spite of some highly inappropriate behavior such as smoking, overeating, or drinking a fifth of alcohol a day. Patients can very effectively block out negative information about their health behavior, and there is often strong reinforcement supporting this denial in the media or in their social environment.

Sophisticated and prevalent cigarette advertisements promising sexual or social rewards for smoking drown out information in the media about the dangers of smoking. Television commercials focusing on the delights of eating one form of "empty" calorie after another create a cloud of delusion about the consequences of eating those empty calories. The social behaviors involved in smoking and drinking and the sedentary life of friends and family produce a false sense of well-being among patients, and the somewhat dissonant message of a friend's heart attack, stroke, or emphysema is quickly blocked with the comforting example of inappropriate behavior on the part of friends and family remaining in the environment.

In order to counteract the enthusiastic dissonance-reduction efforts of patients who evade behavior change, medical care providers must rely upon the available tools. Over the years cognitive dissonance research has indicated some of the techniques that may be useful in creatively producing dissonance in order to successfully guide patients toward the idea that the best way to reduce dissonance, although not the easiest, is to change the objectionable behavior.

The most important lesson to be learned from this aspect of cognitive dissonance research is that the arousal of fear will be effective in producing change only when accompanied by information that convinces the receiver that it is possible to make the changes necessary to alleviate the fear caused by the message. The classic example of the failure of fear campaigns is the World War II army films on venereal disease, which were found to have no effect on either behavior or attitude change toward venereal disease. Another example is a series of films produced to frighten children into appropriate dental hygiene practices. Research on the use of these fear-arousing films on the horrible effects of dental decay indicated that children simply ignored the message unless the productions were coordinated with powerful programs to convince the children that there was a readily available behavior they could use to avoid the situation depicted in the film.

In summary, practitioners must attempt to assess patients' values to enhance their motivation for considering changing behavior and must also increase the extent of their perception of the threats of their existing behavior. These initial steps should be taken in an environment that will be receptive to enhancing patients' potential for moving to the next step of the change process, the *commitment io attempt* a risk reducing behavior change.

GAINING PATIENTS' COMMITMENT
TO *ATTEMPT* BEHAVIOR CHANGE

In seeking the appropriate method to motivate patients to attempt behavior change, all four sets of factors in Figure 2-1 must be brought to bear. The definition and assessment of patients' values certainly must proceed into this step, and exploring the psychological utility of the existing behavior can be very useful in helping patients gain insight into the meaning of their own behavior. Discussions with practitioners and review of the motivation literature both support the view that most patients have little insight into the meaning of their own behavior. Many behavioral self-examination kits are available today that allow patients working alone or with practitioners to explore the psychological utility of their behavior and to plan for dealing with the loss of that utility. The Smoker's Self-Testing Kit, available through the U.S. National Clearinghouse for Smoking and Health (USPHS Pub. No. 1904, 1969), allows patients to identify their smoking type: psychological addiction, habit without affect, reduction of negative affect, accentuation of pleasure, or stimulation smoking behavior. The same kind of material is available to help patients assess their eating behavior, their use of alcohol, or their physical activity pattern. Practitioners should become familiar with those self-assessment materials available to aid patients in the behavior change process.

In addition to the use of behavioral self-assessment kits, medical care practitioners have the advantage of their personal relationship with patients to help them achieve successful behavior change. This personal relationship with patients and knowledge of patients' circumstances and characteristics can be used to design individualized behavior change techniques not available in mass campaigns. A well conceived and organized individual program maximizes the probability of successful behavior change.

The factors characterized as perception of the threat of existing behavior in Figure 2-1 can be used most effectively by medical care practitioners to help patients decide that risk-reducing behavior change is worth trying. Horn reports that the four aspects of this set—the importance of the risk, the potential for personal risk, the value to the individual of making the change, and the individual's capability of making the change—are additive to patients *considering* behavior change but are not additive in the *actual decision* to undertake a change. The national smoking data, says Horn, indicate that the four aspects are equivalent; that is, a single aspect at some critical level is all that is necessary to stimulate a positve *decision* to make a change, and any one of the four aspects at a high enough level can trigger the decision to undertake an attempt at behavior change.

Use of Clinical Data for Heightening Risk Awareness

Medical care practitioners certainly have the opportunity of making health risks real to their patients in order to motivate an attempt at smoking cessation. Practitioners can perform a physical examination to seek cigarette-related physical changes. The presence of oral leukoplakia, a premalignant mucous membrane lesion common to older smokers, and impaired chest expansion are common findings. Additionally, practitioners can order and interpret such tests as pulmonary functions, expired air carbon monoxide content, and blood or saliva thiocyanate levels. An individualized interpretation of the data from these examinations can have a profound effect in making the risk real and personal for patients. And, consistent with Horn's model, this approach frequently triggers an on-the-spot commitment to attempt change. Individual risk assessments can be effective in producing attempts to change eating patterns, physical activity, alcohol consumption, or other risk-producing behaviors.

Many commercial multiple-risk assessment forms and programs are available, but most of them have never been tested in terms of their ability actually to produce change. The unthinking use of a complex, slick health assessment form is probably unwarranted. While these forms have some validity in enhancing the perception of the threat of existing behavior in mass screening programs, such as at county fairs or in large communitywide or organizationwide programs, practitioners can take advantage of the inherent characteristics of their direct relationship with patients to individualize and to focus the attempt at heightening awareness of the threat of existing behavior.

Inference from cognitive dissonance research would indicate that the message from practitioners that the patients' behavior is a threat to life and to health will not be received or processed if the dissonance produced by the message is too great. To improve the effectiveness of the threat message, practitioners can surround the information with significant support messages to enhance patients' perception that they are in control and can make changes in their life, in spite of all their previous evidence to the contrary.

Patients' Potential for Making Life Changes

Patients' perception of their capacity to make risk-reducing change is affected not only by their prior experience with attempts to make the particular change, but also is strongly influenced by their general level of self-esteem and overall sense of self-control. Many patients will be unable to contemplate seriously making behavioral changes because of the lack of the needed perception that changes are possible and because a minimal level of self-regard is required for the development of the perception that specific changes are possible. Practitioners can use this perspective to help patients become committed to attempting change.

Reading this book should motivate medical care providers to renewed effort to create risk-reducing behavior change in their patients and, hopefully, the specific techniques discussed later in this chapter should encourage providers that successful change attempts are possible, if difficult. But providers should keep a balanced perspective about behavior change and should take care to understand the particular social and psychological situation of their patients.

Many patients who will be seen by providers in the 1980s will find their lives in a state of social or psychological disarray. The large number of adult men and women dealing with major life crises at any one time has only recently begun to be discussed in the literature. Problems of parents' relationship to their children, of the strife and dissolution of marriages, and of difficulties in the occupational world overwhelm an increasing number of patients seen in medical care practitioners' offices.

Certainly it is the practitioners' responsibility to point out the risk potential of patients' health-related behavior, to encourage patients to make appropriate risk-reducing modifications in their behavior, and to provide the support and tools required to enhance the potential success of those changes. On the other hand, providers must also remember that patients evaluate their lives in a total fashion and are likely to assess the costs of change in the short term against the benefits in both the short and long term before attempting to make significant changes in their behavior patterns.

The deCharms and Muir review on motivation cited above provides some insight into this particular problem. They review work (for example, Atkinson and Birch, 1970) that points out that the problem in deciphering motivation is to understand the determinants of change in the stream of action, not necessarily to assess what drives impel specific behavior. That approach leads to the dynamic conception of human action as a series of episodes perceived by a patient as extending into the future. Atkinson and Birch argue that motivation for the immediate task must be conceived as a function of how that task is related in the life space of a patient to future events and opportunities.

deCharms and Muir also review the work of Raynor (Atkinson and Raynor, 1975), which expands and broadens this notion of motivation into a framework that would certainly argue for patience on the part of practitioners concerning patients' ability to make behavior change. Raynor argues that motivation is a function, not only of the perceived probability of success and incentive value of the immediate task, but also of the probability of success and the incentives of future tasks and goals, the attainment of which are contingent upon the successful completion of the immediate task. A student's motivation in studying for an exam, for example, relates to the student's perception of the probability of successfully passing that exam, but also relates, in a broader sense, to the impact of that behavior on the probability of passing the course and on the impact of graduating from college and getting a job and starting a career. In like manner, patients' estimates of their probability of successfully making a specific behavior change would relate to their estimate of their potential for making other behavior changes and to the impact and value of those behavior changes in the larger scheme of their lives.

The Practitioner as a Role Model

One element of the behavior of medical care practitioners' behavior that must be taken into consideration in stimulating patients to attempt risk-reducing behavior change is the extent to which practitioners must serve as health behavior role models for patients. Cognitive dissonance theory indicates that inappropriate health behavior on the part of medical care practitioners could have a significant negative effect on their ability to produce behavior change in patients. On the one hand, it is very difficult for clinicians who smoke or are apparently indifferent to their own obesity to produce a convincing behavior change message. But even if the change message is effectively given, it is certainly easier for patients to disregard the message under those circumstances. In fact, it might be argued that patients would be able to disregard any health behavior change messages when faced with clinicians who are apparently not practicing appropriate health behavior themselves.

The degree of concern over role modeling differs widely among medical care practitioners. A recent survey in the Kaiser-Permanente Medical Care Program in Oregon (Greenlick, Freeborn, and Lamb,

1979) indicates a wide difference of opinion about the extent to which a medical care system employee's behavior should serve as a role model to patients. A large proportion of medical care personnel did not consider their behavior to be significant in affecting the behavior of patients. Others know its effect but ignore it.

An anecdote from a health behavior change program in the Kaiser-Permanente system highlights the impact of this negative view on the part of many health professionals. Staff members of this project were interviewing a patient to determine the reasons for his return to cigarette smoking after having been off smoking for several months prior to having a heart attack. The staff was shocked to find the patient's perception that he was encouraged to return to smoking because several nurses took their "cigarette break" in his room of the hospital while they visited with him to help speed his recovery. The extent to which the nurses' smoking behavior actually produced the negative behavior change on the part of the patient may be irrelevant. It is certainly clear that the dissonance produced by the patient's smoking behavior after a heart attack was greatly eased by his reference to the smoking behavior of the nurses.

The health workers involved in this health behavior project, the Portland Center of the National Multiple Risk Factor Intervention Trial (MRFIT), were very impressed by this story. One of the significant intervention techniques used by the multiprofessional staff of the project is to attempt health behavior changes themselves so as to influence the behavior of the participants with whom they work. Most of the staff members have dedicated themselves to a struggle with important health behavior changes, and their ability to interact with otherwise recalcitrant participants has thus been dramatically improved.

In summary, it is suggested that medical care providers interested in helping patients attempt changes in their risk-related health behavior should themselves attempt significant health behavior change. The area and degree of the changes probably is less important than the struggle with difficult changes. It is certainly not necessary for medical care providers to become marathon runners or to lose 75 pounds. It is much more important for them to begin to take seriously the notion of modifying their own behavior to reduce their own risk. The main functions of this activity are to give providers *insight* into the difficulties of behavior change and to allow the opportunity for sharing experiences with patients in order to enable the providers' advice to become more relevant and more real. Empathy and credibility are thus established with patients. Of course, the latent value might be to provide a longer life for providers to stimulate risk reducing behavior among patients.

HELPING PATIENTS *ACHIEVE* SUCCESSFUL RISK-REDUCING BEHAVIOR

To guide providers to understanding the change process and to maximize patients' ability to make successful changes, insight can be gained from Horn's data on predicting short-term success in smoking cessation. While the four aspects of the perception of threat (see Figure 2-1) are additive in predicting the probability of patients *considering* health behavior change and are equivalent in predicting patients' *actual attempts* to change, the situation is more complex in predicting short-term success. Horn reports that each part of the four aspects of the perception of threat (see Figure 2-1) is a necessary condition and must be present above a certain level to predict a high probability of a short-term success in smoking cessation. The absence of a single aspect is sufficient to lower the short-term quit rates significantly. Horn reports that these results are similar to those previously reported as characterizing acceptance of chest x-rays for tuberculosis (Hochbaum, 1958). This finding indicates that it is necessary for practitioners to continue to pay attention to *all four aspects of threat* while dealing with motivation for change, with the psychological factors involved, and with environmental facilitation.

Two considerations should be stressed as background for the discussion of specific behavior change techniques. First, since the general motivation for change is a significant factor in predicting short-term success, it would be well for practitioners to continue to stress the general health values that are beginning to become current in our society. This will assure that the motivation-for-change component depicted in Figure 2-1 remains high enough to produce a significantly high probability of short-term success in risk-reducing behavior.

A second general consideration concerns the fear of many practitioners of creating the sense of failure among patients by stimulating them to attempt to make risk-reducing changes.

The Role of Previous "Failures"

Practitioners are quite familiar with the dismal success rate of many behavior change approaches and may be particularly concerned with perpetuating failure in their patients. For example, it may be inappropriate to stimulate patients to attempt behavior changes unless there appears, in advance, to be a fairly high probability of success. After failing to make changes a number of times, patients may label themselves as "failures."

The current view of most behavioral specialists is that this fear of creating a sense of failure in patients should not prevent practitioners from exerting every effort to motivate their patients to attempt risk-reducing behavior change. First of all, while research (such as Horn's) evaluating the factors influencing successful behavior change have begun to predict on a population basis what factors relate to or are determinants of change, there is no reliable method of predicting, on an individual basis, which patients will be permanently successful in making major changes in their health behavior. Every practitioner has had too many experiences with patients labeled as "hopeless" who make dramatic and permanent changes in their health behavior to become too sanguine about prematurely writing off anyone. At the same time, clinicians who have assessed patients as "sure bets" to achieve behavior change have been proven wrong enough times to cast doubt on their ability to assess change potential in advance.

Perhaps more relevant to this question, however, is the increasing perception that most successful, permanent health behavior change has been preceded by several abortive attempts. Patients appear to try out change behavior and gain some experience with the new behaviors on several occasions before the circumstances become auspicious for the ultimate and permanent change of a specific behavior.

Practitioners are advised, therefore, to view every patient as a "potential success" on the road to becoming an "actual success," rather than to label certain patients as probable failures. Enough is currently known of the clinician–patient relationship to show that the practitioner's perception of the likely success of the patient becomes a powerful influence in the ultimate change process.

While it is critical for practitioners to approach their patients as if they all are "potential successes" on the road to becoming "actual successes," it is equally important that practitioners assure that the locus of control remain within the patient. Practitioners must maintain the position that developing risk-reducing behavior change is the concern of patients and that behavior change belongs to patients and is in their best interest. Practitioners can continue to remind patients of their best interest and continue to provide support and serve as a technical assistant along the road to ultimate success, but they must never allow patients to transfer the locus of control to the practitioner or to anyone else. The patient's spouse, family, or friends should never be allowed to accept the locus of control for what will hopefully become a permanent behavior change on the patient's part.

Community Behavior Change programs

Of prime importance in developing successful behavior change is the selection and application, with patients, of an appropriate behavior change technique. Several techniques will be discussed in this section. Each has its own reports of success. Before discussing behavior change techniques which can be integrated into the practitioners' clinical practice, it would be well to comment on some behavior change programs available in the community. One view holds that busy medical care practitioners are not the appropriate interventionists to make permanent inroads into changing patients' behavior patterns. Thus, it would be well for practitioners, especially those who may believe they are not appropriate change agents, to become familiar with the community resources available to aid patients in making desired or needed behavior changes before attempting systematic change programs in their own office.

Community programs include the Weight Watchers program for obesity control, the Seventh Day Adventist Smoking Program, Alcoholics Anonymous, and commercial programs such as SmokEnders, Schick Smoking Reduction Centers, various commercial alcohol treatment programs, and a variety of exercise programs. Many of these programs appear to have successful long-term results. Weight Watchers, for example, is reported to be the most successful approach to weight reduction that has been subjected to large-scale, long-term evaluation (Stunkard, 1978). By the same token, Alcoholics Anonymous appears to have a longstanding record for the effective treatment of alcohol problems in a particular group of patients.

Practitioners should make a concentrated effort to assess the programs available in their community, to visit with the people responsible for the programs (perhaps visit the programs themselves), to encourage patients who express interest in particular programs to try them and report back, and to evaluate as best they can the experiences of patients with the programs. Practitioners should also petition the local medical society or practice group to do such monitoring of community programs, as well as discuss with colleagues the various programs in the community and do everything possible to take advantage of the technical expertise developed over time as a result of such programs.

Developing Referral Sources

Practitioners might also approach community programs as potential referral sources for specific or overall health behavior changes. Another option is to refer patients to traditional mental health practitioners or clinics for aid in behavior change efforts. Generally speaking, mental health clinics have provided individual and group therapy sessions for dealing with such problems as obesity, smoking, alcohol use, and stress management. Data on the effectiveness of the traditional mental health approach for these problems, however, is not readily available and this approach, as characterized by the traditional therapeutic relationship between mental health professionals and patients, seems not to have produced overwhelming success.

Hypnosis

Hypnosis is a behavioral change technique that gives medical care practitioners the option of referral or of becoming skilled in the use of the techniques themselves. There is a growing literature on the efficacy and safety of hypnosis for assisting people to make basic behavioral changes. Qualified hypnotherapists are now available in most communities, and practitioners can easily find community resources to fill the need when hypnotism is the technique of choice in assisting patients to make long-term behavior changes.

As word of the effectiveness of hypnotism begins to spread through the community, practitioners will be increasingly besieged with demands from their patients to make hypnotism available. Hypnotism is beginning to be used in a rather eclectic way and is being integrated into an overall program of behavioral change on the part of most practitioners. Generally speaking, however, there are two basic approaches to the use of hypnotism in risk-reducing behavior change. The first approach is the relatively direct use of hypnosis using both intra-hypnotic and post-hypnotic suggestion to attempt to eliminate directly an inappropriate behavior pattern or to implant a more appropriate pattern. This approach, which appears to be effective in many situations, appeals to most patients because they like their behavior change program to be simple and easy. The attractiveness of a potential "magic" cure is overwhelming to patients who have unsuccessfully struggled with smoking cessation, weight control, or stress management.

Many hypnotists, however, implement hypnosis as part of an integrated approach to achieving long-term risk-reducing behavior change. The hypnotherapist builds in many imagery techniques, including such approaches as systematic desensitization, and attempts to produce in the patient a sense of mastery and control. This approach generally incorporates training in self-hypnotic techniques which allow patients to become increasingly skilled in their own behavior change and to have at their disposal a tool to be used whenever their life situation requires a reinforcing intervention technique.

A large number of reviews are now available on the use of hypnosis in behavior change (see, for example, the easily read review of Wallace, 1979, or Olness and Gardner, 1978). Perhaps, however, the most effective way for practitioners to evaluate hypnosis as an intervention tool for their own practice would be to explore and perhaps to enroll in one of the many hypnotism training sessions available for medical care practitioners. Most communities have a program available to train practitioners to use various hypnosis techniques within a medical care practice, and the American Society for Clinical Hypnosis provides workshops in several cities in the United States.

As with any of the other behavior change techniques, hypnosis appears to have its place in a well-balanced clinical approach, and most practitioners ultimately learn to feel quite comfortable integrating hypnosis into their practices, either as a tool used directly or through referral.

Behavior Modification

Another set of tools available to practitioners derives from the techniques of behavior modification and behavior therapy. As Pomerleau points out (1979), behavior modification originated with the experimental work of Skinner and his colleagues in the early 1950s and with social learning theory. Behavior modification (as defined by Brown, Wienckowski, and Stolz, 1975) is a special form of behavior influence involving the application of various principles derived from research in experimental psychology to alleviate human suffering and enhance human functioning. It emphasizes a systematic monitoring and evaluation of the effectiveness of these applications and is generally intended to facilitate improved self-control by expanding a patient's skills, abilities, and independence. (Behavior modification is reviewed as part of general behavior therapy by Gomes-Schwartz, Hadley, and Strupp, 1978).

An increasing amount of material and a number of guides are available to help practitioners establish behavior modification programs for their patients. For example, practitioners can find particular reviews of the application of behavior modification for the family physician (e.g., Tapp, Tapp, and Seller, 1979) or a variety of specific behavior modification tools available for weight reduction, smoking, hypertension control, and others (see, for example, Ferguson, 1978, for a practitioner's do-it-yourself kit for a behavior modification program for obesity control).

Incidentally, the Weight Watchers program, which originally focused its activities on specific dietary manipulation and on the reinforcement of frequent visits and group support techniques, has augmented its approach in the last few years by adopting behavior modification techniques. In a review of the effectiveness of behavior modification as a tool for behavior change, Stunkard was hopeful that their results could become even better with the application of behavior modification techniques. (Stunkard, 1978; see also Ferguson, 1978 for a review of the approaches of behavior modification for dietitians.)

Behavioral Self-Management

The particular development in the mid-1970s that may have the most direct applicability in a medical care practitioner's office is the behavioral self-management technique. In the original application of behavior modification, environmental manipulations were used to modify behavior directly. However, with self-management procedures the therapist teaches the person with the problem to change aspects of his or her environment and that in turn is used to modify the problem behavior (Pomerleau, 1979). The therapist's responsibility is to help the patient devise effective behavior change strategies and to maintain the patient's motivation to apply the techniques consistently over a long period of time.

The theoretical perspective underlying behavioral self-management is that most of the behaviors requiring change are maintained by immediate reinforcement, frequently of relatively small magnitude, which maintains the behavior in spite of considerable delayed aversive consequences of a relatively large magnitude, such as the potential of serious illness or death. The basic strategy of behavioral self-management, therefore, is to provide new reinforcing consequences for adaptive behavior and to interfere with or defer the immediate reinforcement for the inappropriate behavior. The techniques of behavioral self-management are relatively straightforward and medical care practitioners can learn, with patience and with practice, to implement them in their clinical practice.

Various reviews of behavioral self-management techniques are available (see, for example, Thoresen and Mahoney, 1974; Mahoney and Thoresen, 1974; Williams and Long, 1975). The essential approach can be summarized in four steps: (1) defining the problem in behavioral terms, (2) developing baseline measurements of the problem behavior, (3) planning and implementing the behavioral change, and (4) obtaining feedback and adjusting the self-management program.[2]

In using behavioral self-management techniques, practitioners should note that the philosophy underlying the approach is that patients can achieve mastery of the approach and, therefore, can learn to understand and to modify their behavior throughout their lives. There are several implications of this perspective. First of all, as with any learning experience, it requires practice using the technique to create a sense of mastery, comfort, and self-control. This means that the effort is frequently slow and will require taking two steps forward and one step back. However, with proper application and a close working relationship between practitioner and patient, it is possible to produce in the patient the feeling of mastery that derives from experience with success in making relevant changes.

In teaching patients to *define the problem* in terms that can be amenable to behavioral self-management, it is necessary to convince them to focus on those proximate behaviors which lead in an inevitable chain to undesirable outcomes. (For example, the focus should be on specific eating behaviors to be changed, and not on weight loss. Weight loss will follow appropriate behavior change.) It is particularly useful to focus on the behaviors within the framework of stimulus and response and to discourage patients from focusing on matters of "will power," personality type, or morality. It is necessary to convince patients that their problems are not a result of their being "bad" or of some inherent weakness in their character. Rather, patients must come to learn that their problems are the result of a series of learned behaviors that can be unlearned and more appropriate behaviors learned as a substitute. The inherent feelings of guilt produced by years of grappling with inherently undesirable behavior frequently make it very difficult for patients to focus on the simple, proximate behaviors that are the antecedents of their inevitable outcome problems.

A most powerful tool that can be used in defining the problem is the careful, highly detailed *baseline measurement of the behavior sets under treatment*. As Thoresen and Mahoney point out (1974, p. 42), self-observation is a highly complex problem that involves both covert and overt behaviors; it does not function in any pure or independent sense because the person "knows that he knows." The differences, however, that result from knowledge from very careful baseline self-

2. This formulation is based on behavioral self-management techniques applied by Vic Stevens and his colleagues at the Portland, Oregon, MRFIT Center.

observation is that much of the behavior exhibited in daily life is automatic and nonconscious. In order to teach patients to self-observe appropriately and, therefore, to begin to develop baseline measurement (whether it is of eating patterns, smoking patterns, or exercise patterns), it is first necessary to teach the process of discrimination. Individuals observing themselves must discern the presence or absence of a particular response. This is not easy or obvious and patients must be provided a great deal of feedback in order for the self-evaluation and baseline measurement to be useful in defining a problem.

An interesting sideline to this baseline measurement problem is that it has become very clear through a number of experiments that the baseline measurement itself causes the behavior to change dramatically. Patients who begin recording all the food they eat, for example, lose weight simply as a result of an honest and diligent recording, which leads to decreased eating. The recording of smoking behavior causes smokers to smoke less, or perhaps forces them to cease smoking, and the careful monitoring of exercise activity seems to increase automatically the amount of physical activity a patient experiences.

In helping patients *plan and implement behavior change* using the behavior self-management technique, the first step is to help them determine a reasonable goal. The behavior change process needs to be a cumulative, long-term process and, therefore, it is necessary to keep several things in mind in determining a goal for each step of the process. The first is that practitioners and patients should understand that the patient's objective should be a permanent change in life pattern. That goal might be defined, for example, as changing patients' permanent eating patterns in such a way as to allow patients to maintain their lifetime weight at an appropriate level. Only after having defined the problem and measured patients' eating patterns over a reasonable baseline period is it possible to pick out a single behavior change goal within that overall pattern. This selection is only one step toward ultimately achieving an appropriate lifelong eating pattern.

The first step must be big enough to make a difference, but small enough to be achievable. Since behavior self-management is essentially a lifetime technique, it should be aplied so that patients learn to derive satisfaction from achieving intermediate goals as part of the program. The first tendency on the part of patients is to attempt to change all patterns at the same time. Since that has failed several times in every person's life, patients should be taught to resist that impulse and to learn rather to develop change strategies that are highly likely to succeed. As the process proceeds, it will be possible to select proximate behavior change goals at any point with reference to the various other change goals that have been selected and perhaps achieved in the past. Patients can learn to define a goal that helps to reinforce the successful behavior change of the past and serves as a guide for a logical next step toward an ultimately successful program. This "shaping" process should be carefully managed. Practitioners can serve as outside observers to the behavioral self-management program and can be very useful as guides and consultants.

A tool to be used in planning and implementing the behavior change program is the use of precommitments. Since many of the maladaptive behaviors to be changed are reinforced by very immediate, although not necessarily very large, rewards, a way to overcome this immediate reinforcer is by achieving a high level of precommitment to the newly defined behavior pattern. Such aids as written meal planning in obesity control, the commitment to social involvement in exercise programs, contracts between practitioner and patient, and public announcements of smoking cessation attempts are examples of precommitments that can serve to overcome the strengths of the immediate reinforcers to the inappropriate behavior problem. Training patients who are learning behavioral self-management techniques to use a variety of precommitment techniques will help insure the success of the program.

One critical precommitment for a successful behavioral self-management program is the commitment to continual record keeping because record keeping itself has been shown to be a powerful tool in behavior change. Various kinds of record keeping systems can serve to focus attention on behavioral goals and can become significant reinforcers in their own right, helping to establish the behavior selected as a goal. It is possible to record various elements of the behavioral self-management program, from goal behaviors themselves to various outcome measures. While change in outcome measures, such as actual weight recorded daily or weekly or the expired-air carbon monoxide level, can be effective reinforcers, it is generally recommended that the record keeping focus on the proximate behavior itself. It is far more effective to define the recording system in terms of, say, the number of calories eaten per day, the minutes of exercise achieved, or the number of puffs of cigarettes taken a day, than it is to record outcome measures. This is certainly true in the beginning of the program because outcome measures show less immediate change to help reinforce the program.

Situational control is another vital part of behavioral self-management. Since this technique derives from the behavioral perspective, it is assumed that a great deal of the behavior to be changed is triggered by environmental or situational stimuli. In many instances, until new behaviors are fully integrated into a person's life pattern, it is appropriate to avoid the stimuli associated with the behavior to be changed. For example, if initial observations show that coffee is strongly associated with cigarette smoking or going to restaurants is strongly associated with overeating, it is well to train patients to manipulate their environment so as to avoid those stimulus-response situations. In instances where it is not possible to avoid the stimulus-response situations (for example, if cigarette smoking is associated with the end of a meal), it is sometimes possible to build substitute responses to the stimuli which can be equally or more strongly reinforcing. In the original baseline measurement and definition of the problem, patients can be trained to identify the stimulus-response situations in their daily environment and to learn to control the situation whenever possible.

A final element in the behavioral self-management technique that is a critical, integral component for planning and implementing the behavior change program is the development of a social support system. (This will be discussed more fully in the section on maintaining successful change.) The reinforcement derived from a strong social support system is a major tool for helping patients maintain their own behavioral self-management programs. The shared posting of behavioral records within groups of significant others is one reinforcement technique. Husbands and wives or groups of friends or co-workers all attempting to make difficult behavioral changes can help each other in their struggle to modify their overall behavior patterns.

The final step in the behavioral self-management program is *the feedback process* (the fine tuning of the program) and the selection of new change goals. As patients become more familiar, and more comfortable, with the use of the behavioral self-management technique, the change from baseline in significant outcome and behavioral measures will increase and the results will encourage participants to move ahead with the program.

Practitioners should legitimize the idea that some of the techniques attempted by patients to change their behavior will be effective and others will not. Patients should be warned not to view this as a success–failure process, but rather as a natural and normal learning process. They should be reminded that it is not possible to attempt a variety of new things without having some of them be more effective than others. Patients will learn to focus on effective techniques and build those techniques into their existing program. The extent to which patients are able to build upon the idea that they are "potential successes" on the way to becoming "actual successes" is the extent to which they can learn to focus on their achievements and not on their failures, thereby encouraging them to move further and to risk more in the program.

This constant feedback/learning experience will enable patients to internalize this very powerful tool for use in analyzing their behavior and for making desired behavior changes throughout their lives. As with any other complex tool, the learning curve is uneven and some people respond much better than others. But those who have learned to implement the program and to use it effectively in their life exhibit a continually growing success over their lifetime in gaining conrol over their health behavior and become more successful in risk-reducing modifications of their health practices.

MAINTAINING SUCCESSFUL CHANGE

In order to gain insight into the problems of maintaining successful behavioral change, it is necessary to go back to the empirical work of Horn (as outlined conceptually in Figure 2-1). Horn reports that there is no relationship between the strength of the cognitive-perceptual variables, the threat variables, and long-term success in smoking cessation. In fact, Horn reports that there even appears to be a negative relationship between the extent to which the threat dimensions motivate the attempt to quit and the ultimate long-term success. It seems that once short-term success has been exhibited by patients, other factors become more critical in maintaining the successful risk-reducing behavior change. Environmental facilitation factors seem to be particularly important. These include the impact of medical care practitioners, the general climate of opinion, the influence of advertising, and most importantly, the influence of key groups of significant others.

The role of the family and similar social support networks in maintaining health has become an area of special interest. Both biological experimentation and social science research among humans document that intimate contacts appear to serve as a buffer against both psychological and physical breakdown from the widest variety of disorders. Kinship or social networks are also an important facilitating factor in achieving and maintaining long-term behavioral change (see, for example, Pilisuk and Froland, 1978).

Because of these findings, practitioners should be alert to family or peer group problems that make it difficult for patients to achieve desired behavior changes. By the same token, practitioners can take advantage of the strengths in the family, all the while maintaining the locus of control in the patient, to help the patient achieve appropriate changes. Practitioners may need to help the family develop a total family program for achieving the desired lifelong health behaviors that are satisfying to all the members of the family. If the patients' social network can be brought to bear, the probability of long-term success will be greatly increased.

With a long-term perspective, practitioners will note that the techniques that appear to be the most successful in the changing of lifelong patterns are techniques that are both slow in gaining initial successes and that require continual monitoring and reinforcement. In accepting that learning curves are very different among different patients, the practitioners should learn to be tolerant and supportive of "slow learners."

In using hypnosis, behavior modification, and, most particularly, behavior self-management techniques, practitioners will find that patients will require frequent follow-up visits or other supportive contacts such as telephone calls for a relatively long period. Continued adherence to the behavior change programs will be strengthened by a precommitment by practitioners to that continual reinforcement. This reinforcement does not necessarily need to be in the practitioners' offices, and, in fact, probably will be most effective through the development of formal or informal long-term networks to produce or maintain the reinforcement patterns. While the family is one possible mechanism for this, practitioners might also tap into community resources or develop their own analogy of the social support systems inherent in Alcoholics Anonymous or Weight Watchers.

Practitioners should also understand that there is a cumulative effect in successful behavior change and that short-term and intermediate successes will help to convince patients that long-term, major changes in their lives are possible. It is very important for practitioners to build on successes and to help produce a long-term change program that will enable patients to achieve successful lifetime change.

Social Policy Considerations

Several final words need to be said concerning the role of practitioners in the maintenance of successful risk-reducing change. Since the behavioral models that appear to be the most useful in understanding health behavior change all focus to some extent on the potential impact of the environment, it might be well for practitioners to consider their role in creating a social environment conducive to healthful living. Until recently, most medical care practitioners have not been as active as they could be in the legislative and public affairs field in attempting to help shape a more healthful environment. Practitioners would probably find it functional for the treatment of their patients if they became advocates in the development of new legislation, in the promotion of existing legislation, and in the general area of the promotion of healthful living.

Public health practitioners have pointed out how laws concerning tobacco use (such laws as tobacco subsidies or public anti-smoking laws) can greatly affect the health of the public. Speed laws, highway safety programs, and seatbelt use also dramatically affect the public's health and create an overall environment for a more or less healthful society. Practitioners might consider dedicating a meaningful portion of their professional activities (possibly through professional organizations) to creating environmental conditions that will foster clinical activities in helping patients achieve their personal goals for as healthy a life as possible.

Finally, if medical care practitioners are to be maximally helpful in facilitating health behavior changes in their patients, it is obvious that many of them will have to change their own behavior more than merely to serve as positive health behavior role models (don't smoke in front of patients, etc.). Many practitioners will have to change their style of work in order to follow the theoretical outlines and behavior change techniques outlined in this chapter. For example, it is clear that it is not possible to give patients attempting risk-reducing behavior changes the time and support they will need if the practitioner has a very full and busy practice that allows only brief, superficial visits. Also, if practitioners are seeing patients for 60 to 80 hours a week, it is obvious that they will not have the time or energy available to acquire the knowledge, insight, and skill required to become effective change agents, to learn about community resources, or to lobby for a healthier environment.

Therefore, the real message of this chapter to practitioners interested in helping their patients attempt risk-reducing behavior change might well be to examine their own style of practice as well as their lifestyles and make a commitment to changing them, if necessary, before undertaking the behavior change strategies outlined in this chapter.

REFERENCES

Atkinson, J.W., and Birch, D.: *The Dynamics of Action*. New York: Wiley, 1970.

Atkinson, J.W., and Raynor, J.O.: *Motivation and Achievement*. Washington, D.C.: Winston, 1975.

Bacon, F.: F.H. Anderson, editor, in *The New Organon and Related Writings*. Indianapolis: Bobbs-Merrill, 1960.

Becker, M.H.: The health belief model and sick role behavior, in M.H. Becker, editor, *The Health Belief Model and Personal Health Behavior*. Thorofare, N.J.: Charles B. Slack, 1974, pp. 82–92.

Becker, M.H., Haefner, D.P., Kasl, S.V., et al.: Selected psychosocial models and correlates of individual health-related behaviors. *Med. Care* 15(5) suppl:27–46, 1977a.

Becker, M.H., Haefner, D.P., Maiman, L.A., et al.: The health belief model and prediction of dietary compliance: A field experiment. *J. Health Soc. Behav.* 18:348–366, 1977b.

Ben-Sira, Z.: Involvement with a disease and health-promoting behavior. *Soc. Sci. Med.* 11:165–173, 1977.

Brehm, J.W., and Cohen, A.R.: *Explorations in Cognitive Dissonance*. New York: John Wiley and Sons, 1962.

Brown, B.S., Wienckowski, L.A., and Stolz, S.B.: *Behavior Modification: Perspective on a Current Issue*. National Institute of Mental Health DHEW Publication No. (ADM) 75-202, 1975.

deCharms, R., and Muir, M.S.: Motivation: Social approaches. *Ann. Rev. Psychol.* 29:91–113, 1978.

Ferguson, J.: Dietitians as behavior-change agents. *J. Am. Dent. Assoc.* 73:231–238, 1978.

Gomes-Schwartz, B., Hadley, S.W., and Strupp, H.H.: Individual psychotherapy and behavior therapy. *Ann. Rev. Psychol.* 29:435–471, 1978.

Greenlick, M.R., Freeborn, D.K., and Lamb, S.: Results of the Kaiser-Permanente Employee Survey. Unpublished, 1979.

Haefner, D.P.: The health belief model and preventive dental behavior, in M.H. Becker, editor, *The Health Belief Model and Personal Health Behavior*. Thorofare, N.J.: Charles B. Slack, 1974, pp. 93–105.

Hochbaum, G.M.: *Public Participation in Medical Screening Programs*. Washington, D.C.: PHS Publication No. 572, 1958.

Horn, D.: A model for the study of personal choice health behaviour. *Intern. J. Health Educ.* 19:89–98, 1976.

Janis, I.: *Psychological Stress* (2nd ed). New York: Academic Press, 1974.

Kasl, S.V.: The health belief model and behavior related to chronic illness, in M.H. Becker, editor, *The Health Belief Model and Personal Health Behavior*. Thorofare, N.J.: Charles B. Slack, 1974, pp. 106–127.

Kasl, S.V., and Cobb, S.: Health behavior, illness behavior and sick role behavior I and II. *Arch. Environ. Health* 12:246–266, 1966 (I); 12:531–541, 1966 (II).

Kirscht, J.P.: The health belief model and illness behavior, in M.H. Becker, editor, *The Health Belief Model and Personal Health Behavior*. Thorofare, N.J.: Charles B. Slack, 1974, pp. 60–81.

Langlie, J.K.: Social networks, health beliefs and preventive health behavior. *J. Health Soc. Behav.* 18:244–260, 1977.

Mahoney, M.J., and Thoresen, C.E.: *Self-Control: Power to the Person.* Monterey: Brooks/Cole, 1974.

Maiman, L.A., and Becker, M.H.: The health belief model: Origins and correlates in psychological theory, in M.H. Becker, editor, *The Health Belief Model and Personal Health Behavior.* Thorofare, N.J.: Charles B. Slack, 1974, pp. 9–26.

Maiman, L.A., Becker, M.H., Kirscht, J.P., et al.: Scales for measuring health belief model dimensions: A test of predictive value, internal consistency, and relationship among beliefs. *Health Education Monographs* 5(3):215–230, 1977.

Olness, K., and Gardner, G.G.: Hypnotherapy in pediatrics. *Pediatrics* 62(2):131–276, 1978.

Pilisuk, M., and Froland, C.: Kinship, social networks, social support and health. *Soc. Sci. Med.* 12B:273–280, 1978.

Pomerleau, O.F.: Behavioral medicine: The contribution of the experimental analysis of behavior to medical care. *Am. Psychologist* 34(8):654–663, 1979.

Rosenstock, I.M.: The health belief model and preventive health behavior, in M.H. Becker, editor, *The Health Belief Model and Personal Health Behavior.* Thorofare, N.J.: Charles B. Slack, 1974, pp. 27–59.

Rosenstock, I.M., Hochbaum, G.M., and Kegeles, S.S.: *Determinants of Health Behavior.* White House Conference on Children and Youth. Washington, D.C., 1960.

Rosenstock, I.M., and Kirscht, J.P.: Practice implications, in M.H. Becker, editor, *The Health Belief Model and Personal Health Behavior.* Thorofare, N.J.: Charles B. Slack, 1974, pp. 143–146.

Stunkard, A.J.: *Personal Communication.* MRFIT Meeting. St. Louis, February 13, 1978.

Tapp, J.T., Kaull, R.S., Tapp, M., and Seller, R.H.: The application of behavior modification to behavior management: Guidelines for the family physician. *J. Fam. Pract.* 6(2):293–299, 1979.

Thoresen, C.E., and Mahoney, M.J.: *Behavioral Self-Control.* New York: Holt, Rinehart and Winston, 1974.

U.S. National Clearinghouse for Smoking and Health. *Smokers' Self-Testing Kit.* USPHS Pub. No. 1904, 1969.

Wallace, B.: *Applied Hypnosis: An Overview.* Chicago: Nelson-Hall, 1979.

White, J.R., and Froeb, H.F.: Small airways dysfunction in nonsmokers chronically exposed to tobacco smoke. *N. Engl. J. Med.* 202(13):720–723, 1980.

Williams, R.L., and Long, J.D.: *Toward a Self-Managed Life Style.* Boston: Houghton Mifflin, 1975.

CHAPTER 3
Hypertension

NEMAT O. BORHANI, M.D., F.A.C.C.

Recent publication of the five-year findings of the Hypertension Detection and Follow-Up Program (HDFP), a community-based randomized trial of the treatment of hypertension (HDFP Cooperative Group, 1979a; 1979b), has brought into focus the necessity for judicious treatment of mild and moderate hypertension (e.g., diastolic blood pressure of 90–104 mm Hg) in prevention of premature mortality. Thus, in a review of the annual progress in disease prevention, hypertension assumes a pivotal point of reference.

Despite the very impressive decline in mortality observed in the United States since 1968, the death rate due to diseases associated with hypertension (e.g., coronary heart disease, stroke, and congestive heart failure) remains high; these diseases constitute a major threat to community health. The threat of these diseases limits our chances for longevity and remains an economic liability which interferes with the realization of human potentials.

Hypertension is one of the most prevalent chronic diseases and is a major independent risk factor for the common adult cardiovascular and renal diseases, including coronary heart disease, stroke, and congestive heart failure. The toll of death and disability inflicted by uncontrolled hypertension, and diseases associated with it, is a challenge to the health profession and to the society as a whole. Further, chronic diseases caused by, or resulting from, uncontrolled hypertension cast a much larger shadow on human potentials than is outlined by their attendant rates of mortality and morbidity. Since mortality and morbidity associated with uncontrolled hypertension increases with age, growing older remains a social and an economic liability rather than a valued confirmation of human potential in our society. On the one hand, we have succeeded in extending the life expectancy by such magnificent achievements as the eradication of small pox and control of other infectious diseases of man. And, on the other hand, our fellow

58

men who have deferred immediate pleasures in favor of a lifetime sense of purpose are too often denied both, because of the diseases caused by hypertension.

Since clinical efficacy of treatment of hypertension is now an established and accepted medical phenomenon, a vigorous and coordinated community health program, aimed at the control of hypertension in the community, must be considered seriously among the first steps in prevention of premature mortality and morbidity. Because the concept of uncontrolled hypertension as a community health hazard, rather than an individual patient's health problem, is a relatively new concept, the magnitude of the problem of hypertension needs to be articulated in its proper perspective, recognizing the epidemiological nature of high blood pressure, its relationship to disease mortality and morbidity, and the fact that hypertension is a disease for which safe and effective treatment is available. Physicians, nurses, and other members of the health profession, as well as the voluntary and public health agencies, must be convinced of the necessity for a comprehensive hypertension education and control program, through a nationally coordinated effort. For if the community hypertension control programs aimed at prevention of premature mortality in this country are to be effective at all, they must have the support of the country's leadership—medical, political, and the public at large.

For this reason the issue of the need for community hypertension control programs must be veiwed in its epidemiological context and the potential impact of its control. In this chapter I shall briefly review (1) the epidemiology of hypertension; (2) the clinical evidence on the safety and efficacy of treatment of uncontrolled hypertension; and (3) the issues that must be carefully considered in planning and implementing community hypertension control programs.

EPIDEMIOLOGY OF HYPERTENSION

Prevalence

Arterial blood pressure is a quantitative biological trait; it has a continuous distribution in population subgroups. The adverse effects of elevated blood pressure are related numerically to the level of blood pressure (Pickering, 1968). The frequency distributions of systolic and diastolic blood pressure in the adult population of the United States are depicted in Figures 3-1 and 3-2. These figures are based on the results of the National Health Examination Survey, conducted in 1960–1962 among a randomly selected sample of the United States population in the age groups of 18–79 years (Blood Pressure of Adults, 1964a; 1964b; Hypertension, 1966). There are certain important features of these two frequency distributions that have significant clinical implications. These features must be considered in planning prevention programs for control of hypertension in the community.

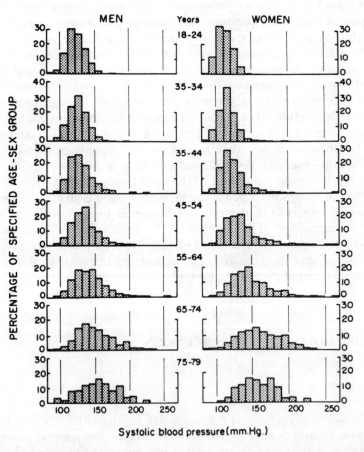

Figure 3-1. Frequency distribution of systolic blood pressure. National Health Examination Survey.

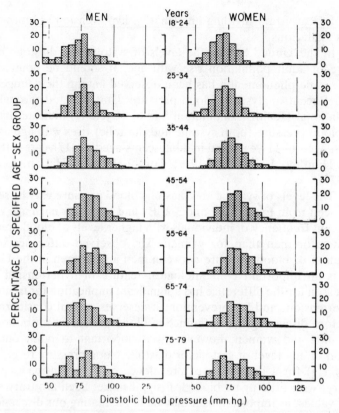

Figure 3-2. Frequency distribution of diastolic blood pressure. National Health Examination Survey.

Foremost among them are the following characteristics:

1. Frequency distributions of both systolic and diastolic blood pressure form a continuous unimodal curve which is skewed slightly to the right; these frequency distributions are log normal; that is, a log transformation of the actual blood pressure readings will produce a Gaussian Normal Distribution. There is no evidence of any break in these distributions to signal a distinction between "normal" and "abnormal" blood pressure levels. In other words, there is no dividing line (cut-off point) above which an individual is at risk and below which he is free from it. Indeed, as pointed out by Sir George Pickering (1968), any consideration of the course and natural history of hypertension in

terms of an arbitrary dividing line (that is, hypertension vs. normotension) is "fallacious."

2. In the United States, the levels of systolic and diastolic blood pressure of adult population rise with age. It should be pointed out that the same phenomenon has been observed among the younger age groups. Recent analysis of blood pressure data collected through the U.S. National Health Examination Survey (Cycle II) indicate that the mean blood pressure (both systolic and diastolic) rises with age among children aged 6–11 years and in adolescents aged 12–17 years (Harlan, Coroni-Huntley, Leaverton, 1979; Coroni-Huntley, Harlan, Leaverton, 1979).

3. The levels of systolic and diastolic blood pressure vary by sex, as can be seen from Figures 3-1 and 3-2. By and large, for each age group the percent frequency of individuals with higher levels of blood pressure is greater for men than for women. The observed difference in the distribution of blood pressure between men and women in the United States is an important epidemiological feature of hypertension. The main reason for the difference has a significant implication for treatment of hypertension, and for prevention; it deserves careful consideration.

Before discussing the difference in blood pressure distribution between men and women, however, it is important to point out that selection of any level of systolic or diastolic blood pressure (e.g., DBP 95 mm Hg) for a discussion of prevalence of hypertension is purely arbitrary, with little or no biological significance. Such arbitrary selection of values, as important as it may be in facilitating our discussion of the magnitude of the problem of hypertension and our understanding of epidemiological features of hypertension, must not be construed as an indication of a dividing line (cut-off point) in the frequency distribution of blood pressure in the community. Nor should it be given any biological significance in prevention. As will be discussed later in this chapter, the desision for treatment of hypertension, and the "ideal" level of blood pressure chosen for prevention of premature mortality, must be based on total health profile, lifestyle, and habits of the people rather than an arbitrary level of blood pressure.

Choosing a diastolic blood pressure of 95 mm Hg as an arbitrary figure for definition of prevalence of hypertension, the National Health Examination Survey of 1960–1962 reported the following prevalence figures: 8.3 percent for white women, 9.1 percent for white men, 21.5 percent for black women, and 22.6 percent for black men (Blood Pressure of Adults, 1964b). Data collected in 1974 by the Hypertension Detection and Follow-Up Program (a program that will be described later in this chapter) reported a similar difference in the prevalence of hypertension between men and women, even though the actual percent of individuals with diastolic blood pressure of 95 mm Hg and above were different between the two reports, mostly due to differences in design, methods, and the age composition of the two samples. The prevalence of hypertension (DBP 95 mm Hg and above) among a sample of population 30–69 years of age in 14 selected communities of the United States, who were screened at home in 1974 for participation in the HDFP, was reported as 8.4 percent for white women, 13.5 percent for white men, 23.1 percent for black women, and 28.1 percent for black men (HDFP Cooperative Group, 1977a), confirming the earlier observations that the prevalence of hypertension is higher among men than women. However, these differences in reported prevalence of hypertension between men and women are misleading.

In reality there is little or no difference in actual prevalence of hypertension in the community between men and women. The difference is in the degree of health care utilization, hence control of hypertension, between men and women. In reviewing the magnitude of the prevalence of hypertension in the community, we should remember that the actual prevalence of hypertension depends on the observed rate of elevated blood pressure in any community at the time of screening and the rate of current use of antihypertensive medication which might produce a lower than actual reading of blood pressure at the time of screening. To assess the total magnitude of the problem of hypertension in the community, we should consider those whose blood pressure is above a certain arbitrary level (e.g., DBP 95 mm Hg) at the time of screening *plus* those who report current use of antihypertensive medication and whose blood pressure may be less than the arbitrary level chosen for screening. We shall refer to these two groups combined as the "actual hypertensives" in the community. Applying this principle to the HDFP data, it was found that, among all persons screened at home, the prevalence of actual hypertension (those with DBP of 95 mm Hg and above and those with DBP below this level but on antihypertensive medication) was 18 percent for white women, 19 percent for white men, 38 percent for black women, and 36 percent for black men. In other words, of all persons screened at home, 37 percent of blacks and 18 percent of whites were found to have actual hypertension, with virtually no difference in total percentages between men and women.

Of all persons with actual hypertension, high blood pressure had been detected, treated, and brought under control, at the time of the survey, in 40 percent of black women, 51 percent of white women, and only 22 percent of black men and in 28 percent of white men. In other words, the percentages of undetected, untreated, and uncontrolled hypertension were 78 percent in black men, versus 60 percent in black women, and 72 percent in white men versus 49 percent in white women (HDFP Cooperative Group, 1977a). Thus, the utilization of health care, hence proper detection and control of hypertension, seems to be higher among women than men, in both races. This difference in the use of medical care and control of hypertension in the United States has led to a spurious observation claiming a difference in the prevalence of hypertension between men and women, when in reality the major portion of this difference, if not all, can be explained by the differences in the rate of detection and treatment of hypertension between men and women.

4. In addition to age and sex, the frequency distribution of blood pressure (both systolic and diastolic) varies by race. As can be seen from the prevalence figures given above, the percentage of those with diastolic blood pressure of 95 mm Hg and above is higher among blacks (both men and women) than whites. The National Health Examination Survey of 1960–1962 reported the prevalence of hypertension (DBP 95 mm Hg and above) in both sexes combined as 22.0 percent for blacks and 8.7 percent for whites (Blood Pressure of Adults, 1964a; 1964b). The HDFP data collected in 1974 reported a prevalence rate of (DBP 95 mm Hg and above) 24.9 percent for blacks and 10.8 percent for whites (HDFP Cooperative Group, 1977a). The observed difference in the prevalence of hypertension between blacks and whites in the United States assumes a significant importance in planning and implementing prevention programs. Two important aspects of this observation deserve special consideration. First, part of the observed difference in the prevalence of hypertension between blacks and whites can be explained on the basis of a differential rate of medical care utilization in the United States between blacks and whites. Unlike the situation in the case of the difference between men and women, however, the effect of medical care utilization, hence the control of hypertension, on the observed difference in the prevalence of hypertension between blacks and whites is very small. For example, when the HDFP data findings are analyzed in terms of the prevalence of actual hypertensives, that is, the percentage of those with a diastolic blood pressure of 95 mm Hg and above at screening plus those whose diastolic blood pressure is below 95 mm Hg but who are under current antihypertensive therapy, the respective prevalence figures become 37 percent for blacks and 18 percent for whites, still a 2:1 ratio between the two races. Second, the observed difference in prevalence of hypertension between blacks and whites varies by the level of blood pressure. For example, as can be seen from data in Figure 3-3, among all hypertensives (those with diastolic blood pressure of 95 mm Hg and above) the black to white ratio in prevalence is 2.1 for males and 2.7 for females. This ratio rises manyfold as the level of diastolic blood pressure increases. At the diastolic blood pressure level of 115 mm Hg and above, the black to white ratio in the prevalence becomes 5.4 for males and 7.1 for females (HDFP Cooperative Group, 1977a; 1977b). This difference in prevalence coupled with the fact that among all blacks with actual hypertension, 78 percent of men and 60 percent of women remain undetected, untreated, and uncontrolled, points out the special need for serious consideration of epidemiological features of hypertension in planning prevention programs in the community.

It should be pointed out that the rate of previously undetected, untreated, and uncontrolled hypertension, although improved considerably during the past few years in the United States, remains unacceptably high at the present time. This rate varies not only by sex and race,

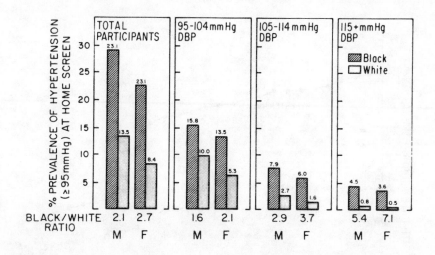

Figure 3-3. Prevalence of hypertension at home screen for total HDFP participants and by selected blood pressure strata [diastolic blood pressure (DBP) ≥ 95 mm Hg]

From the Hypertension Detection and Follow-up Program, *Circulation* 40(5): May 1977. By Permission of the American Heart Association, Inc.

but by age as well; it is highest among young individuals. The stereotype of a young black man is in the worst condition with respect to hypertension, hence at highest risk.

Mortality

Mortality trend for hypertension and hypertensive heart disease, United States 1950–1975, is presented in Figure 3-4. As can be seen, there has been a steady decline in hypertension mortality during the periods of 1950–1958, 1959–1967, and 1968–1975. The assignment of cause of death in each period depicted in Figure 3-4 is according to the International Classification of Diseases, Adapted (ICDA) rubrics in use during that period (i.e., sixth revision of ICD for 1950–1958, seventh revision for 1959–1967, and eighth revision for 1968–1975). The death rate from hypertensive heart disease was 56.0 per 100,000 population in 1950 and declined to 5.1 per 100,000 in 1975; it further de-

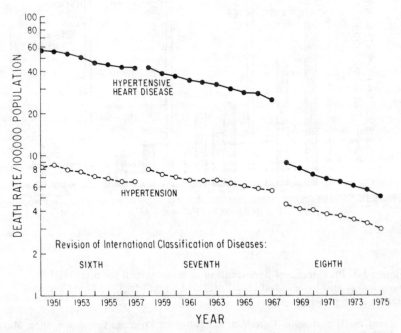

Figure 3-4. Death rates for hypertensive heart disease and hypertension: United States 1950–1975.

clined to 4.8 per 100,000 in 1976. Between 1959 and 1967, the decline in mortality was 31 percent for hypertension and 38.5 percent for hypertensive heart disease. Between 1968 and 1975, the death rate from hypertension declined by an additional 45.5 percent; the respective decline for hypertensive heart disease was 50.8 percent. The decline in mortality from hypertension has occurred consistently among whites and blacks, men and women, and in all age groups.

Although the International Classification of Diseases and Causes of Death has undergone three substantive revisions during the period of 1950–1976 (from sixth revision to seventh and then to eighth), the observed decline in mortality from hypertension and hypertensive heart disease does not seem to be entirely due to changing patterns in diagnosis and coding classification of the cause of death on the death certificate. To measure the degree of change brought about by revisions in the ICD coding procedures, the National Center for Health Statistics has developed comparability ratios for total cardiovascular disease mortality and for its major components. The trend in mortality from 1950 to 1976, therefore, could be constructed after the application of these comparability ratios so that the rates during the period of 1950–1967 would be comparable to the rates between 1968 and 1976, insofar as classification of cause of death is concerned.

Figure 3-5 presents age-adjusted rate of mortality from hypertensive heart disease, with or without renal disease, after the application of the appropriate comparability ratios. The decline in mortality from hypertensive heart disease between 1950 and 1976 is *81 percent*, a phenomenal drop, indeed, in only 26 years. It should be noted that during this period there has also been a concomitant decline in the death rates from cerebrovascular disease (stroke), strongly supporting the notion of a true reduction in the number of deaths due to hypertension, since hypertension is the major factor in stroke mortality. Further, there is no evidence that a shift of diagnosis and/or coding (due to changes that occurred in the eighth revision of the ICD coding system) into the coronary disease category could explain this decline in mortality from hypertension. As can be seen from Table 3-1, a corollary event has been a dramatic decline of *26.5 percent* in mortality from acute myocardial infarction between 1968 (the year that the eighth revision was adopted) and 1976. Corresponding figures in mortality from acute myocardial infarction with and without hypertensive disease respectively are *−17.7* and *−27.4* percent. Thus, the observed decline in mortality from hypertension and hypertensive heart disease is real and not an artifact.

Mortality Trend by Sex. The observed changes in mortality from

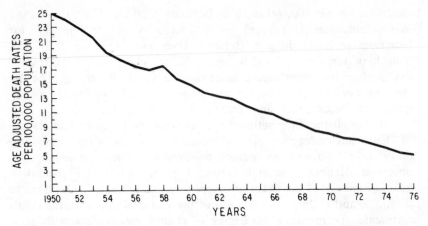

Figure 3-5. U.S. mortality trend from hypertensive heart disease with or without renal disease, and hypertension-adjusted for changes in international classification of diseases (ICD Code Revisions) 1950–1976. Comparability Ratio 8th/7th Revision = 0.398. Comparability Ratio 7th/6th Revision = 1.11.

acute myocardial infarction between 1968 and 1976 were identical for men and women, a reduction of 25.7 percent for men and 26.6 percent for women (Table 3-1). However, the percent changes in mortality from acute myocardial infarction with hypertension differed markedly between the two sexes. As can be seen from Table 3-1, the decline in mortality from myocardial infarction with hypertension was greater in women than in men, 24.8 versus 11.7 percent. The difference in percent change in mortality from acute myocardial infarction with hypertension between men and women emphasizes the difference in the pattern of treatment and control of hypertension between the two sexes, as was stated earlier.

Trend by Race and Sex. Percent changes in mortality from acute myocardial infarction, with and without hypertension, by race and sex are presented in Table 3-2. It can be seen that the percent decline in mortality (between 1968 and 1976) from acute myocardial infarction with hypertension was the largest among white women (25.3 percent) and the smallest in white men (11.3 percent). Among blacks, the rate of decline between 1968 and 1976 was 21.3 percent in women and 13.3 percent in men. It should be noted that in both whites and blacks, men have fared worse than women, confirming further the difference between men and women in the rate of utilization of medical care, hence control of hypertension.

Table 3-1
Percent Changes in Selected United States Age-adjusted Death Rates by Cause and by Sex between 1968 and 1976

Cause of Death ICD, 8th Revision	Both Sexes	Males	Females
Acute MI with Hypertensive Disease (ICD 410.00)	-17.7	-11.7	-24.8
Acute MI Without Hypertensive Disease (ICD 410.9)	-27.4	-26.7	-26.9
Acute Myocardial Infarction (ICD 410.00)	-26.5	-25.7	-26.6

The dramatic decline in mortality from hypertensive disease observed since 1950, and especially changes that have occurred since 1968 (the year of the eighth revision of ICDA), cannot be explained fully on the basis of revisions in the International Classification of Diseases and Causes of Death. If this were the case, it would be unlikely for changes in mortality from hypertensive disease to be accompanied by a concomitant reduction in mortality from coronary heart disease, cerebrovascular disease (stroke), and mortality from all causes, as has been the case. The decline in mortality from hypertension corresponds very well with concomitant decline in mortality from all components of cardiovascular diseases. In addition, mortality from all causes (total mortality) has reached an all-time low in the United States: 8.7 deaths per 1,000 population in 1977. Thus, the evidence suggests that the observed decline in mortality from hypertension and hypertensive heart disease is *real* and *not* an artifact.

Reduction in hypertension mortality must be attributed to, and based on, a factor that can explain at least two important questions. First, why is the downward trend less pronounced in men than in women? And, second, why is the downward trend different between whites and blacks?

To answer these questions, one important fact must be considered; that is, in the absence of any data on incidence, there could be a tendency to attribute the observed decline in mortality to a reduction in prevalence of hypertension. The observed decline in mortality from

Table 3-2
Percent Changes in Age-Adjusted Death Rates in the United States by Cause of Death, Race, and Sex between 1968 and 1976

CAUSE OF DEATH ICD, 8th REVISION	BOTH SEXES		MALES		FEMALES	
	Whites	Non-Whites	Whites	Non-Whites	Whites	Non-Whites
Acute MI With Hypertensive Disease (ICD 410.0)	-17.6	-16.6	-11.3	-13.3	-25.3	-21.3
Acute MI Without Hypertensive Disease (ICD 410.9)	-27.0	-30.1	-26.4	-28.6	-26.4	-31.5
Acute Myocardial Infarction (ICD 410)	-26.2	-28.3	-25.4	-26.8	-26.1	-29.7
Hypertensive Heart Disease With or Without Renal Disease (ICD 402-404)	-50.8					
Hypertension (ICD 400,401,403)	-45.5					

hypertension does not seem to be due to any changes in prevalence. The findings of the National Health Survey Examination indicate that the prevalence of hypertension (diastolic blood pressure of 95 mm Hg and above) in the United States was the same in the 1971–1974 survey (Blood Pressure Levels, 1977) as it was in 1960–1962 (Blood Pressure of Adults, 1964a; 1964b; Hypertension, 1966). The total prevalence rate among U.S. adults aged 18–79 years was 18.1 percent in 1971–1974 (Blood Pressure Levels, 1977); it was 18.2 percent in 1960–1962 (Blood Pressure of Adults, 1964b). Even when adjustment is made to compensate for differences in the age–sex distribution in the United States population between 1960–1962 and 1971–1974 time periods, the projected prevalence rate from the 1960–1962 survey to the present population distribution would be 17.6 percent, just slightly below the rate actually found in the 1971–1974 survey (18.1 percent) but not enough to explain the dramatic decline in mortality between the two points in time, based on any change in prevalence.

The only factor capable of answering the two questions posed above and explaining the secular trend in mortality from hypertension seems to be a true change in case fatality ratio from hypertensive disease, which could be due only to a high rate of medical care utilization, hence control of hypertension. We must, therefore, consider changes in physicians' knowledge about hypertension, changes in physicians' attitude toward treatment of hypertension, and changes in mode of treatment, as well as changes in public attitude, knowledge, and awareness of hypertension as factors which have contributed to a dramatic change in case fatality ratio of hypertension and hypertensive diseases, resulting in the observed favorable trend in mortality.

Two circumstances seem to be most supportive of this interpretation. One is the increased public and professional awareness of the problem of hypertension, and along with it, a new attitude on how to deal with the problem. The other is the emergence of the knowledge about the efficacy of antihypertensive treatment in prevention of mortality from hypertensive disease.

Today, hypertension is recognized as one of the most common causes of death and disability in this country. The degree of public and professional awareness has increased dramatically since government agencies with private industry and voluntary health associations began in earnest a collaborative effort to educate the public and the health profession on the dangers of hypertension and the new methods of detection, treatment, and follow-up of patients with hypertension.

Available evidence indicates that there has been a steady increase in hypertension awareness in this country since 1950. In 1960 the proportion of adults with hypertension who were not aware of their condition (i.e., previously undiagnosed hypertension) was estimated to be about 45 percent. By 1974 the proportion of adults with hypertension who were not aware of their condition had declined to 25 percent (HDFP Cooperative Group, 1977a). Recent data from the Impact of Hypertension Information Study (IHI) indicate a further drop in the proportion of those with hypertension who are now aware of their condition (unpublished data). Changes in the status of detected, treated, and adequately controlled hypertension among white women, given only as an example, are depicted in Figure 3-6. As can be seen, the proportion of white women with hypertension who were not aware of their condition was 18 percent in 1973–1974; it declined to 12 percent in 1977–1978. Likewise, the proportion of those whose hypertension has been adequately controlled had risen from 51 percent in 1973–1974 to 69 percent in 1977–1978. Similar changes have occurred among other race–sex groups.

These dramatic changes in awareness and control of hypertension are reflected in a shift to the left in the distribution of blood pressure by age among all adults (whites and blacks) of both sexes and are corroborated by an increase in the percent of patient visits to physicians for hypertension and hypertensive heart disease. While the in-

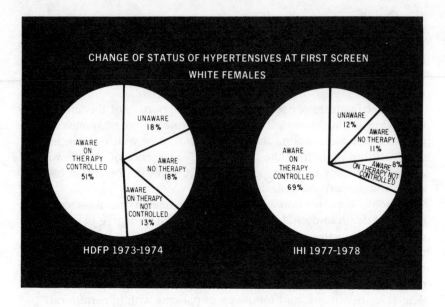

Figure 3-6. Change of status of hypertensives at first screen (white females).

crease over 1971 for all patient visits to physicians was 3.4 percent in 1972 and rose to 4.9 percent in 1976, the corresponding increase in visits for hypertension and hypertensive heart disease over 1971 was 7.9 percent in 1972 and rose to 48.5 percent in 1976. Visits to physicians for hypertension during a two-year period (1975–1976) comprised *4 percent* of the *1.1 billion visits,* and ranked *first* among visits for all morbid events in the United States. These changes are consistent with current epidemiological features of hypertension and percent decline in mortality from it. The difference in the prevalence of actual hypertension between men and women, the difference in the percent reduction in mortality from hypertension between men and women, and, to some degree, the difference in the prevalence of hypertension between blacks and whites, all can be explained on the basis of a differential in the degree of awareness of hypertension and the rate of utilization of medical care aimed at controlling hypertension for prevention of premature mortality.

Hypertension as a Risk Factor in Mortality and Morbidity

Despite the recent decline in its mortality, hypertension remains as a major risk factor associated with, or contributing to, most of the major components of cardiovascular disease mortality, e.g., coronary heart disease, stroke, and death from all causes.

In considering the relationship between hypertension and mortality (mortality from all causes and from cardiovascular diseases) four important epidemiological features of hypertension must be emphasized, as illustrated by data presented in Tables 3-3 and 3-4, derived from the 1950–1960 longitudinal study of the San Francisco Longshoremen (Borhani, Hechter, and Breslow, 1963). These features are:

1. Both measured blood pressure components (i.e., systolic and diastolic) contribute significantly and independently to the risk of mortality. The probability of death rises significantly with increments in the levels of either systolic or diastolic blood pressures, even in the range not considered abnormal in clinical practice (e.g., SBP 130–150 mm Hg and DBP 80–90 mm Hg).

2. The positive and sustained relationship between the level of blood pressure and mortality has been demonstrated consistently by the findings of prospective epidemiological studies, using only a casual reading of blood pressure. Thus, a casual reading of blood pressure is just as predictive of the subsequent risk of mortality as are measure-

Table 3-3
Death Rates for All Causes in Smokers and Nonsmokers, Grouped According to Systolic Blood Pressure

Age Group	Systolic Blood Pressure (mm Hg)	Death rates per 10,000	
		Smokers	Nonsmokers
45 to 54	Less than 130	91	46
	130 to 149	131	72
	150 to 169	189	76
	170 and more	353	223
55 to 64	Less than 130	159	71
	130 to 149	290	125
	150 to 169	324	160
	170 and more	534	304

From Borhani et al. (1963).

Table 3-4
Death Rates for All Causes in Smokers and Nonsmokers, Grouped According to Diastolic Blood Pressure

Age Group	Diastolic Blood Pressure (mm. Hg)	Death rates per 10,000 Smokers	Death rates per 10,000 Nonsmokers
45 to 54	Less than 80	79	47
	80 to 89	128	54
	90 to 99	135	119
	100 and more	424	137
55 to 64	Less than 80	179	104
	80 to 89	243	118
	90 to 99	403	145
	100 and more	623	325

From Borhani et al. (1963).

ments obtained under basal conditions. This observation has an important implication for planning community prevention programs and should not be dismissed lightly, despite the known variability of blood pressure measurements.

3. The relationship between the level of blood pressure and mortality is continuous. The higher the level of blood pressure, the greater the risk of mortality. There is no cut-off point or threshold, no apparent critical blood pressure level above which people are at risk of mortality and below which they are free from it. Systolic and diastolic levels of blood pressure should be considered independent biological variables that influence the risk of mortality at all levels. The traditional distinction, in relation to the risk of mortality, between "hypertension" and "normotension" is arbitrary and fallacious; it should be abandoned by the health profession.

4. There is a considerable interaction between the level of blood pressure as a force of mortality and other risks of death. In addition to age, this interaction is most prominent with the habit of cigarette smoking, as can be seen from data in Tables 3-3 and 3-4. The findings of practically all epidemiological studies conducted since then have consistently confirmed this important epidemiological feature of hypertension in terms of its relationship with mortality.

In terms of morbidity, the association between the level of blood pressure and the incidence of coronary heart disease and stroke is the most significant aspect of the epidemiology of hypertension and should be considered in further detail. The strongest evidence demonstrating an association between the level of blood pressure and the incidence of coronary heart disease and stroke is derived from the results of prospective population-based epidemiological studies conducted in the United States and elsewhere during the last 30 years. The basic strategy of these epidemiological studies is the characterization of individuals by casual measurement of blood pressure levels, excluding those with any evidence of overt disease at entry into the study, meticulous follow-up over the years for the discovery of new events (e.g., acute myocardial infarction), and assessment of the incidence rate of the disease under study (e.g., coronary heart disease) in relation to the initial casual blood pressure levels at entry into the study. All such studies, conducted in the United States and in other countries, have reported hypertension as a major risk factor associated with the incidence of coronary heart disease and stroke.

Recently, data from the major United States prospective epidemiological studies of coronary heart disease have been pooled together, analyzed collectively, and reported as the U.S. Pooling Project (1978). Obviously, the pooling of these data increases the number of observations and thus provides additional confidence in the strength of the association between the level of blood pressure and the incidence of coronary heart disease. Data from the U.S. Pooling Project indicate that the incidence of first event of coronary heart disease (fatal and nonfatal myocardial infarction and sudden death due to coronary heart disease) increases proportionally, in a positive stepwise gradient, with the levels of systolic and diastolic blood pressure at entry into the study, even in the range not generally considered extremely high by clinical criteria; e.g., diastolic blood pressure of 85–94 mm Hg (U.S. Pooling Project, 1978). The association between diastolic blood pressure at entry into the study and the first major coronary event (fatal and nonfatal myocardial infarction and sudden CHD death) is presented graphically in Figure 3-7. As can be seen, in every age group the mean diastolic blood pressure at entry into the study was higher among those men who subsequently experienced an event of fatal or nonfatal coronary heart disease than among those who did not experience such an event during the years of follow-up. All differences in mean blood pressure in each age group between men who experienced the event and those who did not are statistically significant ($p \leq .01$). It should be noted that every level of diastolic blood pressure depicted in the Figure 3-7 is below 95 mm Hg, the arbitrary level chosen earlier in this chapter to describe the magnitude of the prevalence of hypertension in the community.

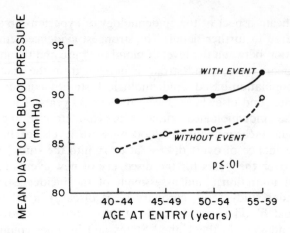

Figure 3-7. Mean diastolic blood pressure (mm Hg) in men experiencing a first major coronary event (fatal and nonfatal myocardial infarction and sudden CHD death) and men not experiencing an event, by age at entry.

From the Hypertension Detection and Follow-up Program, *Circulation* 40(5): May 1977. By Permission of the American Heart Association, Inc.

In addition to the actual level of blood pressure as measured casually at the time of entry into these prospective studies, there is evidence that subsequent changes in blood pressure influences significantly the occurrence of subsequent events among the cohort under observation. For example, it has been reported recently that although longitudinal studies demonstrate an increase in the level of blood pressure among the members of a cohort over time (mostly due to increase in age and changes in other determinants of blood pressure such as body weight), a greater positive change (i.e., an increase) in blood pressure over time is found among those who subsequently develop new events of coronary heart disease than among those who remain free of any manifestations of new events of coronary heart disease (Rabkin, Matthewson, and Tate, 1979). The implications of this important epidemiological observation in clinical management of hypertension and in prevention of premature mortality are obvious.

In addition to coronary heart disease, hypertension is a risk factor in stroke. In fact, hypertension is regarded as a major risk factor in stroke, both hemorrhagic and thrombotic (Borhani, 1966; Chapman, 1966; Kannel, 1970). Based on consistent findings of all prospective epidemiological studies conducted in the United States and throughout the world, there is evidence of a strong, positive, and stepwise association between the level of blood pressure and subsequent incidence of new cases of thrombotic and hemorrhagic stroke. Further, the available data on the decline in mortality from stroke, and, more important, the evidence on the changing pattern in stroke concomitant with an increased level of awareness and effective control of hypertension, provide the most convincing evidence of a causal relationship between hypertension and stroke. There is evidence that the markedly increased proportion of patients with mild or moderate hypertension who were under treatment and control during the period of 1970–1974 may have contributed to the accelerated rate of decline in the incidence of cerebral infarction (Garroway et al., 1979). In addition, the results of clinical trials in treatment of hypertension (which will be discussed later in this chapter) clearly demonstrate the necessity of hypertension control in prevention of stroke.

Determinants of Hypertension

There is marked variation in blood pressure during a 24-hour period. Also, there is marked intra-individual variation in blood pressure response to a host of physiologic and environmental stimuli. Sir George Pickering has demonstrated this important phenomenon quite eloquently, and has argued convincingly that blood pressure varies widely in a single day depending on what the subject does and that hypertension is a quantitative disease in which the deviation of blood pressure from normal is a deviation of degree and not of kind (1968). Environmental and genetic factors constantly influence the level of blood pressure and may cause a deviation from normal under different circumstances. The quantitative relationship between the level of blood pressure and clinical manifestation of disease is the more remarkable when one considers the numerous factors that influence it, favorably or adversely, in a 24-hour period. The lowest level of blood pressure is recorded during sleep and the highest in response to severe environmental stimuli (e.g., fear and pain). Elevated blood pressure is, therefore, dependent upon the circumstances that affect the casual reading, in the office, at home, at rest, standing, sitting, facing the physician, the nurse, or the technician. In making a judgment on the deviation of blood pressure from normal, the circumstances under which blood pressure had been measured must be considered and carefully evaluated.

By and large, determinants of hypertension are either genetic or environmental. There is no question that inheritance makes a contribution to the level of blood pressure. Studies among first-degree relatives of patients with hypertension and among twins have demonstrated that the degree of genetic contribution to the variance of blood pressure can be estimated by a regression that may vary from 0.25 to 0.64 (Pickering, 1968; Borhani et al., 1976). It should be pointed out, however, that the inheritance of hypertension is, in all probability, multifactoral (polygenic) and that there is a significant interaction between genetic and environmental factors as they influence the level of blood pressure. For example, the relationship between blood pressure of first-degree relatives almost disappears in the highest level of blood pressure, indicating, perhaps, a severe interference by environmental factors responsible for high levels of blood pressure. Similarly the response to a given environmental factor (e.g., salt intake) varies significantly among population groups with different genetic susceptibility to hypertension.

One of the most illustrative examples of genetic and environmental interaction in blood pressure is the rise of blood pressure with age. It is an accepted fact that in Western societies blood pressure rises with age. Yet there are many societies in which blood pressure does not rise significantly with age. Although there is some genetic influence in the rise of blood pressure with age, presumably the rise with age is influenced largely by environmental factors. Whatever the environmental factors may be which influence the level of blood pressure, or its rise with age (e.g., dietary sodium and sociopsychological stress), the genetic factor, at a given age, seems to determine the arterial blood pressure response to it. Further, there is good evidence that the pattern of blood pressure response to environmental stimuli starts with childhood; tracking of susceptible children is demonstrated in recent studies, even though the nature of genetic defects remains illusive. According to Sir George Pickering, what is inherited " . . . may be a structural or biochemical peculiarity of vessels which may influence their response to stimuli" (1977). Despite many hypotheses about the mechanism and numerous arguments about the role of inheritance and/or environment in the genesis of hypertension, we are almost totally ignorant today in understanding the extent, the nature, and the interaction between genetic and environmental factors in hypertension.

Among the most prominent environmental factors known to influence the level of blood pressure, body weight, excessive dietary intake of salt, glucose, and certain trace metals (e.g., cadmium), oral contraceptives, and sociopsychological and physical stimuli should be considered as relevant in the context of planning hypertension control programs for purposes of prevention.

Body Weight and Hypertension. Many epidemiological studies have demonstrated a positive relationship between body weight and the level of blood pressure. Data from the National Health Survey Examination indicate that systolic and diastolic blood pressure were associated with body weight among the adult population of the United States, aged 18–79 years. Table 3-5 presents data from a randomly selected sample of the general population of Alameda County, California (Borhani, 1969), which demonstrate the relationship between the level of blood pressure and body weight. Other epidemiological studies in the United States and elsewhere have confirmed these findings.

Salt Intake and Hypertension. Dahl's classic experimental studies have provided a sound scientific base on which the issue of salt question in hypertension must rest (Dahl, Heine, Tassinari, 1962). Briefly, epidemiological studies have demonstrated a good correlation between the variance in blood pressure distribution among different countries of the world and the level of salt intake; prevalence of hypertension is highest in northern Japan, where the average daily intake of NaCl is as high as 30 gm, and lowest among Eskimos in Alaska whose daily intake of NaCl averages about less than 5 gm. In some primitive communities, in villages of New Guinea and Solomon Islands, a relative absence of hypertension has been demonstrated to be associated with low intake of salt in the inhabitants' daily diet. Also, regional differences in blood pressure distribution in Japan have been explained by a difference in the rate of daily intake of salt in Japanese diet. Difference in the average daily intake of salt between southern Japan (with

Table 3-5
Correlation Coefficients of Systolic and Diastolic Blood Pressure and Selected Body Weight Indicators

Age	Ponderal Index		Relative Body Weight		Metropolitan Index	
	SBP	DBP	SBP	DBP	SBP	DBP
20-34	-.235	-.140	.305	.206	.302	.190
35-44	-.376	-.280	.438	.349	.452	.364
45-54	-.216	-.251	.304	.302	.299	.297
55-64	-.218	-.118	.253	.188	.247	.187
P Value	< .01		< .01		< .01	

From Borhani (1969).

low prevalence of hypertension) and northern Japan (with high prevalence of hypertension) is approximately 10–15 gm.

In his classic laboratory experiments, Dahl demonstrated that, among rats, a significant variation in response to salt feeding exists. Some animals do not respond at all while some develop malignant hypertension. He hypothesized that such disparate responses among animals on the same salt intake may suggest differences in genetic susceptibility in blood pressure response to salt intake among experimental laboratory animals. By selective breeding, in successive generations of rats Dahl inbred what he called "susceptible" and "resistant" rats and demonstrated clearly the interaction between genetic susceptibility and response to excessive salt intake for development of hypertension (Dahl et al., 1962). He concluded that the genetic substrate is a critical determinant in whether or not experimental hypertension develops in experimental animals after excessive intake of salt. He proposed that a similar interaction operates in humans (Dahl, 1977). Beneficial effect of salt restriction in treatment of hypertension (whether be it through weight loss due to caloric restriction or the salt restriction per se) has been demonstrated in numerous clinical observations and confirmed in laboratory by metabolic studies; since the introduction of thiazide diuretics in 1957, salt elimination has become recognized as the mainstay of treatment of hypertension. Further, there is evidence that a sudden and large increase in salt intake raises the level of extracellular fluids, hence increases plasma volume and cardiac output. These hemodynamic changes lead to a rise in blood pressure. Thus, despite the controversy surrounding the issue of salt in hypertension, it seems prudent to view excessive intake of salt as an important determinant of hypertension, especially in children and young adults in whom clinical manifestation of the disease may set in long after exposure.

Glucose Intake and Hypertension. Data from the National Health Survey Examination indicate that carbohydrate intake, especially glucose, is associated significantly with the level of blood pressure among adult populations of the United States, aged 18–79 years. Of course, it is a known clinical fact that hypertension is quite frequent among diabetics; as much as 80 percent of diabetics have been reported to suffer from hypertension. Also, some population epidemiological studies have demonstrated high prevalence of hypertension among diabetics (Ostrander et al., 1965). This relationship appears to be independent of the association between body weight and hypertension.

Oral Contraceptives and Hypertension. Based on epidemiological data, the relationship between oral contraceptives and hypertension has been established; it is confirmed clinically and supported by laboratory studies on the effect of hormones (e.g., progesterone) on hypertension. Thus, it is not an exaggeration to state that newly discovered hypertension or an accelerated course of the disease in a previously known hypertensive young woman should raise suspicion for the use of oral contraceptives as a culprit. Fortunately, the cessation of the use of contraceptive pills will result in lowering blood pressure. The obvious importance of the observed association between the use of oral contraceptives and hypertension cannot be overemphasized, especially since it is estimated that as many as 5 percent of women using oral contraceptive pills may develop, sometime during the course of usage, moderate to severe hypertension. Because of the magnitude of the problem, and because of the catastrophic consequences of hypertension, planners for programs on prevention must seriously consider this relationship.

Trace Metals and Hypertension. Great controversy exists regarding the relationship between trace metals (studied mostly in the form of water hardness) and hypertension. Despite some tantalizing reports from the United States and elsewhere, it is fair to conclude that no firm relationship between trace metals (either water hardness or specific trace elements, e.g., cadmium) and hypertension has been established. The epidemiological data reported thus far lack consistency and strength (Comstock, 1979).

Sociopsychological Factors in Hypertension. The concept that sociocultural, psychological, and emotional factors play an important role in the genesis of hypertension is an old one. Based on the reported findings of numerous studies in this field, sociopsychological factors are viewed by some as important determinants of hypertension. Unfortunately, there is a great deal of controversy on the mechanism of these factors influencing the development of a new case of hypertension or the course of existing hypertension. Sociocultural factors have been regarded as a phenomenon of civilization, affecting the level of blood pressure and indeed the rise of blood pressure with age. In support of this argument is the fact that the rise of blood pressure with age does not occur in primitive people in Africa and Pacific Islands. But when these people move to cities, as in the case of the African Nomadic Warriors serving in the Army in Kenya, then their blood pressure does rise with age (Sharper et al., 1969). Sir George Pickering believes that the most likely explanation for the observed influence of sociocultural factors on blood pressure is what he describes as the security of life in the primitive tribal life and the resulting insecurity when the primitive people are exposed to the daily pressure of civilization. This seems to be the best explanation. But whatever the reason, there is no denying the fact that changes in sociocultural environment influence blood pressure, and health in general. From the point of view of planning prevention programs these important factors must be considered in earnest.

Psychological factors can be divided into three distinct categories (Gluck and Leonard, 1957):

1. Those emphasizing the whole configuration of characteristics making up the hypertensive personality
2. Those considering specific psychologic conflicts as the central features
3. Those dealing with conditions of psychologic stress

Perhaps one of the important points to consider in evaluating the role of psychological factors in hypertension is the interaction of these factors with obesity. It has been demonstrated that obesity, a determinant of hypertension, is linked with decreased intellectual productivity, which is used as a psychological variable in testing for psychological factors in relationship with hypertension (Thomas and Kendrick, 1962). Further, it should be pointed out that most of the data on the relationship between psychological factors and hypertension are collected retrospectively. Thus, it is difficult to determine whether the psychological factors are indeed predictors of hypertension or result from it. In an excellent review of the subject, Weiner points out the methodological problems that exist in unravelling the true relationship between psychological factors and hypertension (1977). He concludes that although we have learned a great deal from previous studies on the relationship between psychological factors and hypertension, our ability to study variations in blood pressure over long periods of time and in life situations would have to be deferred until the development of a method for continually measuring blood pressure and relating changes in blood pressure to everyday events (Weiner, 1977), such as studies conducted by Sokolow and his colleagues, who reported a correlation between blood pressure level and its variation, and anxiety, depression, hostility, and pressure of time and deadline (Sokolow et al., 1970).

CLINICAL TRIALS ON THE EFFICACY OF TREATMENT

The evidence on the relationship between hypertension and mortality is based on data derived from nonexperimental observational studies. As impressive as these data are, in terms of their consistency, strength of association, and reproducibility of observation, they do not by themselves justify community intervention programs for treatment and control of hypertension. From clinical and epidemiological perspectives, we must consider the evidence derived from experimental studies designed to test the hypothesis that judicious treatment of hypertension is feasible and safe and that it would result in a significant reduction in mortality. Foremost among the clinical trials conducted during the past decade on the efficacy of antihypertensive treatment is the well known Veterans Administration Cooperative Study (1967; 1970; 1972).

Veterans Administration Study

In 1967, 1970, and 1972 the Veterans Administration Cooperative Study reported on the efficacy of antihypertensive therapy in reducing mortality and morbidity from hypertension. The Veterans Administration Cooperative Study was a prospective randomized double-blind therapeutic clinical trial conducted among male veterans with a mean age of 57 years. Patients selected for the study had sustained elevated blood pressure (diastolic blood pressure of 90–129 mm Hg) in and out of the hospital, and a high prevalence of cardiovascular and renal damage at entry into the study. Results of the VA Study are summarized in Table 3-6.

Briefly, a total of 523 patients were selected for the study and were randomized into placebo and active drug therapy. The study population included two groups of patients. Group I (143 patients) had a diastolic blood pressure of 115–129 mm Hg. Group II (380 patients) had a pretreatment diastolic blood pressure of 90–114 mm Hg. Active treatment consisted of combinations of thiazide diuretics, adrenergic blockers (e.g., reserpine), and vasodilators (e.g., hydralazine). In the severe hypertensives (Group I) the study recorded significantly lower incidence of morbid events among treated patients as compared with controls, who received placebo. The difference in incidence of morbid events between treated and control groups was so great, and the rate of morbid events in control group was so high, that the investigators decided, on ethical grounds, to terminate the study prematurely and place the placebo group on active therapy (Veterans Administration Cooperative Study, 1967). The study also recorded a significant reduction in morbid events among Group II (DBP 90–114 mm Hg) patients by the end of the trial (VA Cooperative Study, 1970). The VA Study provided evidence that treatment of hypertension with antihypertensive agents reduces the risk of mortality and morbidity, especially

Table 3-6
Summary of Results of the Veterans Administration Cooperative Study on Antihypertensive Agents

| | Diastolic Blood Pressure 90-115 mm Hg | | | | Diastolic Blood Pressure 115-129 mm Hg | | | |
| | Control Group | | Treatment Group | | Control Group | | Treatment Group | |
	Number	Percent	Number	Percent	Number	Percent	Number	Percent
Terminating Morbid Events:								
Death	19	9.8	8	4.3	4	5.7	0	---
Morbid Events	9	4.6	0	---	10	14.3	0	---
Treatment Failures	7	3.6	1	0.5	7	10.0	1	1.4
Nonterminating Events:	21	10.8	13	7.0	6	8.6	1	1.4
Terminations Due to Blood Pressure	20	10.3	0	---	2	2.9	0	---
Free of All Assessible Events	118	60.8	164	88.2	41	58.6	71	97.3
Total Study Group:	194	99.9	186	100.0	70	100.1	73	100.1

From Veterans Administration Study (1967; 1970; 1972).

among patients with severe hypertension, e.g., DBP 105–114 and 115–129 mm Hg. However, the results were not significantly different between placebo and treated group in patients with less severe hypertension, e.g., DBP 90–104 mm Hg. Further, the VA study left unanswered many important questions; foremost among them are the following questions:

1. Is treatment of hypertension as effective among the young and in women?
2. Can the results of the VA Study be replicated at the community level?
3. Do the advantages of therapy exceed possible undesirable effects among people with mild hypertension, DBP 90–104 mm Hg?
4. Can hypertensives detected in a general community screening program be brought under therapeutic management and kept under control?
5. Will treatment of hypertension, especially mild hypertension (DBP 90–104 mm Hg) in the community reduce significantly the rate of mortality?

These and many more questions left unanswered by the results of the VA Study were considered by a panel of experts appointed by the National Heart, Lung and Blood Institute (NHLBI), to review the problem of hypertension in the United States. In 1970 this panel recommended:

> The first priority need is to determine the effectiveness of antihypertensive therapy in reducing mortality and morbidity from hypertension in the general population. Such a study should include both sexes, all races in a community, and younger (adults) as well as middle age people. Such a study would not have a placebo group but could allow randomization of subjects for comparison of optimum drug regimens versus the customary medical care in the community.

Acting on these recommendations the NHLBI initiated plans for a multicenter prospective cooperative community trial which became known as the Hypertension Detection and Follow-Up Program.

The Hypertension Detection and Follow-Up Program

The Hypertension Detection and Follow-Up Program (HDFP) was the largest randomized clinical trial ever undertaken. In 14 communities across the United States, more than 178,000 households were identified as the target areas. Of these more than 84 percent were enumerated, resulting in the identification of 441,846 persons of whom 178,009 were age eligible for entry into the study (i.e., 30–69 years of age). A total of 158,906 completed the first screen at home, and at the end of a two-stage screening, a total of 10,940 were found eligible for entry into the study, with a mean diastolic blood pressure of 90 mm Hg and above, and were designated as the HDFP participants and followed for five years (HDFP Cooperative Group, 1977a; 1977b; 1979a; 1979b). The great majority of these participants (71.5 percent) had a diastolic blood pressure in the range of 90–104 mm Hg.

After completion of the baseline examination, participants were divided randomly into two groups. In one group (N = 5,455), the participants were referred to their usual source of medical care in the community, called the Referred Care Group. In the other (N = 5,485), antihypertension therapy was provided in the HDFP clinics according to a standardized protocol; this group was called the Stepped Care Group. Both groups were comparable with regards to all demographic and other characteristics; the mean blood pressure (systolic and diastolic) was the same in both groups, indicating the effectiveness of the randomization procedure, as can be seen from Table 3-7 (HDFP Cooperative Group, 1979a; 1979b).

Table 3-7
Comparability of Stepped Care (SC) And Referred Care (RC) Groups, HDFP 1974

Selected Group Characteristics	Stepped Care Group	Referred Care Group
Age-Sex-Race:		
Mean Age (Years)	50.8	50.8
Percent White Men	34.5	34.1
Percent White Women	21.6	21.2
Percent Black Men	19.4	19.9
Percent Black Women	24.5	24.8
Blood Pressure at Entry:		
Mean Systolic BP (mm Hg)	159.0	158.5
Mean Diastolic BP (mm Hg)	101.1	101.1
Others:		
Percent Smoking Cigarettes	25.6	26.2
Mean Serum Cholesterol (mg/dl)	235.0	235.4
Mean Serum Creatinine (mg/dl)	1.1	1.1

The therapeutic regimen adopted for the Stepped Care Group (SC) is outlined in Table 3-8. It aimed at achieving a diastolic blood pressure in a predetermined goal range, by maximizing treatment effect while minimizing undesirable side effects, by constant monitoring and meticulous follow-up. The treatment schedule is called Stepped Care because therapy was adjusted progressively in a step-wise fashion until the goal blood pressure was achieved. The goal blood pressure was set at 90 mm Hg for those with a diastolic blood pressure of 100 mm Hg or above at entry, and 10 mm Hg reduction for those with diastolic blood pressure of 90–99 mm Hg at entry into the study. Movement through therapeutic steps was controlled by response to therapy and/or achievement of goal blood pressure. The percent of participants receiving antihypertensive medication increased each year for both groups. It was consistently higher, however, for the Stepped

Table 3-8
Suggested Stepped Care Treatment Schedule

STEP	DRUGS*	DURATION
Step 0	Hygienic Advice e.g., Weight Control	--
Step 1	Thiazide Diuretics**	4 to 12 weeks
Step 2	Thiazide plus Adrenergic Blockers	4 to 12 weeks
Step 3	Thiazides plus Adrenergic Blockers plus Vasodilators	4 to 12 weeks
Step 4	Add Additional Drugs as may be indicated, e.g., Guanethidine	

*In each step use the smallest recommended dose of each drug.
**Long-acting diuretics are preferred, in small doses once a day.

Care Group than for the Referred Care Group. Similarly, a higher proportion of the Stepped Care Group achieved goal blood pressure than did the Referred Care Group.

Data in Table 3-9 present a summary of the results of the HDFP. Mortality from all causes (total mortality was 17 percent less among the Stepped Care Group as compared to the Referred Care Group, a significant difference, between the two groups, in five-year mortality ($p < .01$). Among those participants with diastolic blood pressure of 90–104 mm Hg, the five-year mortality was 20 percent lower in the Stepped Care Group than in the Referred Care Group (HDFP Cooperative Group, 1979a). With regard to cause-specific mortality, the number of deaths from cerebrovascular diseases was smaller by 45 percent in Stepped Care Group than in the Referred Care Group. And there were 26 percent fewer deaths from acute myocardial infarction among the Stepped Care Group as compared to the Referred Care Group (HDFP Cooperative Group, 1979a).

The results of the five-year follow-up among the HDFP participants provide, for the first time, convincing evidence on the efficacy of

Table 3-9
Summary of Final Results of the Hypertension Detection and Follow-Up Program

	Stepped Care Group (SC)		Referred Care Group (RC)	
	Number	Percent	Number	Percent
Total	5,485	100	5,455	100
B.P. Status:				
At or Below Goal	3,560	64.9	2,378	43.6
Treated	4,267	77.8	3,180	58.3
Average Diastolic Blood Pressure	84.1 (mm Hg)		89.1 (mm Hg)	
Mortality:				
All Causes	349	6.4	419	7.7
All Cardiovascular	195	3.5	240	4.4
Cerebrovascular	29	0.5	52	0.9
Myocardial Infarction	51	0.9	69	1.3
Hypertensive Disease	9	0.2	14	0.3
Other CVD	26	0.5	26	0.5
All Non Cardiovascular	154	2.8	179	3.3

From HDFP Final Results (1979a; 1979b).

a systematic and judicious treatment of hypertension in the community, including treatment of mild hypertension (i.e., diastolic blood pressure 90–104 mm Hg). Further, the findings of the HDFP provide affirmative answers to the key questions left unanswered by the VA Study, as enumerated above. The results of the HDFP provide evidence that systematic and Stepped Care approach to treatment of hypertension, compared to the routine care in the community, is feasible and safe. Further, these data provide evidence that such systematic treatment reduces mortality significantly, from all causes and from cardiovascular diseases. In addition, the results of the HDFP provide evidence that benefits of antihypertensive therapy exceed severe toxicity in mild hypertension (DBP 90–104 mm Hg) as well as in the more severe hypertension strata (DBP 105 mm Hg and above).

In terms of planning hypertension control programs in the community for the purpose of prevention of premature deaths, especially among individuals with mild hypertension who are asymptomatic but at high risk of mortality nevertheless, the results of the HDFP are of tremendous significance. They provide a mandate for prevention programs to improve the nation's health, with a great potential for saving additional lives, by identifying all persons with high blood pressure in the community and treating them systematically and effectively, especially those with mild hypertension (DBP 90–104 mm Hg).

COMMUNITY HYPERTENSION CONTROL PROGRAM

The findings of the VA Cooperative Study on the efficacy of antihypertensive treatment and the recently published results of the HDFP provide the needed scientific conditions prerequisite to launch a massive prevention program against the threat of hypertension (often referred to as a silent killer). Epidemiologic data demonstrate that hypertension is a major risk of premature mortality and morbidity. The results of clinical trials and experimental studies indicate that hypertension can be treated safely and without undue toxicity, and that systematic treatment reduces significantly the rate of mortality from all causes and from cardiovascular diseases. It is essential, therefore, that present knowledge of the epidemiology of high blood pressure be utilized in the orderly planning and implementation of a wide and massive public health program for detection and proper treatment of hypertension. The most important criterion to consider is to plan and implement, concurrently with all community hypertension programs, a program of evaluation that permits accurate assessment of prevention.

From an epidemiological point of view, hypertension must be considered a community rather than individual health problem. Thus, the basic elements of a hypertension control program must be defined and articulated in precise terms in advance. As a minimum, the following steps must be taken in the design and operation of a community hypertension control program. These steps are set out schematically in Figure 3-8, which is a flow diagram representing the passage of population cohorts through each step (the term *cohort* refers to a group of individuals classified together by virtue of the presence of a particular characteristic).

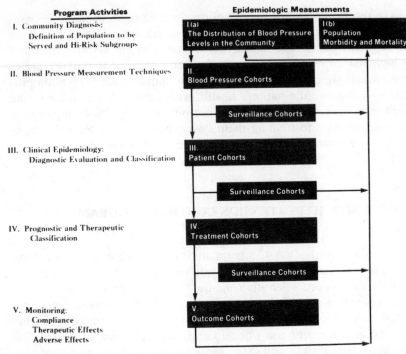

Figure 3-8. A suggested model for community blood pressure intervention programs.

Definition of the Target Population

The population to be served by the community hypertension control program, that is, population at risk, must be defined in precise terms and articulated in advance. Ideally, the target population should be the entire population of the community, but limited resources may not allow such an ideal course of action. For this reason, it is absolutely necessary to define the target population which will be selected for hypertension detection and treatment on the basis of its epidemiological characteristics and vulnerability to the ravages of hypertension. The high-risk subgroups within the selected population must also be identified prior to the design of the program, to allow specific stratification of the selected population on the basis of their risk of mortality. For example, in the United States the young-black-male subgroup of the total population in the community seems to be at highest risk. Thus, identification of such a subgroup would allow the administrators of the program to plan additional safeguards in the operational phase of the program to guarantee complete follow-up, surveillance, and adherence to the program regimen.

Concurrently with the identification of target populations, epidemiological measures should take place, as indicated in 1 (a) portion of Figure 3-8. Central to this concept is a defined population whose blood pressure is measured at one initial point, that is, *baseline,* along with ascertainment of subsequent mortality and morbidity [1(b) Figure 3-8]. It is important to emphasize that, at the very least, the identification and precise definition of the target population must produce a quantitative description of the distribution of blood pressure among members of the cohort thus identified, and the relationship of the described blood pressure distribution with the existing morbidity. The precise description of this baseline information will allow subsequent assessment of the program's effectiveness and success.

Accurate Blood Pressure Measurement

Because of the nature of blood pressure and its inherent biological variability, it is important to take every step necessary to minimize the observer variability in a community hypertension control program. Usually, the systolic and the fifth phase diastolic (i.e., disappearance of sound) are recorded, with participant seated comfortably, with the arm at the adjoining table in a resting position. Every attempt should be made to insure that the participant is comfortable and is rested quietly at least five to ten minutes before the first measurement is taken. By and large, two or three consecutive measurements should be recorded, at five-minute intervals. The blood pressure cuff *must be* the correct size, and the mercury sphygmomanometer should be in perfect operating condition. A standard mercury sphygmomanometer is preferable over aneroid or automatic sphygmomanometers. If a program administrator wishes to use either aneroid or automatic sphygmomanometers, he must guarantee the proper calibration and thorough staff training so that they become familiar with the operation procedures of these equipments.

A concurrent epidemiological step is the identification of blood pressure cohort among the target population. Groups thus classified as blood pressure cohort can then be conveniently substratified into participants cohort by subsequent diagnostic and therapeutic classifications, and into outcome cohorts by epidemiologic monitoring of compliance, side effects, morbidity, and mortality.

All program personnel who measure blood pressures must be trained adequately and certified to make the measurement. For community hypertension control programs to be successful, periodic recertification of the program personnel is necessary to guarantee the accuracy of the measured blood pressure among the cohort under surveillance and follow-up. It should be pointed out that involvement and cooperation of the target population in the successful operation of the program depends heavily on the attitude and expertise of the program staff. Thus, training programs for the staff, especially those who measure blood pressure, must include a comprehensive curriculum that deals with the objectives and mission of the program, the nature and demographic characteristics of the target population, the epidemiology of blood pressure, and the specific points of the design of the hypertension control program which are considered important in terms of meeting the needs of the target population. The staff must be convinced of their contribution to community health and their importance in the program. The attitude of the staff toward their job, and toward the program as a whole, will have a significant effect on the accuracy of the measurements they record as well as on the success of the entire program. A positive and cheerful attitude of the staff, coupled with adequate training in the techniques of blood pressure measurement and data collection, as well as training in proper methods of dealing with people, will enhance smooth operation of the program and success in compliance by participants. Accuracy in blood pressure measurement and other data collection procedures will provide a further opportunity to learn additional scientific information from a community hypertension control program in terms of specific aspects of the care for hypertensive individuals which are hitherto unknown or not well understood, for example, compliance and patient behavior, while simultaneously the program itself will proceed toward its main objective of reducing the risk of mortality from uncontrolled hypertension.

Definition of Diagnostic, Therapeutic, and Referral Methods

The basic elements, premise, and methods for eligibility to participate in the program, ancillary diagnostic criteria, referral procedures, and treatment schedule must be clearly formulated in advance, articulated, and strictly observed throughout the duration of the program. Concurrently, and from the epidemiological perspective, based on the diagnostic evaluations performed in this phase of the program, the participants can be further classified into surveillance cohorts, patient cohorts, and treatment cohorts. These cohorts are represented in Figure 3-8, as they are identified at each point in the flow, while noncompliers and inadequately treated participants will be identified as losses from the main flow. Description of the criteria for such a classification and adherence to them will provide an opportunity for accurate assessment of the loss to follow-up, hence additional information may be gained on the nature (and problems) of community hypertension programs.

It is important to emphasize that these criteria must be developed with consultation with practicing physicians in the community and the officials of the voluntary and public health agencies. Physicians in the community should be willing to agree with these criteria, because they will end up implementing them by accepting the referrals into their private practice. They will not accept the diagnostic or other criteria if they were not consulted in advance in their formulation. Also, physicians and other sources of medical care in the community should know in advance that they will be asked to follow patients referred to them from the hypertension control program. All aspects of the program must be discussed with them, and indeed developed with their input and promise of full cooperation. It should be emphasized to them that hypertension detection without proper development of a workable system for adequate comprehensive diagnostic, therapeutic, and follow-up care is a *disservice* to the community rather than a public health asset.

The criteria for diagnostic, referral, and follow-up procedures must also take into consideration the detection of cumulative effects of long-term antihypertensive therapy in large groups of people. Thus, the refined epidemiological criteria for surveillance and monitoring should be developed concurrently with diagnostic and other clinical criteria. Obviously, accompanying these clinical and epidemiological activities will be administrative and logistical problems that must be resolved. Long-term follow-up of hypertensive patients will undoubtedly uncover new problems that must be dealt with. These problems should be anticipated in advance; plans for their resolution must be developed, articulated, and understood by all.

Epidemiologic Surveillance of the Program

It should be understood that participants in a hypertension control program are a cohort of people followed over time, noting the occurrence of a disease, or death, among them. Criteria for such a follow-up are very specific and must be defined in advance as they meet the needs of that particular community in which the program is being developed. Specific epidemiological activities such as death surveillance system, computer-based retrieval system of morbidity information, establishment of a registry, locating the loss to follow-up, and many more are inherent in a comprehensive hypertension control program; they must be identified precisely in terms of the need in the community and the resources available to it, and once identified they must be implemented with the same rigor and precision applied to the rest of the program. The need for objective assessment of the beneficial effects of the program (e.g., positive cost-benefit ratio) requires that surveillance procedures be defined, in precise terms, in advance of the operational phase of the program. In addition, considerations of these points will indicate the importance of surveillance activities for advancing knowledge along with improving community health.

In the final analysis, the most important objective of any community hypertension control program must be to achieve a significant reduction in mortality and morbidity that could be attributed directly to the program's activities, and that this reduction in mortality would not have occurred without the program. For this reason, the criteria for surveillance and assessment of the results of the program must be developed according to epidemiological principles that will lend themselves to mathematical derivation of the accrued benefits. The end points that will be used for this purpose (or the scoring system) must be defined *before* the program begins and should not be revised during the operation of the program. If new knowledge develops in the interim that would, if applied, strengthen the already developed criteria, it should be used with clear understanding that the revision of such criteria in midstream has added rigor to the evaluation of the benefits of the program.

REFERENCES

Blood Pressure of Adults, by Race and Area, United States 1960–62: Report of the National Center for Health Statistics, Series 11, No. 4, 1964a.
Blood Pressure of Adults by Age and Sex, United States 1960–62: Report of the National Center for Health Statistics, Series 11, No. 4, 1964b.
Blood Pressure Levels of Persons 18–79 Years, United States 1971–74: National Health Survey, Series II, No. 203, 1977.
Borhani, N.O.: Magnitude of the problem of cardiovascular-renal diseases, in

A. Lilienfeld, editor, *Chronic Disease and Public Health.* Baltimore, MD.: Johns Hopkins Press, 1966.

Borhani, N.O.: Alameda County blood pressure study. Berkeley, Calif.: University of California Press, 1969, pp. 1–216.

Borhani, N.O., Feinleib, M., Garrison, R.J., Christian, J.C., and Rosenman, R.H.: Genetic variance in blood pressure. *Acta Genet. Med. Gemellol.* (Roma) 25:137–144, 1976.

Borhani, N.O., Hecter, H.H., Breslow, L.: Report of a ten year follow-up of San Francisco longshoremen. *J. Chron. Dis.* 16:1251–1260, 1963.

Chapman, J.: Epidemiology of vascular lesions affecting the central nervous system. *J. Public Health* 56:191–201, 1966.

Comstock, G.: Review and commentary; water hardness and cardiovascular diseases. *Am. J. Epidemiol.* 110:375–400, 1979.

Coroni-Huntley, J., Harlan, W.R., and Leaverton, P.E.: Blood pressure in adolescence, the national health examination survey. *Hypertension* 1:566–571, 1979.

Dahl, L.K.: Salt intake and hypertension, in H. Genest, E. Koiw, and O. Kuchel, editors, *Hypertension.* New York: McGraw-Hill, 1977.

Dahl, L.K., Heine, M., and Tassinari, L.: Role of genetic factors in susceptibility to experimental hypertension due to chronic salt ingestion. *Nature* 194:480–501, 1962.

Garroway, W.M., Whisnant, J.P., Kurland, L.T., and O'Fallon, W.M.: Changing pattern of cerebral infarction: 1945–1974. *Stroke* 10:657–663, 1979.

Gluck, C., and Leonard, H.: Studies in hypertension, psychologic factors in hypertension. *J. Chron. Dis.* 5:174–201, 1957.

Harlan, W.R., Coroni-Huntley, J., and Leaverton, P.E.: Blood pressure in adolescence, the national health examination survey. *Hypertension* 1:559–565, 1979.

HDFP Cooperative Group: Blood pressure studies in 14 communities, A two stage screen for hypertension. *JAMA* 237:2385–2391, 1977a.

HDFP Cooperative Group: A progress report. *Circ. Res.* (Suppl. I) 40:I-106–I-109, 1977b.

HDFP Cooperative Group: Five Year Findings of the Hypertension Detection and Follow-Up Program: I. Reduction in Mortality of Persons with High Blood Pressure, Including Mild Hypertension. *JAMA* 242:2562–2571, 1979a.

HDFP Cooperative Group: Five Year Findings of the Hypertension Detection and Follow-Up Program: II. Mortality by Race, Sex and Age. *JAMA* 242:2572–2577, 1979b.

Hypertension and Hypertensive Heart Disease in Adults, United States 1960–62: Report of the National Center for Health Studies, Series 11, No. 13, 1966.

Impact of Community Based Hypertension Programs on Blood Pressure. HDFP-IHI Cooperative Group. Unpublished data.

Kannel, W.: Epidemiologic assessment of the role of blood pressure in stroke. *JAMA* 214:301–310, 1970.

Ostrander, L., Francis, T., Hayner, N., Kjelsberg, M., and Epstein, F.: The relationship of cardiovascular disease to hyperglycemia. *Ann. Intern. Med.* 62:1188–1198, 1965.

Pickering, G.: *High Blood Pressure.* New York: Grune and Stratton, 1968.

Pickering, G.: Personal views on mechanism of hypertension, in H. Gevest, E. Koiw, and O. Kuchel, editors, *Hypertension.* New York: McGraw-Hill, 1977.

Rabkin, S.W., Matthewson, F.A.L., and Tate, R.B.: Longitudinal blood pressure measurements during a 26 year observation period and the risk of ischemic heart disease. *Am. J. Epidemiol.* 109:650–662, 1979.

Shaper, A.G., Leonard, P.J., Jones, K.W., and Jones, M.: Environmental effects on the body build, blood pressure and blood chemistry of nomadic warriors serving in the army in Kenya. *East Afri. Med. J.* 46:282–289, 1969.

Sokolow, M., Werdigar, D., Perloff, D., Cowan, R., and Brenenstuhl, H.: Preliminary studies relating portably recorded blood pressure to daily life events in patients with essential hypertension. *Bibl. Psychiatry* 144:164–170, 1970.

Thomas, C.B., and Kendrick, M.A.: The relationship of intellectual productivity as measured by the Rorschach test to body weight. *Ann. Intern. Med.* 56:107–114, 1962.

U.S. Pooling Project Research Group: Relationship of blood pressure, serum cholesterol, smoking habit, relative weight and ECG abnormalities to incidence of major coronary events: Final report of the Pooling Project. *J. Chron. Dis.* 31:201–206, 1978.

Veterans Administration Cooperative Study Group on Antihypertensive Agents: Effects of treatment of morbidity in hypertension: Results in patients with diastolic blood pressure averaging 115 through 129 mm Hg. *JAMA* 202:1028–1034, 1967.

Veterans Administration Cooperative Study Group on Hypertensive Agents: Effects of treatment on morbidity in hypertension: II. Results in patients with diastolic blood pressure averaging 90 through 114 mm Hg. *JAMA* 213:1143–1152, 1970.

Veterans Administration Cooperative Study Group on Antihypertensive Agents: Effects of treatment on morbidity in hypertension: III. Influence of age, diastolic pressure, and prior cardiovascular disease; further analysis of side effects. *Circulation* 45:991–1004, 1972.

Weiner, H.: Personality factors and the importance of emotional stresses, in J. Genest, E. Koiw, and O. Kuchel, editors, *Hypertension.* New York: McGraw-Hill, 1977.

CHAPTER 4

Physical Activity in the Prevention of Coronary Heart Disease: An Update, 1981

ARTHUR S. LEON, M.S.,
M.D., F.A.C.C., F.A.C.S.M.

HENRY BLACKBURN, M.S.,
M.D., F.A.C.C.

Physical inactivity because of sedentary living habits is postulated to be a factor in Western life which contributes to mass atherosclerosis and coronary heart disease (CHD) through associated metabolic maladaptations, while regular vigorous physical activity is hypothesized to have cardioprotective effects. Though scientific uncertainty and controversy surround these interpretations, there is little question about the beneficial effect of regular exercise and physical fitness on general well-being, psychological outlook, and cardiovascular function. The benefits of exercise have been increasingly accepted by the American public, as shown by the findings of a 1977 Gallup Poll that the number of people who exercise regularly and vigorously has almost doubled since 1960 and is now close to 50 percent of the adult population. The estimated number of recreational runners ("joggers") now stands at over 20 million, swimmers at 15 million, regular cyclists at 15 million, tennis players at 29 million (Thomas, 1979), and regular walkers at 45 million (Davis, 1979). It has been speculated that this mass exercise phenomenon is a contributing factor to the recent decline in death rates from CHD (Paffenbarger, 1979). These remarkable social changes underscore the importance of updating and reevaluating the epidemiologic information on associations of physical activity with CHD and evidence about the cardiovascular and metabolic consequences of physical activity, which are the objectives of this report. A rational basis for preventive medical practice and the public health policy on fitness and health depend on these sorts of evidence, because of the unlikelihood of an appropriate controlled, large-scale primary prevention trial or demonstrations of the effects on CHD rate of regular exercise and physical activity. A prototype collaborative pilot study involving several hundred middle-aged men at hisk risk for CHD, coordination from the Minnesota Laboratory of Physiological Hygiene in the late 1960s, illustrated the difficulties: high dropout rate, great cost per experimental subject, and control of factors other than exercise (Taylor, Buskirk, and Remington, 1973). In the absence of experimental "proof" by a definitive trial, careful analysis of epidemiological studies among "natural experiments" offers insights about the relationship of physical inactivity to CHD, particularly if confounding risk factors are considered.

More that 75 retrospective and prospective studies of the past 25 years have recently been reviewed elsewhere (Leon and Blackburn, 1977a1; Blackburn, 1977, 1978a1; Froelicher, 1978; Pate and Blair, 1978; Clarke, 1979). These studies have involved large populations, including occupational groups, regional samples, hospitalized patients, insurance plans, and former college students. They have correlated habitual physical activity levels in health with subsequent CHD incidence and mortality rates.

METHODS OF ASSESSMENT OF HABITUAL PHYSICAL ACTIVITY

In the earlier studies, physical activity classification of light, medium, and heavy work categories was based on occupational requirements judged by job title or by questionnaire. The Health Insurance Plan of New York Study (Frank et al., 1966) was among the first to consider leisure time physical activity from responses to questions on the frequency and nature of sports, walking, and working around the home. The Tecumseh (Michigan) Community Study (Montoye, 1975) also analyzed both job and leisure time characterized by a questionnaire which considered intensity, duration, and frequency of exercise. Morris and colleagues (1973) and Chave and co-workers (1978) considered only leisure activities of male civil service officers, all of whom engaged in sedentary or light occupations. Vigorous exercise involved an energy expenditure of 7.5 kCal. per minute or more, a standard definition of heavy industrial work. Paffenbarger and colleagues (1977) used a self-administered questionnaire to consider flights of stairs climbed, blocks walked, and sports played weekly. An interviewer-administered questionnaire developed in this Laboratory assesses annual energy expenditure according to light, moderate, and heavy leisure time activity. It has been validated in several studies and is currently used in the National Heart, Lung, and Blood Institute (NHLBI) Multiple Risk Factor Intervention Trial (MRFIT) (Taylor et al., 1978). Andersen and co-workers (1978) recently reviewed other questionnaires and techniques for assessing habitual physical activity.

RECENT EPIDEMIOLOGICAL STUDIES
IN HEALTHY MEN

Many but not all earlier population studies reveal an inverse relationship between habitual physical activity levels and CHD incidence and mortality. The findings of more recent studies are also inconsistent. In an update of the Framingham Study (Kannel, 1978), CHD morbidity and mortality and overall mortality were all inversely related to the level of physical activity. This effect was modest as compared to other risk factors, but persisted when they were taken into account analytically. Paffenbarger and colleagues (1977), in a 22-year follow-up of 3,686 San Francisco longshoremen, found a strong inverse relationship between vigorous job-related activity and fatal CHD. Higher energy output on the job (1,875 kCal. over basal output per eight-hour workday) was associated with reduced risk of fatal heart attacks, especially sudden death. Less active workers in all age classes had a three times greater risk of sudden death and 1.3 times more total deaths than the very active. Allowances made for job transfer affecting energy output (transfers from high-to-low energy jobs) were insufficient to account for the observed differences in heart attack rate. The reduced risk for the vigorous workers persisted with adjustment for cigarette smoking, systolic blood pressure, serum cholesterol level, a history of diagnosed heart disease, relative weight, glucose tolerance, and race. The combination of low-energy occupation, heavy cigarette smoking, and elevated blood pressure increased risk by as much as 20 times.

In contrast, the ten-year results of a long-term prospective study from Finland failed to reveal differences in CHD mortality or sudden death in lumberjacks, who expend 4,500 to 8,000 kCal. per day, compared to men who perform moderate or low-intensity work or are sedentary (Punsar and Karvonen, 1976). A greater frequency of resting ECG abnormalities was found in the lumberjacks and of exercise-induced ischemic ECG changes in the sedentary men. The possibility was raised that higher levels of other risk factors may have "overwhelmed" protective effects of vigorous activity. For example, the lumberjacks consumed more calories from fat, smoked slightly more, and were of lower socioeconomic status. Similarly, the Finnish population in the Seven Countries Collaborative Study (Keys, 1970, 1980) had a very high CHD rate despite a high level of habitual physical activity. This was attributed in part to mass hypercholesterolemia in a population with a very high dietary intake of saturated fat.

Wilhelmsen and colleagues (1976), in an eight-year follow-up of 973 middle-aged men originally examined in 1967 in Göteborg, Sweden, found no relationship with occupational activity level among 49 documented CHD events. However, there was decreased risk among men active during leisure for the year prior to the event, but this relationship disappeared after multivariate analysis including age, serum cholesterol, smoking habits, and blood pressure. The association between increased leisure activity and decreased CHD rate could be explained by the negative association between leisure activity and cigarette smoking. Furthermore, the lack of an association between the men's job activity and CHD was in part explained by the finding that the more physically active workers tended to smoke more. These investigators raised, as have others, the important possibility that an insufficient gradient between activity levels may negate the possibility of detecting an effect.

Lie and Erikssen (1978), in a cross-sectional study compared 149 highly trained cross-country skiers, age 26 to 64 with healthy, sedentary men in Norway and found a similar age-specific prevalence of ischemic exercise ECG changes and blood cholesterol levels in the two groups. It is generally concluded from these and other studies that other risk factors are of greater importance than physical inactivity at least in high risk Western cultures (Keys, 1970; Punsar and Karvonen, 1976; Wilhelmsen et al., 1976; Kannel, 1978; Lie and Erikssen, 1978).

In a study of 17,000 Harvard University male alumni, Paffenbarger and colleagues (1978) attempted to assess CHD risk across a wider range of physical activity. They found that the risk of initial heart attack was inversely related to the level of energy expenditure obtained by questionnaire. Men with a physical index below 2,000 kCal. per week were at 64 percent higher risk than their classmates with higher indices. Ex-varsity athletes were at lower risk only if they maintained a high physical activity index after graduation. Risk was further increased by cigarette smoking, hypertension, diabetes, obesity, and parental history of heart attacks or hypertension; however, none of these other risk factors could explain the differences between groups. It should be noted that serum cholesterol level was not measured nor were the questionnaires independently validated.

Morris and co-workers (1973) and Chave and colleagues (1978) reported that male executive grade civil servants in the United Kingdom who performed vigorous exercise in leisure had lower risk of CHD morbidity and mortality than sedentary colleagues. In a later follow-up, Epstein and co-workers (1976) evaluated a sample of 509 of the original cohort of approximately 17,000 men to include leisure-time activity (125 of the subjects or about 25 percent exercised vigorously), smoking history, relative weight, skinfold thickness, blood pressure, total serum cholesterol, and resting ECG. No statistically significant differences in CHD risk factors were noted between the physically active and inactive groups except for frequency of resting ECG findings; 11 percent of men reporting vigorous exercise had one or more noteworthy ECG abnormalities compared to 22 percent of men not reporting vigorous exercise. In both groups the excess of ECG abnormalities increased with increasing blood pressure but remained lower in the more active group. The results of the study are in agreement with Rose (1969) who found an inverse relationship between duration of walk to work and prevalence of resting ECG evidence of ischemia in British civil service workers and with Blackburn, Parlens and Keys, (1967) who found ischemic resting and exercise ECG findings concentrated in men in sedentary occupations in the Seven Countries Study.

Hennekens and co-workers (1977) collected retrospective information from wives of 568 men from two Florida countries, age 30 to 70, who died of CHD and a matched sample of living neighborhood controls. Physical activity was classified according to the Health Insurance Plan of New York criteria (Frank, 1966). Increased leisure physical activity, but not job activity, was associated with a decreased risk of CHD death. This difference persisted when cigarette smoking and elevated blood pressure were accounted for. A potential source of bias is that wives may not accurately report physical activity status of their deceased husbands.

Cooper and colleagues (1976) correlated physical fitness levels with CHD risk factors in approximately 3,000 middle aged men in Dallas, judged by age-adjusted duration of a maximal treadmill test. A consistent inverse relationship was found between fitness categories and resting heart rate, vital capacity, relative weight, percent body fat, systolic blood pressure, and serum levels of cholesterol, triglyceride, and glucose. The more physically fit men were at lower estimated risk of future CHD. Cantwell, Watt, and Piper (1979) also found among 184 men seen in their clinical practice that the more physically-fit (based on maximal oxygen uptake) had lower coronary risk profiles than less fit men of the same age. In contrast, CHD risk factors, singly as well as in a derived composite risk score, were higher for men from a group of 2,635 federal employees with heavy as compared to sedentary or moderate habitual physical activity; however, this appeared to be a spurious association from differences in socioeconomic status (Rosenman, Bawol, and Oscherwitz, 1977). A higher CHD risk profile was significantly associated with lower socioeconomic status. Montoye, Block, and Gayle, (1978) performed treadmill tests on 1,060 men and 119 women age 10 to 69, in Tecumseh, Michigan, and failed to find a relationship between maximal oxygen consumption or work capacity and non-fasting levels of serum cholesterol and triglycerides after removing the effects of age, weight, and body fatness.

POSTMYOCARDIAL INFARCTION STUDIES

Over the past 25 years, early mobilization and exercise rehabilitation of carefully selected groups of patients after myocardial infarction has been shown to be safe in well designed and careful trials and rehabilitation programs, and to result in lower reinfarction and mortality rates than in unmatched groups of patients not taking part (Hellerstein, 1968; Gottheimer, 1968; Rechnitzer et al., 1972; Kellermann, 1977; Leon and Blackburn, 1977b; Wenger, 1977). The overall average mortality rate is 4 to 5 percent per year among functional class one and two patients who would be considered acceptable candidates for exercise programs. However, the Coronary Drug Project (1972) revealed a subgroup of 5 to 10 percent of infarction survivors, with good functional capacity and stable clinical and ECG status, have a mortality rate as low as 1 to 2 percent per year. This renders the effectiveness of uncontrolled exercise rehabilitation programs impossible to evaluate with confidence.

Another major problem in carrying out large-scale secondary prevention trials of conditioning exercise has been the high drop-out rate. Bruce and co-workers (1976) reported a 58 percent loss from 603 long-term patients in the Seattle CAPRI program. Wilhelmsen and colleagues (1975) initiated a randomized prospective trial starting with 158 hospitalized patients in Göteborg, Sweden, but found 25 percent to be ineligible because of contraindications. They experienced a 40 percent drop-out rate the first year and 75 percent loss by the fourth year, greatly limiting conclusions from the study. Two long-term prospective investigations of the effect of conditioning on the recurrence rates of myocardial infarction are underway, one in Canada (Rechnitzer et al., 1975) and the other in the United States (Naughton, 1978). Although the statistical power of these trials is low, due to small samples, they should yield useful information on trends.

LIMITATIONS OF EXERCISE STUDIES

Major problems in interpretation of exercise studies have recently been reviewed (Leon and Blackburn, 1977a; Milvy, Forbes, and Brown, 1977; Blackburn, 1977) and will be only briefly summarized here:

1. There is inevitable self-selection in comparison of people engaged in different levels of work or recreational activity. Their inherent physiological constitutional characteristics may have an independent influence on the course of CHD.
2. Confounding coronary risk factors may have a more potent influence on the progress of CHD than physical activity level.
3. Change from more active to less activity occupational and recreational activities may occur because of health reasons, leaving later comparisons biased.
4. Reliability, validity, and precision in assessing physical activity levels are major methodological limitations.
5. Physical activity gradients are not large in the occupations of affluent society.
6. Standard physiological measurements of fitness, i.e., exercise test duration or maximal oxygen uptake, are influenced at least as much by natural endowment as by habitual physical activity levels.
7. The diagnosis of CHD has its own set of errors.
8. Studies after death are limited by the unknown validity of assessing physical activity status after death and comparing such data to that from the living.
9. Sample size, drop-out rate, design, and operational problems in the few reported exercise intervention studies reduce their power to answer questions about the protective effect of exercise against CHD.

CARDIOVASCULAR ADAPTATIONS TO EXERCISE

Physiological changes resulting from exercise training have indirect relevance to CHD risk characteristics and possible protective mechanisms. They have been studied in detail in recent years in athletes, healthy nonathletes of all ages, patients with CHD, and in laboratory animals (Leon, 1972; Froelicher, 1972, 1978; Clausen, 1976, 1977; Degré et al., 1977; König, 1977; Scheuer and Tipton, 1977; Adams, McHenry, and Barnauer, 1977; Kellermann et al., 1977), and the results are briefly summarized here in respect to their potential relationship to protection against CHD. Two experimental approaches have been utilized to evaluate conditioning effects in humans and animals: (1) repeat evaluations of the same subjects before and after a period of training; and (2) cross-sectional studies comparing trained and untrained subjects. Variability in circulatory adjustment to training may result from prior physical condition, the type of exercise employed, the intensity, duration, and frequency of exercise, and the length of the program. Exercise studies in women and the elderly, though few, suggest that relative training effects do not vary much with sex and age.

Training effects are anatomic, physiologic, and metabolic adaptations resulting from regular, rhythmic, isotonic contractions of large muscle groups such as occurs with running, bicycling, or swimming. Cardiorespiratory performance improves in most people with three to five sessions a week for at least 30 to 40 minutes per session at an intensity of at least 50 percent of maximal oxygen consumption (VO_2 max), which corresponds to about 60 percent of the maximal heart rate (Pollock, 1973; American College of Sports Medicine, 1978). The improvement in VO_2 max can apparently be maintained by two such sessions per week. Most of the cardiovascular adaptations are lost within ten weeks after cessation of exercise and much more rapidly at bed rest.

MAXIMAL OXYGEN UPTAKE (VO_2) AND OXYGEN TRANSPORT

The improvement in work capacity and fitness obtained by training is usually expressed by an increase in VO_2 max, that is, the highest oxygen uptake that can be achieved during exercise. Longitudinal and cross-sectional studies have revealed exercise-induced increases in VO_2

max, maximal cardiac output, and maximal systemic arteriovenous oxygen difference (A-VO$_2$ max). The limiting factor appears to be oxygen supply to the working muscle (Clausen, 1977).

Recent studies indicate that the increase in A-VO$_2$ max with training is associated with increased oxygen extraction by working muscles. Oxygen uptake also rises to meet oxygen demand more rapidly in the trained than the untrained state (Hickson, Bomze, and Holloszy, 1978). An increased carrying capacity for oxygen in the blood and a decrease in oxyhemoglobin affinity have been postulated as contributing to the increase in A-VO$_2$ max, although the evidence for this is meager (Scheuer and Tipton, 1977). Exercise-induced increases in blood volume are accounted for by an increase in plasma volume with less change in red blood cell volume or hemoglobin concentration. Studies have reported that training may result in higher oxygen tension when 50 percent of the hemoglobin is saturated (P$_{50}$) and/or increase of red blood cell 2-3, diphosphoglycerate. However, it appears unlikely that the changes are physiologically significant in increasing oxygen delivery to tissues during physical activity (Scheuer and Tipton, 1977).

SKELETAL MUSCLE ADAPTATIONS

Widening of the A-VO$_2$ max difference with training appears to be primarily due to adaptations in trained skeletal muscles, including increases in oxygen extraction, muscle myoglobin concentration, and mitochondrial density and associated oxidative and respiratory chain enzymes (Holloszy, 1975; 1977; Holloszy and Booth, 1976; Scheuer and Tipton, 1977; Gollnick and Sembrowich, 1977). The resulting increase in muscle oxidative capacity may occur even with low-intensity training insufficient to increased VO$_2$ max (Orlander et al., 1977). Enzymatic adaptations also help explain the decreased lactate production from trained muscles. The exercise-induced increase in myoglobin content facilitates diffusion of oxygen through the cytoplasm to the mitochondria. An increase in skeletal muscle capillary density and capillary-to-fiber ratio initially demonstrated in animals with training has recently been confirmed in humans and probably contributes to increased oxygen extraction by working muscles (Brodal, Ingjer, and Hermansen, 1977). Thus, in the trained state there is good evidence for increased efficiency in oxygen delivery, extraction, uptake, and utilization by skeletal muscle.

MYOCARDIAL STRUCTURAL
AND FUNCTIONAL CHANGES

Exercise training also results in central cardiovascular adaptations with direct effects on the myocardium. Athletes have lower heart rates at rest and at given amount of exercise than healthy sedentary individuals of the same age. So do wild animals compared to domestic animals of the same or similar species. Heart rate reduction at rest and during submaximal exercise usually occurs with short-term training in animals and humans while the heart rate at VO_2 max is usually either the same or less in the trained state. Recent studies indicate that two mechanisms contribute to the reduced heart rate after training: (1) peripheral changes in conditioned muscle decreases sympathetic stimulation of the heart; and (2) the balance shifts between sympathetic and parasympathetic activity in the heart toward dominance of the parasympathetic component (Scheuer and Tipton, 1977). In addition to decreasing myocardial work and oxygen requirements, cardiac slowing increases the duration of the diastolic phase of coronary flow. The diastolic pressure time index at any submaximal work level, an estimate of subendocardial blood supply, also increases with training (Barnard et al., 1977). Thus, training may enhance coronary blood flow without directly affecting coronary anatomy and thereby improve the myocardial supply/demand balance, reducing risk of ischemia.

Active and former athletes of all ages generally have higher stroke volumes, maximal cardiac outputs, and heart volumes than nonathletes at rest and at any level of exercise (Leon, 1972). An increased stroke volume has also been demonstrated after exercise conditioning in healthy subjects of all ages and in some CHD patients. A concomitant increase in heart volume is usually confined to the young. Cardiac output during submaximal exercise is usually unchanged by training because of the associated reduction in heart rate. Nevertheless, cardiac output at VO_2 max is generally increased despite the lack of change or decreased maximal heart rate, because of the increased maximal stroke volume (Clausen, 1976; Scheuer and Tipton, 1977). Approximately 50 percent of the increased VO_2 max in healthy subjects is due to change in maximal stroke volume. In CHD patients with substantial myocardial damage or ischemia in whom stroke volume fails to improve with training, increased VO_2 max is entirely due to increased peripheral extraction of oxygen (Clausen, 1976).

Studies of the effects of chronic exercise on intrinsic contractile properties of the myocardium in experimental animals have recently been reviewed (Scheuer and Tipton, 1977). Improved contractility and pumping performance has generally been observed even in the presence of reduced arterial pO_2 (hypoxia) or pressure overload, although this is not a universal finding. Penpargkul and Scheuer (1970) suggest, based on animal work, that the greater mechanical reserve of the conditioned heart results from improved oxygen delivery (i.e., increased coronary flow). Improved contractility may also be related to adaptative changes in the myofibrillar protein systems responsible for contraction. This includes an increase in myosin ATPase activity found in trained rat hearts in many (but not all) studies and enhanced $Ca++$ interaction with the contractile apparatus (Wilkerson and Evonuk, 1971; Bahan and Scheuer, 1975; Scheuer, Penpargkul, and Bahan, 1977; Tibbits et al., 1978). Recently echocardiographic examination has been used to confirm increased intrinsic myocardial contractility with exercise training in man (Parker et al., 1978) and in the dog (Wyatt and Mitchell, 1974).

Cardiac hypertrophy occurs with short-term training in the rat (Leon, 1972; Froelicher, 1972; Clausen, 1977; Scheuer and Tipton, 1977) and probably in the dog (Wyatt and Mitchell, 1974). In humans, comparisons between well-trained endurance athletes and sedentary subjects including X-ray determination of heart volume, echocardiographic, and postmortem findings have demonstrated increased cardiac ventricular volume and wall thickness in the athletes after at least a year's exposure to heavy exertion (Clausen, 1977; Scheuer and Tipton, 1977). It is still controversial whether short-term training also produces myocardial hypertrophy. It is generally believed that physiological hypertrophy is a useful adaptive mechanism to improve contractile force and increase cardiac work capacity.

MYOCARDIAL VASCULARITY

In animal studies, an increase in size of the coronary artery tree and its principal vessels has repeatedly been demonstrated in the exercise-trained rat (Leon, 1972; Froehlicher, 1972; Leon and Bloor, 1976; Scheuer and Tipton, 1977). The extent of the coronary capillary bed is a vital factor in determining oxygen supply to myocardial cells. Capillary density, that is, capillaries per unit volume of ventricle, as well as total number of myocardial capillaries, and capillary-to-fiber ratio are also increased in the rat within 4 to 10 weeks of regular exercise (Leon and Bloor, 1968; 1976; Tomanek, 1969; Ljungquist and Unge, 1977; McElroy, Gissen, and Fishbein, 1978; Ljungquist, Tornling, and Adolfsson, 1979), and can be maintained by as little as 30 minutes of exercise a week (Leon and Bloor, 1976). An increase in capillary density with training has also been reported in other species. McElroy and colleagues (1978) demonstrated that rats with an exercise-induced increase in capillary-to-fiber ratio have smaller myocardial infarctions when their left coronary artery is ligated than sedentary controls.

In the dog, gradual narrowing of a coronary artery stimulates development of intercoronary collaterals after substantial reduction of artery lumen size (Elliot et al., 1971). In a classical study, Eckstein (1957) showed that the addition of daily exercise also produced an increase in collateral circulation in dogs with only slight or moderate coronary artery constriction and further augmented collateral development in those with substantial constriction. In pigs, exercise plus occlusion increased coronary collateral development as demonstrated by tracer microspheres more than occlusion alone (Sanders et al., 1979). However, other studies in dogs using angiography have failed to support the concept that exercise has an additive effect to ischemia in development of coronary collateral vessels (Kaplinsky et al., 1968; Cobb, Ruby, and Fariss, 1968). Differences in methodology for demonstrating collaterals may account for these discrepancies. Daily vigorous exercise in the absence of constriction does not appear to increase collateral development in either dogs or pigs (Burt and Jackson, 1965; Sanders et al., 1979).

In squirrel monkeys on an atherogenic diet for three years, concurrent exercise, two hours daily, resulted in significantly less intramyocardial artery atherosclerosis and coronary artery obstruction, and improved cardiac performance, but little improvement in development of coronary collateral vessels (Bond et al., 1973; Bond, Manning, and Clarkson, 1975).

In man, there are few data on the effects of physical activity on the coronary artery tree. Rose and colleagues (1967) found at necropsy a significant increase in cross-sectional area of the main coronary arteries among men physically active at work compared to light workers, and smaller coronary arteries in those with infarction compared to those without. Methods do not exist for studying changes in myocardial capillary density with training in man. In man, as in experimental animals, myocardial hypoxia and ischemia appear to be major factors stimulating coronary collateral development and flow. It is unknown whether relative hypoxia associated with exercise promotes collateral development in healthy humans or furthers the development in those with CHD, because of insufficient autopsy studies and the ethical problems associated with repetitive coronary arteriograms in life. Furthermore, there are difficulties in delineating coronary collaterals by angiograms since only those vessels 100 microns or more in diameter can be visualized in the living heart. Most of such collateral are in the 40 to 100 micron range and are devoid of significant flow in the unstressed heart, while post-mortem studies show that 80 to 90 percent of hearts with myocardial infarction have well-developed collaterals in this size range (Hellerstein, 1977). In the angiograms of living patients intra-arterial/inter-arterial collaterals become more abundant the greater the severity of occlusive coronary disease, and they do not appear to contribute to an improvement in myocardial function, symptomatology, or prognosis in CHD patients (Hellerstein, 1977; Wenger, 1977). Several studies in which serial coronary arteriograms were performed on patients with angina pectoris or post-infarction in supervised exercise programs have revealed only sporadic improvement in collaterals despite demonstrated physiological and metabolic improvements (Bemis et al., 1973; Kattus and Grollman, 1972; Ferguson et al., 1974, 1978; Kennedy et al., 1976; Conner et al., 1976); however, it cannot be excluded that exercise promoted development of functional collaterals of a smaller diameter. Such change could lead to a more favorable redistribution of flow not reflected by total flow. In addition, Selvester and colleagues (1977) demonstrated by serial coronary angiograms over a 20-month period in 104 post-infarction patients that the more physically active ones had less progression of coronary atherosclerosis than those who were inactive; however, there were more heavy cigarette smokers in the inactive group, and subjects self-selected themselves for exercise.

Since myocardial O_2 consumption increases during exercise in relation to heart rate and systolic blood pressure (HR × SBP), changes in myocardial O_2 consumption can be estimated from the easily obtained HR × SBP product (Jorgensen et al., 1977). The demonstration of a higher double product after training in some patients with pathologically limited maximal coronary blood flow, prior to the development of angina or ST-T displacement on the ECG, suggests that a few may attain increased myocardial oxygen supply and coronary blood flow (Redwood, Rosing, and Epstein, 1972; Sims and Neill, 1974). However, conditioning in CHD patients more commonly results in a lower HR × SBP value for a given work load (Neill, 1977). This indicates lower myocardial O_2 consumption because of improved cardiovascular efficiency.

CARDIAC EXCITABILITY AND EXERCISE

Acute exercise increased myocardial oxygen demands, which in the presence of coronary artery disease enhances risk of instantaneous coronary death by ventricular fibrillation (Bruce and Kluge, 1971; Friedman et al., 1973; Thompson et al., 1979). In the presence of experimentally produced coronary occlusion in dogs, exercise is more likely to provoke ventricular fibrillation than coronary occlusion alone (Thompson and Lown, 1976; Dawson and Leon, 1978; Dawson, Leon, and Taylor, 1979). However, in the absence of ischemia, moderate exercise does not increase vulnerability to ventricular fibrillation in the dog (Dawson et al., 1979). In clinically normal men ventricular premature constriction (VPCs) are not uncommon during isotonic (McHenry et al., 1972, 1976; Viitaslos et al., 1979) or isometric exercise (Mullins and Blomquist, 1973).

These findings support current recommendations to the public for cardiac evaluation, including exercise ECG tests for those middle-aged and older who wish to do strenuous exercise, especially those with coronary risk factors (American Heart Association, 1972; American College of Sports Medicine, 1978).

Increased sympathetic nervous system activity and associated catecholamine release appear to contribute to development of ventricular ectopic rhythms during physical or emotional stress (Raab, 1970; Leon and Abrams, 1971). A reduction in sympathetic tone of the heart is postulated to result from exercise training (Lin and Horvath, 1972; Scheuer and Tipton, 1977); the supporting evidence, however, is equivocal. In support of this hypothesis were the demonstrations of reduced uptake and turnover of norepinephrine in hearts of conditioned animals and reduced urinary excretion rates of catecholamines in trained rats (Scheuer and Tipton, 1977). De Schryver and colleagues (1969; 1972) also found a decrease in cardiac norepinephrine contents in the heart of exercise-trained rats, but this was not confirmed by other investigators (Ostman and Sjöstrand, 1971; Leon et al., 1975). In human studies, reduced plasma catecholamine secretion after training was recently reported in healthy men and CHD patients (McCrimmon et al., 1975; Cousineau et al., 1977), which differ from later studies (Scheuer and Tipton, 1977). More work is needed to clear up these discrepancies.

In this laboratory exercise training in dogs was found to raise the ventricular fibrillation threshold (Dawson, Taylor, and Bacaner, 1973). An earlier study from this laboratory also suggested that exercise-induced VPCs might be reduced by exercise training in clinically healthy men (Blackburn et al., 1973); however, in a more recent study (DeBacker et al., 1979), six weeks of multiple-factor hygenic intervention including exercise and abstinence from caffeine and smoking in healthy men failed to suppress persistent ventricular premature contractions (VPCs) during rest, isotonic and isometric exercise, and other stresses. Additional studies are needed to elucidate the relationship of exercise training and cardiac excitability.

BLOOD PRESSURE CHANGES

Hypertension has been reported to occur less frequently and at later ages in physically active compared to sedentary persons (Leon, 1972; Scheuer and Tipton, 1977). Reductions after isotonic exercise training in systolic and disatolic blood pressure, especially in hypertensives, have also been found, although this is not a consistent finding (Choquette and Ferguson, 1973; Scheuer and Tipton, 1977; Blackburn, 1978b). Some of these studies were not optimally controlled, and familiarization, weight loss, changes in sodium balance, and other intervention may have contributed to blood pressure reduction. In favor of a direct blood pressure lowering effect of exercise is the significant drop in systolic pressure induced by training in the normotensive and the spontaneously hypertensive rat (SHR), a model for essential hypertension (Scheuer and Tipton, 1977; Tipton et al., 1977; Edwards and Diana, 1978). An associated drop in precapillary resistance was noted in the SHR by Edwards and Diana (1978) and probably contributed to the fall in blood pressure. Exercise training has previously been demonstrated in man to reduce peripheral vascular resistance, leading to relatively higher splanchnic-hepatic blood flow during exercise (Clausen, 1977). Decreased sympathetic activity may play a role.

EFFECTS ON BLOOD COAGULABILITY

It has been hypothesized that a disturbance in the equilibrium between coagulation and fibrinolysis may be associated with atherosclerosis and thrombosis formation, and, in turn, it has been documented that acute and chronic physical activity affect both blood coagulation and fibrinolysis. This topic has recently been reviewed in detail by Lee and colleagues (1977) and Astrup (1973) and will be summarized only briefly here. Acute exercise enhances blood coagulability and is associated with an increased factor VIII activity. Strenuous (but not milder) exercise also increases the number of circulating blood platelets. Platelet adhesiveness is decreased by mild exercise and is unaffected by strenuous exertion. Platelet aggregation is either decreased or unaltered by mild exercise, while a variable response occurs with strenuous exercise. However, in CHD patients exercise is reported to promote platelet aggregation (Levites and Haft, 1975). The hypercoagulable state associated with acute exercise is "counteracted" by an increase in fibrinolytic activity through either increased plasminogen activator or reduced anti-activator or antiplasminogen. CHD patients are reported to have a significantly smaller increase in fibrinolytic response than normal people (Khanna et al., 1975). Physical conditioning appears to diminish the increased coagulability, acceleration of clotting factors, and thrombocytosis induced by exercise while maintaining reactivity of the fibrinolytic system, and not affecting resting fibrinolytic activity. Thus, conditioning may reduce risk of vascular thrombosis and possibly contributions of blood coagulation to development of atherosclerosis.

PSYCHOSOCIAL EFFECTS OF EXERCISE

It has been postulated that psychological stress plays a significant role in the etiology of CHD. The predominant epidemiological view is that if so, and if important, it enhances risk in individuals and cultures having a high burden of atherosclerosis and is not a primary factor in pathogenesis. The reported psychological effects of exercise training have recently been reviewed (Heinzelmann, 1973; Folkins and Amsterdam, 1977; Morgan and Pollock, 1978). Psychological benefits include a feeling of well-being, reduced anxiety and depression, improved self-concept and body image, and sometimes favorable alterations in detrimental health habits, including diet and cigarette smoking. There have been few long-term follow-up studies of the effects of physical activity interventions on health habits. Ilmarinen and Fardy (1977) reevaluated lifestyle habits of 166 middle-aged, high-risk men in Finland three years after an 18-month exercise program and found little impact on current exercise and other lifestyle habits.

METABOLIC EFFECTS OF EXERCISE

Obesity

Obesity has little demonstrable *independent* contribution to CHD incidence, except for angina pectoris (Keys, 1975; Gordon et al., 1977). Obesity is, however, frequently associated with elevated plasma levels of total cholesterol and triglycerides and decreased levels of high-density lipoprotein (HDL) cholesterol, elevated blood pressure, and maturity onset diabetes, and thereby it increases coronary proneness. An inverse relationship between excess body fat, energy intake, and physical activity levels has been repeatedly demonstrated in individuals and in whole cultures (Mayer, 1968; Keys, 1970). The Seven Countries Study suggests that the population "control" of obesity occurs somewhere between 15 and 20 kCal/kg of daily average energy expenditure (Keys, 1970). Increased physical activity has been demonstrated in human and animal experiments to promote loss of weight and body fat (Björntorp, 1973; Horton, 1973; Oscai, 1973; Booth, Booth, and Taylor, 1974; Clarke, 1975; Gwinup, 1975; Lewis et al., 1976; Stalonas, Johnson, and Christ, 1978; Leon et al., 1979). It may be that rapid proliferation of adipose tissue cells in early life predisposes to development of obesity later in life (Stern and Johnson, 1978). Evidence that exercise may modify this early process consists of the demonstration of effects on the rate of adipose cell accumulation in young rats, resulting in reduced adipose cellularity and lower levels of body fat later in life (Oscai, Babirak, and Spirakis, 1974; Stern and Johnson, 1978). However, chronic exercise in adult rats reduces fat cell size but not number (Booth et al., 1974).

Lipid Metabolism

Even mild exercise if regularly performed may alter lipid metabolism. Metabolic studies in rats and man recently reviewed by Simko (1978) have demonstrated that during exercise cholesterol catabolism and its conversion to bile salts increases. Physical activity also increases secretion of bile with an increase concentration in bile salts and cholesterol, promoting fecal loss of sterols. Exercise training also increases plasma levels of lecithin cholesterol acyltransferase activity (LCAT), which works in conjunction with high-density lipoproteins (HDL) in promoting transfer of cholesterol from peripheral tissues to the liver (Lopez-S.

et al., 1974; Miller and Miller, 1975; Simko, 1978). These metabolic changes explain the decrease in peripheral tissue cholesterol in man and rats associated with regular exercise, which should be beneficial in retarding or reversing the atherosclerotic process.

The available literature on the effects in man of well-controlled exercise training studies on serum levels of total cholesterol and its lipoprotein carriers is relatively controversial, and as a whole inconclusive (Leon, 1972; Lopez-S., 1976; Naito, 1976; Clarke, 1979). It is difficult in most studies to differentiate the effects of exercise from the effects of weight loss and dietary changes. Differences in exercise levels and seasonal fluctuations in serum cholesterol levels add to the variability in results. Most studies have reported no changes or only a slight reduction in serum total cholesterol levels as a consequence of regular physical activity, which is more likely to occur in those with high initial levels exercising vigorously (Naito, 1976). Intriguing recent data indicates that it is more likely that exercise causes shifts in cholesterol levels in lipoproteins which may not be reflected in serum total cholesterol levels. Wood and colleagues (1976, 1979) demonstrated that physically active people have higher HDL cholesterol than others of the same age and sex who are sedentary. Several studies have shown that exercise training with or without associated weight loss increases HDL, HDL cholesterol, and HDL to low-density lipoprotein (LDL) cholesterol ratio (Altekruse and Wilmore, 1973; Lopez-S. et al., 1974; Leon et al., 1979; Squires et al., 1979; Weltman et al., 1978). However, several recent studies failed to find such changes (Melisch et al., 1978; Lipson et al., 1979; Moss and Bonner, 1979). Further research is needed to resolve the discrepancies since it appears that plasma HDL levels are negatively related to CHD incidence, particularly in elderly people in affluent societies, while LDL levels are positively associated with risk of CHD (Rhoads, Gulbrandsen, and Kagan, 1976; Gordon et al., 1977; Castelli et al., 1977).

Evidence of the serum triglyceride (TG) lowering effect of exercise in man and laboratory animals has recently been reviewed by Terjung (1978) and Lopez-S. (1976). This is most apparent in humans or perhaps is limited to those with initially elevated TG levels, such as those with type IV hyperlipoproteinemia or endogenous hypertriglyceridemia (Gyntelberg et al., 1977; Lampman et al., 1978). A lowering effect on TG may become apparent after a single exercise session or several daily sessions and persist for several days following cessation of training (Carlson and Mossfeldt, 1964; Holloszy et al., 1964). Most of the diminution of the TG is in the very-low-density lipoprotein (VLDL) fraction. This fraction is the major source of TG in fasting plasma and has recently been postulated to play a role in the atherosclerotic process through conversion to LDL in the arterial wall (Zilvermat, 1975). An inverse correlation between plasma TG and HDL cholesterol has also been reported for both normal and hyperlipoproteinemic subjects (Schaefer et al., 1978). Reduced postprandial chylomicronemia also results from exercise training which may reduce changes for coronary thrombosis (Leon, 1972). The basis for the TG lowering effect of exercise has not as yet been fully established. It probably includes increased muscle lipoprotein lipase activity, enhanced TG clearance and utilization by skeletal muscle, and decrease in TG synthesis in the liver because of peripheral utilization of glucose for muscle and liver glycogen synthesis; exercise-induced increases in blood levels of catecholamines, thyroid hormone, and glucagon and a decrease in plasma insulin (a lipogenic agent); and associated weight loss (Terjung, 1978).

Glucose Metabolism

Diabetes mellitus appears to enhance significantly risk of CHD both directly and indirectly through its frequent association with an abnormal blood lipid profile (increased TG and VLDL and reduced HDL levels), elevated blood pressure and serum uric acid, and obesity (Bierman and Brunzell, 1978; Kannel and McGee, 1979). Hyperinsulinemia appears to be another CHD risk factor (Pyörälä, 1979), perhaps through a direct effect on the arterial wall accelerating the atherosclerotic process (Bierman and Brunzell, 1978). Hyperinsulinemia may result from insulin oversecretion in response to cellular insensitivity, a frequent finding in maturity-onset diabetics and obese people (Lockwood, Livingston, and Amatruda, 1975; Harrison and King-Roach, 1976; Olefsky, 1976; Reaven and Olefsky, 1978; Berger, Muller, and Reynolds, 1978), and can be induced by weight gain (Sims, Horton, and Salans, 1971) or bed rest (Lipman et al., 1972; Vermikos-Danellis et al., 1976; Dolkas and Greenleaf, 1977). The effects of exercise on glucose metabolism, cellular sensitivity to insulin, and diabetic control has recently been investigated and results extensively reviewed (Björntorp, 1976; Holm, Björntorp, and Jagenburg, 1978; Wahren, Felig, and Hagenfeldt, 1978; Vranic and Berger, 1979; Vranic, Horvath, and Wahren, 1979; Ruderman, Ganda, and Johansen, 1979; Saltin et al., 1979; Leon et al., 1979). An increase in rate of glucose utilization occurs during exercise and persists after cessation of exercise during resynthesis of depleted glycogen stores in muscle and the liver (Newsholme, 1979; Wahren, 1979). Enhanced sensitivity to endogenous insulin, which may occur with acute exercise (Pruett, 1970), and reduced adiposity with exercise training appear to act in conjunction to lower plasma insulin concentration and improve glucose tolerance. In insulin-dependent diabetics with mild or moderate hyperglycemia, glucose tolerance and diabetic control are enhanced by exercise training; however, in those with marked hyperglycemia and ketonemia, a further rise in both blood glucose and ketone bodies may result from exercise (Wahren, 1979; Ryan et al., 1979). This indicates the importance of adequate insulin administration in connection with exercise in uncontrolled diabetics.

CONCLUSIONS AND RECOMMENDATIONS

Epidemiologic Studies

Despite their limitations, careful analysis of epidemiologic studies supports the concept that regular vigorous physical activity offers some protection against CHD. In contrast, there is little evidence that regular and vigorous habitual physical activity is harmful with the possible exception of men who perform extremely heavy levels of physical activity for long hours, such as lumberjacks, in whom the presence of other CHD risk factors probably contribute to a higher age-specific mortality rate than among laborers in the same culture who do lighter work. Anecdotal reports of sudden death during jogging are not amenable to analysis; however, Thompson and co-workers (1979) have collected a number of such cases and report that most had evidence of prior heart disease.

The available epidemiologic evidence also suggests that physical inactivity is probably not as powerful an individual risk factor as elevated serum cholesterol levels, hypertension, and cigarette smoking, and that any protective effects of exercise may be "overwhelmed" by them. This is borne out by studies of individual risk factors within populations as well as in comparisons of active and inactive populations. But relative importance of risk factors is not an easy matter to determine.

Physically active people generally have lower blood pressure and plasma triglyceride and cholesterol levels, and higher plasma HDL levels, probably related in part to lower body weight and body fat. When exercise programs are associated with weight reduction, other CHD risk factors are more likely to be reduced.

Future epidemiological studies will focus on leisure time physical activity because labor saving devices, automated occupations, and transport reduce previous high levels of physical activity, and insufficient gradients of physicial activity exist for useful studies within most industries. Validated questionnaires and other methods for assessing habitual leisure activity are needed, along with simpler methods for determining cardiorespiratory fitness in populations. New studies require that other coronary risk factors be quantitatively measured, including smoking dosage, and data should be subjected to several analytical techniques, simple and multivariate.

A randomized clinical trial for testing the activity hypothesis in primary prevention of CHD does not appear feasible because of difficulties in design, size, participation, and costs of such an undertaking. The clear opportunities for such a trial in the Armed Forces have never been sufficiently entertained. The most feasible and acceptable study design at this time might therefore be to test the contribution of exercise over and above multiple risk factor intervention in a high-risk population such as maturity-onset diabetics. Even here, the numbers and cost may be prohibitive. Smaller-scale, controlled clinical trials are also needed to assess further the independent effects of exercise and weight loss on blood lipid, lipoprotein, and insulin levels; the effects of control of hypertension, diabetes, and cigarette smoking; and the optimal amounts of exercise required for cardiovascular and metabolic effects.

Uncontrolled studies have demonstrated the relative safety of long-term exercise rehabilitation programs for selected post-myocardial infarction patients and their possible value in secondary prevention; however, the results of randomized trials currently in progress are needed to ascertain long-term benefits.

Cardiovascular and Metabolic Studies

Physiologic research in humans and experimental animals confirms the value of regular rhythmic endurance-type (aerobic) exercise in improving cardiac function and thereby contributing to reduction in symptoms and certain potential risks in clinical CHD. It has been established that physical activity increases the capacity of the cardiorespiratory system to deliver and perform work, through central cardiac and peripheral adaptive changes. Probably of greater importance in those with relatively advanced coronary atherosclerosis is an associated improved efficiency of the cardiovascular system, which reduces myocardial oxygen and blood flow requirements during submaximal effort. It would apear from animal studies that the capacity of the coronary tree can also be expanded by exercise conditioning, but this is difficult to confirm in man. Effects of exercise on blood coagulability suggest the possibility of reduced risk of thrombus formation in narrowed coronary arteries especially during physical exertion.

Metabolic adaptations of chronic exercise appear primarily to result from the mobilization (lipolysis) of adipose stores for use as fuel and decreased triglyceride formation in the liver and adipose cells. Hormonal changes appear to be involved, particularly reduced insulin secretion in response to improved cellular sensitivity. The end result may be lower fat weight, improved carbohydrate tolerance, and reduced total blood lipid levels with an increase in the proportion of cholesterol carried in the HDL fraction. The net expected effect would be to retard or reverse the atherosclerotic process; however, confirmation of this awaits additional studies.

Psychological Effects

Psychological benefits of regular exercise are difficult to measure; there is little doubt, however, that exercise makes one feel better. It probably relieves anxiety and muscular tension, improves sleep, and alleviates depression, and it may help in motivation to improve other health habits. These effects should improve the quality of life and perhaps reduce CHD risk.

Implications for Preventive Strategies

Insistence on final experimental proof prior to prudent practice or vigorous public health policy on physical inactivity, or for that matter any of the other CHD risk factors, indicates problems in understanding the nature of scientific proof and the evidence required for most health actions. Such insistence leads to inaction in the face of a major public health problem which apears potentially amenable to preventive measures. There is substantial agreement in official recommendations such as the Report of the Joint Working Party of the Royal College of Physicians and British Cardiac Society report (1976; Morris, 1977), the HEW Goals for Prevention and Health Promotion (1979), and the American Public Health Association policy statement (1979), that in any strategy for health promotion and disease prevention in modern affluent society, increased and regular leisure time physical activity should be recommended and prescribed. Reasons given for this include the following:

1. The available evidence is sufficient that increased physical activity in high-risk populations may reduce the risk of heart attack, obesity, and other maladaptations of sedentary man, and will result in an overall improvement in health and vigor.
2. The benefits of regular exercise appear to outweigh the risks of continued inactivity for most people.
3. The need for exercise is universal in sedentary cultures because of the physiological, metabolic, and psychological concomitants of sedentariness.
4. Goals of more regular exercise are appropriate as a public health measure and realizable and compatible with the growing public interest and knowledge about exercise, physical fitness, disease prevention, and quality of life, and the absence of special interest groups against it.
5. Promotion of regular exercise imposes little extra burden on health services and can be carried out at relatively low cost to the individual, to industry, and to municipalities and all levels of government.

Some strategies for increasing physical activity levels in the United States are discussed below.

Since failure during youth to obtain proper attitudes toward physical activity and skills for exercise performance is likely to lead to a lifetime of inactivity, encouragement of a physically active lifestyle should begin during early childhood so that it is more likely to become part of a lifetime behavioral pattern. In school physical education programs, emphasis should be to provide skills in healthful sports and activities for all students that can be continued throughout life, such as running, swimming, cycling, and racquet games rather than on only team sports and development of elite athletes.

Adults of all ages and both sexes should be encouraged to walk more, including at least part of the way to work, and in general to take advantage of opportunities to be more active throughout the working day. Higher levels of aerobic physical activity such as jogging or cycling should be instituted slowly and gradually by the neophyte or long sedentary person and should be noncompetitive in nature. Medical evaluation is recommended with an individualized exercise prescription prior to initiating high-intensity activites for those over age 40, the grossly obese, and for those with a history of cardiovascular disease or at high risk due to risk factors for CHD. Selected activities should be ones that an individual enjoys and is willing and able to pursue regularly, several times a week, for life.

Exercise should be promoted by government at the federal, state, and local levels and more research funds appropriated for studying still unanswered questions about exercise effects. The President's Council on Physical Fitness encourages children to exercise through youth fitness tests and the Presidential Physical Fitness Award Program, and the general public via public service announcements, television, and magazines. Recently the Stanford Three Community Study (Blackburn and Farquhar, 1977) has demonstrated that such a health education campaign can influence risk factors and health behaviors in a target population. A mass-media campaign to promote exercise as proposed in Canada (Lalonde, 1975, 1977; Gellman, Lachaine, and Law, 1977) should be part of any major public exercise promotion effort to educate the public on the need for exercise and how to start. Current public service announcements on television and in magazines of the United States President's Council should be increased substantially through government and industrial support. A substantial increase in credibility would be added to the campaign through co-sponsorship or direct promotion of exercise by local medical societies, the American Medical Association, the American Heart Association, and other community service agencies. Public running, walking, and cross-country skiing events sponsored by health-oriented agencies are helpful in promoting physical fitness; however, either they should be noncompetitive in nature or careful precompetition medical screening should be required for middle-aged or high-risk participants to screen out those with latent myocardial ischemia or other contraindications to high-intensity exercise.

There is much room for improvement at the state level, since generally little is done to promote exercise and fitness except for a few states with Governor's Councils on Physical Fitness and state park systems. Legislation is required to increase the number of state-mandated physical education programs and to encourage the development of physical fitness activities and facilities, particularly in urban areas. At the local level, communities should develop more hiking, cycling, jogging, cross-country skiing and nature trails (some of which can be used for commuting to work or school), parks, tennis courts, and swimming pools and offer more adult sports and physical fitness programs using public schools and parks.

Recently many private businesses and industries have begun to offer employees exercise facilities and programs on company time, and over 300 companies now employ full-time fitness directors (Thomas, 1979). However, only a small percentage of the American working force currently has access to such programs. Other companies are contracting with local facilities such as the Y.M.C.A. and Community Centers to provide services to their employees, though programs for motivating employees to use available facilities and services are little developed. Tax incentives should be helpful in encouraging private industries to develop and maintain fitness facilities and programs. Reduced rates on health and life insurance for regular exercisers, after verification, has also been proposed and is being tried by a few companies as a means of promoting physical fitness (Yenkel, 1979).

Exercise should be prescribed by physicians as part of a comprehensive preventive medicine practice and health promotion strategy to include elimination of smoking, weight normalization, lowering of cholesterol by diet, and control of blood pressure. This requires that information on exercise physiology, the health benefits of regular exercise, and basic skills and guidelines to help change behavior be included in medical school and continuing medical education curricula and that physicians serve as role models by being physically active themselves. It is this combination of public education, participation of the health professions, community organization, and government, and changes in the environment which is likely to most effectively enhance the activity and health of our people.

REFERENCES

Adams, W.C., McHenry, M.M., and Barnauer, E.M.: Long-term physiologic adaptations of exercise with special reference to performance and cardiovascular functions in health and disease, in E.A. Amsterdam, J.H. Wilmore, and A.N. DeMaria, editors, *Exercise in Cardiovascular Health and Disease.* New York: Yorke Medical Books, 1977, pp. 322–343.

Altenkruse, E.B., and Wilmore, J.G.: Changes in blood chemistry following a controlled exercise program. *J. Occupational Med.* 15:110–113.

American College of Sports Medicine: *Guidelines for Graded Exercise Testing and Exercise Prescription.* Philadelphia: Lea and Febinger, 1975.

American College of Sports Medicine: Position statement on the recommended quantity and quality of exercise for developing and maintaining fitness in healthy adults. *Sports Med. Bull.* 13:1, 4, 1978.

American Heart Association Committee on Exercise: *Exercise Testing and Training of Apparently Healthy Individuals: A Handbook for Physicians,* AHA, 1972.

American Public Health Association: Position statement on physical fitness as a public health issue. *Am. J. Public Health* 61:308–309, 1979.

Andersen, K.L., Masironi, R., Rutenfranz, J., and Seliger, V.: *Habitual Physical Activity and Health.* Copenhagen: WHO, 1978, pp. 105–159.

Astrup, T.: The effects of physical activity on blood coagulation and fibrinolysis, in J.P. Naughton and H.K. Hellerstein, editors, *Exercise Testing and Exercise Training in Coronary Heart Disease.* New York: Academic Press, 1973, pp. 169–192.

Bahan, A.K., and Scheuer, J.: Effects of physical training on cardiac myosin ATPase activity. *Am. J. Physiol.,* 228:1178–1182, 1975.

Barnard, R.J., MacAlpin, R., Kattus, A.K., and Buckberg, G.D.: Effect of training on myocardial oxygen supply/demand balance. *Circulation* 56: 289–291, 1977.

Bemis, C.M., Gorlin, R., Kemp, H.G., and Herman, M.V.: Progression of coronary artery disease: A clinical anteriographic study, 1973. *Circulation* 47:455–464, 1973.

Berger, M., Muller, W.A., and Reynolds, A.E.: Relationship of obesity to diabetes: Some facts, many questions, in H.M. Katzen and R.J. Mahler, editors, *Diabetes, Obesity, and Vascular Disease. Metabolic and Mollecular Interrelationships.* Part 1. New York: John Wiley and Sons, 1978, pp. 211–228.

Bierman, E.L., and Brunzell, J.D.: Interrelations of atherosclerosis, abnormal lipid metabolism and diabetes mellitus, in H.M. Katzen and R.J. Mahler editors, *Diabetes, Obesity, and Vascular Disease. Metabolic and Mollecular Interrelationships.* Part 1. New York: John Wiley and Sons, 1978, pp. 187–210.

Björntorp, P.: Effects of physical conditioning in obesity, in G. Bray, editor, *Obesity in Prospective,* Fogarty International Center Series on Preventive Medicine, Vol. 2, Part 2. NIH. Bethesda MD.:DHEW Publication No. (NIH) 75-708, 1973, pp. 397–408.

Björntorp, P.: Effects of exercise and physical training on carbohydrate and lipid metabolism in man. *Adv. Cardiol.* 18:158–166, 1976.

Blackburn, H.: Physical activity as a preventive measure in coronary disease, in M.K. Wenger, editor, *Critical Evaluation of Cardiac Rehabilitation.* Basel: Karger, 1977, pp. 19–25.

Blackburn, H.: Physical activity and cardiovascular health. The epidemiological evidence, in F. Landry and W.A.R. Orban, editors, *Physical Activity and Human Well-Being,* Vol. 1. Miami: Symposium Specialists, 1978a, pp. 129–137.

Blackburn, H.: Non-pharmacologic treatment of hypertension. Discussion. *Ann. N.Y. Acad. Sci.* 304:236–242, 1978b.

Blackburn, H., and Farquhar, J.W.: Community implementation, in A.T. Hansen, P. Schnohr, and G. Rose, editors, *Ischemic Heart Disease. The Strategy for Prevention.* Chicago: Year Book Medical Publishers, 1977, pp. 227–256.

Blackburn, H., Parlen, R.W., and Keys, A.: The inter-relationship of electrocardiographic findings and physical characteristics of middle-aged men, in A. Keys, editor, *Epidemiological Studies Related to Coronary Heart Disease: Characteristics of Men Aged 40–59 in Seven Countries. Acta Med. Scand.* 316 (Suppl): 316–341, 1967.

Blackburn, H., Taylor, H.L., Hamrell, B., Buskirk, E., Nicolas, W.C., and Thorsen, R.D.: Premature ventricular complexes induced by stress testing. *Am. J. Cardiol.* 31:441–449, 1973.

Bond, R.F., Manning, E.S., Clarkson, T.B., and Parker, R.E.: Effects of exercise on cardiac performance of atherosclerotic squirrel monkeys (abstr). *Circulation* 13 (Supple. 4):10, 1973.

Bond, R.F., Manning, E.S., and Clarkson, T.B.: The effects of physical conditioning on cardiac performance of squirrel monkeys with atherosclerosis. *J. Am. Osteopath. Assoc.* 74:673, 1975.

Booth, M.A., Booth, M.J., and Taylor, A.W.: Rat fat cell size and number with exercise training, detraining, and weight loss. *Fed. Proc.* 33:1959–1963, 1974.

Brodal, P., Ingjer, F., and Hermansen, L.: Capillary supply of skeletal muscle fibers in untrained and endurance-trained men. *Am. J. Physiol.* 232: H705–H712, 1977.

Bruce, R., and Kluge, W.: Defibrillatory treatment of exertional cardiac arrest in coronary disease. *JAMA* 216:653–658, 1971.

Bruce, E.H., Frederick, R., Bruce, R.A., and Fisher, L.D.: Comparison of active participants and dropouts in CAPRI cardiopulmonary rehabilitation programs. *Am. J. Cardiol.* 37:53–60, 1976.

Burt, J.T., and Jackson, R.: The effects of physical exercise on the coronary collateral circulation in dogs. *J. Sports Med.* 4:203–206, 1965.

Cantwell, J.D., Watt, E.W., and Piper, J.H., Jr.: Fitness, aerobic points, and coronary risk. *Physician Sportsmed.* 7:79–84, 1979.

Carlson, L.A., and Mossfeldt, F.: Acute effects of prolonged heavy exercise on plasma lipids and lipoproteins in man. *Acta Physiol. Scand.* 62:51–59, 1964.

Castelli, W.P., Doyle, J.T., Gordon, T., Hanes, C.G., Hjortland, M.C., Hulley, S., Kagan, A., and Zukel, W.J.: HDL Cholesterol and other lipids in coronary heart disease. The cooperative lipoprotein phenotyping study. *Circulation* 55:767–772, 1977.

Chave, S.P.W., Morris, J.N., Moss, S., and Semmence, A.M.: Vigorous exercise in leisure time and the death rate: A study of male civil servants. *J. Epidemiol. Community Health* 32:239–243, 1978.

Choquette, G., and Ferguson, R.J.: Blood pressure reduction in "borderline" hypertensives following physical training. *Can. Med. Assoc. J.* 108:699–703, 1973.

Clarke, H.H.: Exercise and fat reduction. *Physical Fitness Research Digest* Vol. 5, No. 2, President's Council on Physical Fitness and Sports, Washington, D.C., 1975.

Clarke, H.H.: Update: Physical activity and coronary heart disease: An update; and, Exercise and some risk factors. *Physical Fitness Research Digest* Vol. 9, No. 2 and No. 3, President's Council on Physical Fitness and Sports, Washington, D.C., 1979.

Clausen, J.P.: Circulatory adjustments to dynamic exercise and effects of physical training in normal subjects and in patients with coronary artery disease. *Prog. Cardiovasc. Dis.* 18:459–494, 1976.

Clausen, J.P.: Effect of physical training on cardiovascular adjustments to exercise in man. *Physiol. Rev.* 57:779–815, 1977.

Cobb, F.R., Ruby, R.L., and Fariss, B.L.: Effects of exercise on acute coronary occlusion in dogs with prior partial occlusion (abstr). *Circulation* 38:104, 1968.

Conner, J.F., LaCamera, F., Jr., Swanick, E.J., Oldham, M.J., Holaaefee, D.W., and Lyczkowskyj, O.: Effects of exercise on coronaryl collateralization—angiographic studies of six patients in a supervised exercise program. *Med. Sci. Sports* 8:145–151, 1976.

Cooper, K., Pollock, M.L., Martin, R.P., White, S.R., Linnerud, A.C., and Jackson, A.: Physical fitness levels vs. selected risk factors: A cross-sectional study. *JAMA* 236:166–169, 1976.

Coronary Drug Project Research Group: The prognostic importance of the ECG after myocardial infarction. *Ann. Intern. Med.* 77:677–682, 1972.

Cousineau, D., Ferguson, R.J., DeChamplain, J., Gauthier, P., Cote, P., and Bourassa, M.: Catecholamines in coronary sinus during exercise in man, before and after training. *J. Appl. Physiol.* 43:801–806, 1977.

Davis, J.T.: *Walking.* Kansas City: Andrews and McMeal, 1979, p. 1.

Dawson, A.K., and Leon, A.S.: Effect of cardiac work loads on vulnerability to fibrillation in the ischemic canine ventricle: The role of heart rate, in P.J. Schwartz et al., editors, *Nerve Mechanisms in Cardiac Arrhythmia.* New York: Raven Press, 1978, pp. 283–286.

Dawson, A.K., Taylor, H.L., and Bacaner, M.: Effect of physical training on canine ventricular fibrillation threshold (abstr.). *Physiologist* 16:295, 1973.

Dawson, A.K., Leon, A.S., and Taylor, H.L.: Effect of submaximal exercise on vulnerability to fibrillation in the canine ventricle. *Circulation* 59:798–804, 1979.

DeBacker, G., Jacobs, D., Prineas, R., Crow, R., Villandre, J., Kennedy, H., and Blackburn, H.: Ventricular premature contractions: A ramdomized non-drug intervention trial in man. *Circulation* 59:762–769, 1979.

Degré, S.C., Degré-Coustry, C., Hoylaerts, M., Grevisse, M., and Denolin, H.: Therapeutic effects of physical training in coronary heart disease. *Cardiology* 62:206–217. 1977.

DeSchryver, C., and Mertens-Strythagen, J., Intensity of exercise and heart tissue catecholamine content. *Pflueger Arch.* 336:345–354, 1972.

DeSchryver, C., Mertens-Strythagen, J., Becsei, I., and Lammerant, J.: Effect of training on heart and skeletal muscle catecholamine content in rats. *Am. J. Physiol.* 217:1589–1597, 1969.

Dolkas, C.B., and Greenleaf, J.E.: Insulin and glucose responses during bed rest with isotonic and isometric exercise. *J. Appl. Physiol* 43:1033–1038, 1977.

Eckstein, R.W.: Effect of exercise and coronary artery narrowing on coronary collateral circulation. *Circ. Res.* 5:230–235, 1957.

Edwards, M.T., and Diana, J.N.: Effect of exercise on pre- and post-capillary resistance in the spontaneous hypertensive rat. *Am. J. Physiol.* 234:H439–H446, 1978.

Elliot, E.C., Bloor, C.M., Jones, E.L., Mitchell, W.J., Gregg, D.E.: Effect of controlled coronary occlusion on collateral circulation in the conscious dog. *Am. J. Physiol.* 220:857–861, 1971.

Epstein, L., Miller, G.T., Sitt, F.W., and Morris, J.N.: Vigorous exercise in leisure-time, coronary risk-factors, and resting electrocardiogram in middle aged civil servants. *Br. Heart J.* 38:403–409, 1976.

Ferguson, R.J., Petitclerc, R., Choquette, R., Chanotis, L., Gauthier, P.,

Huot, R.F., Allard, C., Jankowski, L., and Campeau, L.: Effect of physical training on treadmill exercise capacity, collateral circulation, and progression of coronary disease. *Am. J. Cardiol.* 34:674–769, 1974.

Ferguson, R.J., Cote, P., Gauthier, P., and Bourass, M.G.: Changes in exercise coronary sinus blood flow with training in patients with angina pectoris. *Circulation* 58:41–47, 1978.

Folkins, C.H., and Amsterdam, E.A.: Control and modification of stress emotions through chronic exercise, in E.A. Amsterdam, J.H. Wilmore, and A.N. DeMaria, editors, *Exercise in Cardiovascular Health and Disease.* New York: Yorke Medical Books, 1977, pp. 280–294.

Frank, C.W., Weinblatt, E., Shapiro, S., and Sager, R.V.: Physical inactivity as a lethal factor in myocardial infarction among men. *Circulation* 34:1022–1033, 1966.

Friedman, M., Manwaring, M.J.H., Rosenman, R.H., Donlon, G., Ortega, P., and Grube, S.M.: Instantaneous and sudden death. Clinical and pathological differentiation in coronary artery disease. *JAMA* 225:1319–1328, 1973.

Froelicher, V.F.: Animal studies of effects of chronic exercise on the heart and atherosclerosis: A review. *Am. Heart J.* 84:496–506, 1972.

Froelicher, V.F.: Exercise and the prevention of coronary atherosclerotic heart disease, in N.K. Wenger, editor, *Exercise and the Heart.* Philadelphia: F.A. Davis, 1978, pp. 13–23.

Gellman, D.D., Lachaine, R., and Law, M.M.: The Canadian approach to health policies and programs. *Prev. Med.* 6:265–275, 1977.

Gollnick, P.D., and Sembrowich, W.L.: Adaptation in human skeletal muscles as a result of training, in E.A. Amsterdam, J.H. Wilmore, and A.N. DeMaria, editors, *Exercise in Cardiovascular Health and Disease.* New York: Yorke Medical Books, 1977, pp. 70–94.

Gordon, T., Castelli, W.P., Hjortland, M.C., Kannel, W.B., and Dawber, T.R.: Predicting coronary heart disease in middle aged and older persons. The Framingham Study. *JAMA* 238:497–499, 1977.

Gottheimer, V.: Long-range strenuous sports training for cardiac reconditioning and rehabilitation. *Am. J. Cardiol.* 22:426–435, 1968.

Gwinup, G.: Effect of exercise alone on the weight of obese women. *Arch. Intern. Med.* 135:675–680, 1975.

Gyntelberg, F., Brennan, R., Holloszy, J.O., Schonfeld, G., Rennee, M.J., and Weidman, S.W.: Plasma triglyceride lowering by exercise despite increased food intake in patients with type IV hyperlipoproteinemia. *Am. J. Clin. Nutr.* 30:716–720, 1977.

Harrison, L.C., and King-Roach, A.P.: Insulin sensitivity of adipose tissue in vitro and the response to exogenous insulin in obese human subjects. *Metabolism* 25:1095–1101, 1976.

Heinzelman, F.: Social and psychological factors that influence the effectiveness of exercise programs, in J.P. Naughton and H.K. Hellerstein, editors, *Exercise Testing and Exercise Training in Coronary Heart Disease.* New York: Academic Press 1973, pp. 275–288..

Hellerstein, H.K.: Exercise therapy in coronary disease. *Bull. N.Y. Acad. Sci.* 44:1028–1047, 1968.

Hellerstein, H.K.: Acceleration of collaterals due to physical activity—dogmas or fact. A misguided goal or unrealized objective, in H.K. Wenzel, editor,

Critical Evaluation of Cardiac Rehabilitation. Basel: Karger, 1977, pp. 125–135.

Hennekens, C.H., Rosner, B., Jesse, M.J., Drolette, M.E., and Splizer, F.E.: A retrospective study of physical activity and coronary deaths. *Internatl. J. Epidemiol.* 6:243–246, 1977.

HEW: Goals for Prevention and Health Promotion for 1990. *Physical Fitness and Exercise,* 1979.

Hickson, R.C., Bomze, H.A., and Holloszy, J.O.: Faster adjustment of O_2 uptake to the energy requirements of exercise in the trained state. *J. Appl. Physiol.* 614:877–881, 1978.

Holloszy, J.O.: Adaptation of skeletal muscle to endurance exercise. *Med. Sci. Sports* 7:155–164, 1975.

Holloszy, J.O.:Adaptations of muscular tissue to training, in E.H. Sonnenblick and M. Lesch, editors, *Exercise and Heart Disease.* New York: Grune and Stratton, 1977, pp. 25–38.

Holloszy, J.O., and Booth, F.W.: Biochemical adaptations to endurance exercise in muscle. *Ann. Rev. Physiol.* 38:273–291, 1976.

Holloszy, J.O., Skinner, J.S., Toro, G., and Cureton, T.K.: Effects of a six month program of endurance exercise on the blood lipids of middle aged men. *Am. J. Cardiol.* 14:753–760, 1964.

Holm, G., Björntorp, D., and Jagenburg, R.: Carbohydrate, lipid and amino acid metabolism following physical exercise in man. *J. Appl. Physiol.* 45:128–131, 1978.

Horton, E.G.: The role of exercise in prevention and treatment of obesity, in G.A. Bray, editor, *Obesity in Prospective.* Fogarty International Center Series on Preventive Medicine. Vol. 2, Part 1. NIH, Bethesda, Md., DHEW Pub. No. (NIH) 75–708, 1973, pp. 62–66.

Ilmarinen, J., and Fardy, P.S.: Physical activity intervention for males. *Prev. Med.* 6:416–425, 1977.

Jorgensen, C.R., Gobel, F.L., Taylor, H.L., and Wang, Y.: Myrocardial blood flow and oxygen consumption during exercise. *Ann. N.Y. Acad. Sci.* 301:213–223, 1977.

Kannel, W.B.: Recent findings of the Framingham Study. *Resident and Staff Physician* 24:56–71, 1978.

Kannel, W.B., and McGee, D.L.: Diabetes and glucose tolerance as risk factors for cardiovascular disease. The Framingham Study. *Diabetes Care* 2:120–126, 1979.

Kaplinsky, E., Hood, W.B., Jr., McCarthy, B., McCombs, H.L., and Lown, B.: Effects of physical training on dogs with coronary artery ligation. *Circulation* 37:556–565, 1968.

Kattus, A.A., and Grollman, J.: Patterns of coronary collateral circulation in angina pectoris: Relation of exercise, in M. Russek and B.L. Zohman, editors, *Changing Concepts in Cardiovascular Disease.* Baltimore: Williams and Wilkins, 1972, pp. 352–358.

Kellermann, J.J.: Exercise as preventive measure: A controversion, in N.K. Wenger, editor, *Critical Evaluation of Cardiac Rehabilitation.* Basel: Karger, 1977, pp. 30–36.

Kellermann, J.J., Ben-Ari, E., Chayet, M., Lapidot, C., Drory, Y., and Fisman, E.: Cardiocirculatory responses to different types of training in patients with angina pectoris. *Cardiology* 62:218–231, 1977.

Kennedy, C.C., Spiekerman, R.E., Lindsay, M.I., Jr. and Manken, H.J.: One year graduated exercise program for men with angina pectoris. *Mayo Clinic Proc.* 51:231–236, 1976.

Keys, A., editor: Coronary heart disease in seven countries. *Circulation* 41 (Supple 1), 1970.

Keys, A.: Coronary heart disease. The global picture. *Atherosclerosis* 22:149–192, 1975.

Keys, A.: *Seven Countries—Deaths and Coronary Heart Disease in Ten Years.* Cambridge: Harvard University Press, 1980.

Khanna, P., Hari, N.S., Balasubramanian, V., and Hoon, R.S.: Effect of submaximal exercise on fibrinolytic activity in ischaemic heart disease. *Br. Heart J.* 37:1273–1276, 1975.

König, K.: Changes in physical capacity, heart size, and function in patients after myocardial infarction, who underwent a 4 to 6 week physical training program. *Cardiology* 62:232–246, 1977.

Lalonde, M.: *A New Perspective on the Health of Canadians.* Ottawa: Information Canada, 1975.

Lalonde, M.: Beyond a new prospective. *Am. J. Public Health* 67:357–360, 1977.

Lampman, R.M., Santings, J.T., Bassett, D.R., Mercer, N.M., Block, W.D., Flors, J.D., Foss, M.L., and Thorland, C.G.: Effectiveness of unsupervised and supervised high intensity physical training in normalizing serum lipids in men with type IV hyperlipoproteinemia. *Circulation* 57:172–180, 1978.

Lee, G., Amsterdam, E.A., DeMaria, A.M., Davis, G., LaFave, T., and Mason, D.T.: Effects of exercise on hemostatic mechanisms, in E.A. Amsterdam, J.H. Wilmore, and A.N. DeMaria, editors, *Exercise in Cardiovascular Health and Disease.* New York: Yorke Medical Book, 1977, pp. 122–136.

Leon, A.S.: Comparative cardiovascular adaptation to exercise in animals and man and its relevance to coronary heart disease, in C.M. Bloor, editor, *Comparative Pathophysiology of Circulatory Disturbances.* New York: Plenum Publishing, 1972, pp. 143–173.

Leon, A.S., and Abrams, W.B.: The role of catecholamines in producing arrhythmias. *Am. J. Clin. Sci.* 262:9–13, 1971.

Leon, A.S., and Bloor, C.M.: Effects of exercise and its cessation on the heart and its blood supply. *J. Appl. Physiol.* 23:485–490, 1968.

Leon, A.S., and Bloor, C.M.: The effect of complete and partial deconditioning on exercise-induced cardiovascular changes in the rat. *Adv. Cardiol.* 18:81–92, 1976.

Leon, A.S., and Blackburn, H.B.: The relationship of physical activity to coronary heart disease and life expectancy. *Ann. N.Y. Acad. Sci.* 301:361–578, 1977a.

Leon, A.S., and Blackburn, H.: Exercise rehabilitation of the coronary heart disease patient. *Geriatics* 32:66–67, 1977b.

Leon, A.S., Horst, W.D., Spirt, N., Wiggan, E.B., and Womelsdorf, A.H.: Heart norepinephine levels after exercise training in the rat. *Chest* 67:341–343, 1975.

Leon, A.S., Conrad, J., Hunninghake, D.B., and Serfass, R.: Effects of vigorous walking on body composition, and carbohydrate and lipid metabolism in obese young men. *Am. J. Clin. Nutr.* 32:1776–1787, 1979.

Levites, R., and Haft, J.I.: Effects of exercise-induced stress on platelet aggregation. *Cardiology* 60:304–314, 1975.

Lewis, S., Haskell, W.B., Wood, P.D., Manoogian, N., Bailey, J.E., and Pereira, M.: Effects of physical activity on weight reduction in obese middle-aged women. *Am. J. Clin. Nutr.* 29:151–156, 1976.

Lie, H., and Erikssen, J.: ECG aberration, latent coronary heart disease and cardiopulmonary fitness in various age groups of Norwegian cross-country skiers. *Acta Med. Scand.* 203:503–507, 1978.

Lin, Y., and Horvath, S.M.: Autonomic nervous control of cardiac frequency in the exercise-induced rat. *J. Appl. Physiol.* 33:796–799, 1972.

Lipman, R.L., Raskin, P., Love, T., Triebwasser, J., Lecocaq, F.R., and Schure, J.J.: Glucose intolerance during decreased physical activity in man. *Diabetes* 21:101–107, 1972.

Lipson, L.C., Bonow, R.O., Schaefer, E., Brewer, H.B., Lingren, F., and Epstein, S.E.: Effect of exercise on plasma lipoproteins (abstr.) *Am. J. Cardiol.* 43:409, 1979.

Ljungquist, A., and Unge, G.: Capillary proliferative activity in myrocardium and skeletal muscle of exercised rats. *J. Appl. Physiol.* 43:306–307, 1977.

Ljungquist, A., Tornling, G., and Adolfsson, J.: The proliferative activity of myocardial capillary wall cells in variously aged swimming-exercised rats. *J. Acta Pathol. Microbiol. Scand.* 87:15–17, 1979.

Lockwood, D.H., Livingston, H.N., and Amatruda, J.M.: Relation of insulin receptors to insulin resistance. *Fed. Proc.* 34:1564–1568, 1975.

Lopez-S., A.: 1976. Effect of exercise on serum lipids and lipoprotein, in C.E. Day and R.S. Levy, editors, *Low Density Lipoproteins*. New York: Plenum, 1976, pp. 135–148.

Lopez-S., A., Vise, R., Balart, L., and Arroyave, G.: Effect of exercise and physical fitness on serum lipids and lipoproteins. *Atherosclerosis* 20:1–9, 1974.

Mayer, J.: *Overweight Causes, Cost and Control*. Englewood Cliffs, N.J.: Prentice-Hall, 1968, 69–83.

McCrimmon, D.R., Cunningham, D.A., Rechnitzer, P.A., and Griffiths, J.: Effect of training on plasma catecholamines in postmyocardial infarction patients. *Med. Sci. Sports* 8:152–156, 1975.

McElroy, C.L., Gissen, S.A., and Fishbein, M.C.: Exercise-induced reduction in myocardial infarct size after coronary artery occlusion in the rat. *Circulation* 57:958–962, 1978.

McHenry, P.L., Fisch, C., Jordon, J.W., and Corys, R.: Cardiac arrhythmias observed during treadmill exercise testing in clinically normal men. *Am. J. Cardiol.* 29:331–336, 1972.

McHenry, P.L., Faris, J.V., Jordan, J.W., and Morris, S.N.: Comparative study of cardiovascular function and ventricular premature complexes in smokers and nonsmokers during maximal treadmill exercise. *Am. J. Cardiol.* 39:493–498, 1976.

Melisch, J., Bronstein, D., Gross, R., Dann, D., White, J., Hunt, H., and Brown, W.V.: Effect of exercise training in type II hyperlipoproteinemia (abstr.). *Circulation* 58 (Suppl. 2): 38, 1978.

Miller, G.J., and Miller, N.E.: Plasma high density lipoprotein concentration and development of ischemic heart disease. *Lancet* 1:16–19, 1975.

Milvy, P., Forbes, W.F., and Brown, K.S.: A critical review of epidemiological studies of physical activity. *Ann. N.Y. Acad. Sci.* 301:519–549, 1977.

Montoye, J.H.: *Physical Activity and Health: An Epidemiological Study of an Entire Community.* Englewood Cliffs, N.J.: Prentice-Hall, 1975, pp. 8–9.

Montoye, H.J., Block, W.D., and Gayle, R.: Maximal oxygen uptake and blood lipids. *J. Chron. Dis.* 31:111–118, 1978.

Morgan, W.P., and Pollock, M.L.: Physical activity and cardiovascular health: Physiological aspects, in F. Landry and W.A.R. Orban, editors, *Physical Activity and Human Well-being,* Vol. 1. Miami: Symposia Specialists, 1978, pp. 163–184.

Morris, J.N.: Current objectives in prevention: Physical exercise, in A.T. Hansen, P. Schnohr, and G. Rose, editors, *Ischemic Heart Disease. The Strategy for Prevention.* Chicago: Year Book Medical Publisher, 1977, pp. 89–103.

Morris, J.W., Adams, C., Chave, S.P.W., Sirey, C., Epstein, L., and Sheeham, D.J.: Vigorous exercise in leisure-time and the incidence of coronary heart disease. *Lancet* 1:333–339, 1973.

Moss, R.F., and Bonner, H.: The effect of a five week monitored training program on fasting levels of serum cholesterol and triglyceride in college males maintained at normal weight (abstr.). *Med. Sci. Sports* 11:108, 1979.

Mullins, C.B., and Blomquist, G.: Isometric exercise and the cardiac patient. *Texas Med.* 69:53–58, 1973.

Naito, H.K.: Effects of physical activity on serum cholesterol metabolism. *Clev. Clin. Q.* 43:21–49, 1976.

Naughton, J.: The National Exercise and Heart Disease Project, in N.K. Wenger, editor, *Exercise and the Heart.* Philadelphia: F.A. Davis, 1978, pp. 205–222.

Neill, W.A.: Coronary and systemic circulatory adaptation to exercise training and their effects on angina pectoris, in E.A. Amsterdam, J.H. Wilmore, and A. DeMaria, editors, *Exercise in Cardiovascular Health and Disease.* New York: Yorke Medical Books, 1977, pp. 137–146.

Newsholme, E.A.: The control of fuel utilization by muscle during exercise and starvation. *Diabetes* 28 (Suppl. 1): 1–7, 1979.

Olefsky, J.M.: The insulin receptor: Its role in insulin resistance of obesity and diabetes. *Diabetes* 25:1154–1162, 1976.

Orlander, J., Kiessling, K.H., Karlsson, J., and Ekblom, B.: Low intensity training, inactivity and resumed training in sedentary men. *Acta Physiol. Scand.* 101:351–362, 1977.

Oscai, L.B.: The role of exercise in weight control, in J. Wilmore, editor, *Sports Science Review,* Vol. 1. New York: Academic Press, 1973, pp. 103–123.

Oscai, L., Babirak, S.P., and Spirakis, C.N.: Effect of exercise on adipose tissue cellularity. *Fed. Proc.* 33:1956–1958, 1974.

Ostman, I., and Sjöstrand, M.O. Effect of prolonged physical training on the catecholamine levels of the heart and adrenals in the rat. *Acta Physiol. Scand.* 82:202–208, 1971.

Paffenbarger, R.S., Jr.: Counter currents of physical activity and heart attack trends, in R.H. Havlik and M. Feinleib, editors, *Proceedings of the Conference on the Decline in Coronary Heart Disease Mortality.* Bethesda, Md.: USDHEW, NIH Pub. No. 79-610, 1979, pp. 298–311.

Paffenbarger, R.S., Jr., Hale, W.E., Brand, R.J., and Hyde, R.T.: Work-energy level, personal characteristics, and fatal heart attack: A birth-cohort effect. *Am. J. Epidemiol.* 105:200–213, 1977.

Paffenbarger, R.S., Jr., Wing, A.L., and Hyde, R.T.: Physical activity as an index of heart attack risk in college alumni. *Am. J. Epidemiol.* 108:161–175, 1978.

Parker, B.M., Londeree, B.L., Cupp, G.V., and Dubiel, J.P.: The noninvasive cardiac evaluation of long-distance runners. *Chest* 73:376–381, 1978.

Pate, R.R., and Blair, S.M.: Exercise and the prevention of atherosclerosis: Pediatric implications, in W.B. Strong, editor, *Atherosclerosis: Its Pediatrics Aspects.* Philadelphia: Grune and Stratton, 1978, pp. 251–286.

Penpargkul, S., and Scheuer, J.: The effect of physical training upon the mechanical and metabolic performance of the rat heart. *J. Clin. Invest.* 49:1858–1868, 1970.

Pollock, M.L.: The quantification of endurance training programs, in J. Wilmore, editor, *Exercise and Sports Reviews.* New York: Academic Press, 1973, pp. 155–188.

Pruett, E.D.R.: Plasma insulin concentration during prolonged work at near maximal oxygen consumption. *J. Appl. Physiol.* 29:155–158, 1970.

Punsar, S., and Karvonen, M.: Physical activity and coronary heart disease in populations from east and west Finland. *Adv. Cardiol.* 18:196–207, 1976.

Pyörälä, K.: Relationship of glucose tolerance and plasma insulin to the incidence of coronary heart disease: Results from two population studies in Finland. *Diabetes Care* 2:131–141, 1979.

Raab, W.: *Preventive Myocardiology.* Springfield: Charles C. Thomas, 1970, p. 227.

Reaven, G.M., and Olefsky, J.M.: Role of insulin resistance in the pathogenesis of hyperglycemia, in H.M. Katzen and R.J. Mahler, editors, *Diabetes, Obesity and Vascular Disease. Metabolic and Molecular Interrelationships,* Part 1. New York: John Wiley and Sons, 1978, pp. 229–266.

Rechnitzer, P.A., Pickard, H.A., Paivo, A.V., Yuhasz, M.S., and Cunningham, D.: Long-term following study of survival and recurrence rate following myocardial infarction in exercising and control subjects. *Circulation* 45:853–857, 1972.

Rechnitzer, P.A., Sangal, S., Cunningham, D.A., Andrew, G., Burke, C., Jones, H.L., Kavanagh, T., Parker, J.O., Shepard, R.J., and Yukaz, M.S.: A controlled prospective study of the effects of endurance training on the recurrence rate of myocardial infarction. A description of the experimental design. *Am. J. Epidemiol.* 102:358–364, 1975.

Redwood, D.R., Rosing, D.R., and Epstein, S.E.: Circulatory and symptomatic effects of exercise training in patients with coronary heart disease and angina pectoris. *N. Engl. J. Med.* 286:959–965, 1972.

Report of a Joint Working Party of the Royal College of Physicians and the British Cardiac Society: Prevention of Coronary Heart Disease. *J. R. Coll. Physicians Lond.* 10:213–275, 1976.

Rhoads, G.G., Gulbrandsen, C.L., and Kagan, A.: Serum lipoproteins and coronary heart disease in a population study of Hawaiian-Japanese men. *N. Engl. J. Med.* 294:293–298, 1976.

Rose, G.: Physical activity and coronary heart disease. *Proc. R. Soc. Med.* 62:1183–1188, 1969.

Rose, G., Prineas, R.J., and Mitchel, J.R.A.: Myocardial infarction and the intrinsic caliber of coronary arteries. *Br. Heart J.* 29:548–552, 1967.

Rosenman, R.H., Bawol, R.D., and Oscherwitz, M.: A 4-year prospective study of the relationship of different habitual vocational physical activity to risk and incidence of coronary heart disease in volunteer federal employees. *Ann. N.Y. Acad. Sci.* 301:627–641, 1977.

Ruderman, N.B., Ganda, O.P., and Johansen, K.: The effect of physical training on glucose tolerance and plasma lipids in maturity-onset diabetes. *Diabetes* 28 (Suppl. 1):89–92, 1979.

Ryan, A.J., Leon, A.S., Etzwiler, D., Costell, D., and Zinman, D.L.: Diabetes and exercise. *Physician Sportsmed.* 7:49–52, 55–61, 64, 1979.

Saltin, B., Lindgarde, F., Houston, M., Horlin, R., Nygaard, E., and Gad, P.: Physical training and glucose tolerance in middle-aged men with chemical diabetes. *Diabetes* 28 (Suppl. 1):30–32, 1979.

Sanders, M.F., White, F., Peterson, T., Sisson, S., and Bloor, C.: Coronary collateral development with exercise and coronary occlusion in pigs (abstr.). *Med. Sci. Sports* 11:87, 1979.

Schaefer, E.J., Levy, R.I., Anderson, D.W., Danner, R.N., Brewer, H.B., Jr., and Blackwelder, W.C.: Plasma-triglycerides in regulation of H.D.L.-cholesterol levels. *Lancet* 2:391–392, 1978.

Scheuer, J., and Tipton, C.M.: Cardiovascular adaptation to physical training. *Ann. Rev. Physiol.* 39:321–351, 1977.

Scheuer, J., Penpargkul, S., and Bahan, A.K.: Experimental observations on the effects of physical training upon intrinsic cardiac physiology and biochemisry, in E.A. Amsterdam, J.H. Wilmore, and A.M. DeMaria, editors, *Exercise in Cardiovascular Health and Disease.* New York: Yorke Medical Books, 1977, pp. 108–121.

Selvester, R., Camp, J., and Sanmarco, M.: Effects of exercise training on progression of documented coronary atherosclerosis in men. *Ann. N.Y. Acad. Sci.* 301:495–508, 1977.

Simko, V.: Physical exercise and the prevention of atherosclerosis and cholesterol gall stones. *Postgrad. Med. J.* 54:270–277, 1978.

Sims, D.N., and Neill, W.A.: Investigations of the physiological basis for increased exercise threshold for angina pectoris after physical conditioning. *J. Clin. Invest.* 54:763–770, 1974.

Sims, E.A.H., Horton, E.S., and Salans, L.B.: Inducible metabolic abnormalities during the development of obesity. *Annu. Rev. Med.* 22:235–250, 1971.

Squires, W.G., Hartung, G.H., Welton, D., Young, J., Jessup, G., and Zinkgraf, S.: The effects of exercise and diet modification on blood lipids level (abstr.). *Med. Sci. Sports* 11:109, 1979.

Stalonas, P.M., Jr., Johnson, W.G., and Christ, M.: Behavior modification for obesity: The evaluation of exercise, contingency management and program adherence. *J. Consult. Clin. Psychol.* 46:463–469, 1978.

Stern, J.S., and Johnson, P.R.: Size and number of adipocytes and their implications, in H.M. Katzen and R.J. Mahler, editors, *Diabetes, Obesity, and Vascular Disease.* New York: John Wiley and Sons, 1978, pp. 303–340.

Taylor, H.L., Buskirk, E.R., and Remington, R.D., Exercise in controlled trials of the prevention of coronary heart disease. *Fed. Proc.* 32:1623–1627, 1973.

Taylor, H.L., Jacobs, D.R., Jr., Schucker, B., Knudsen, J., Leon, A.S., and Debacker, G.: A questionnaire for the assessment of leisure time physical activity. *J. Chron. Dis.* 31:741–755, 1978.

Terjung, R.L.: Physical activity and cardiovascular health: biochemical aspects, in F. Landry and W.A.R. Orban, editors, *Physical Activity and Human Well-Being.* Vol. 1. Miami: Symposium Specialists, 1978, pp. 151–162.

Thomas, G.S.: Physical activity and health: Epidemiologic and clinical evidence and policy implications. *Prev. Med.* 8:89–103, 1979.

Thompson, P.D., Stern, M.P., Williams, P., Duncan, K., Haskell, W.P., and Wood, P.D.: Death during jogging or running: A study of eighteen cases. *JAMA* 242:1265–1267, 1979.

Thompson, P.L., and Lown, B.: Coronary occlusion before, during, and after strenuous exercise. *Cardiovase. Res.* 10:385–388, 1976.

Tibbits, G., Koziol, J., Roberts, N.K., Baldwin, K.M., and Barnard, R.J.: Adaptation of the rat myocardium to endurance training. *J. Appl. Physiol.* 44:85–89, 1978.

Tipton, C.M., Matthes, R.D., Callahan, A., Tcheng, T.K., and Lais, L.T.: The role of chronic exercise on resting blood pressures of normotensive and hypertensive rats. *Med. Sci. Sports* 9:168–177, 1977.

Tomanek, R.J.: Effects of age and exercise on the extent of the myocardial capillary bed. *Anat. Rec.* 167:55–62, 1969.

Vermikos-Danellis, J., Leach, C.L., Winget, C.M., Goodwin, A.C., and Rambaut, P.G.: Changes in glucose, insulin, and growth hormone levels associated with bed rest. *Aviation Space Environ. Med.* 47:583–587, 1976.

Viitaslos, M.T., Kals, R., Eisalo, A., and Halonen, P.I.: Ventricular arrhythmias during exercise testing, jogging, and sedentary life. *Chest* 76:21–26, 1979.

Vranic, M., and Berger, M., Exercise and diabetes mellitus. *Diabetes,* 28 (Suppl. 1):147–167, 1979.

Vranic, M., Horvath, S., and Wahren, J.: Exercise and diabetes: An overview. *Diabetes* 28 (Suppl. 1):107–110, 1979.

Wahren, J.: Glucose turnover during exercise in healthy men and in patients with diabetes mellitus. *Diabetes* 28 (Suppl. 1):82–88, 1979.

Wahren, J., Felig, P., and Hagenfeldt, L.: Physical exercise and fuel homeostatis in diabetes mellitus. *Diabetologia,* 14:213–222, 1978.

Weltman, A., Stamford, B.A., Levy, R.S., Matter, S., Short, C., and Fulco, C.: Diet, exercise and lipoprotein cholesterol (abstr.). *Circulation* 58 (Suppl. 2): 204, 1978.

Wenger, M.K.: Does exercise training enhance collateral development? in M.K. Wenger, editor, *Critical Review of Caradic Rehabilitation.* Basel: Karger, 1977, pp. 143–145.

Wilhelmsen, L., Sanne, H., Elmfeldt, D., Grimby, G., Tibblin, G., and Wendel, H.: A controlled trial of physical exercise on risk factors, nonfatal myocardial infarction and death. *Prev. Med.* 4:491–508, 1975.

Wilhelmsen, L., Tibblin, G., Aurell, M., Bjure, J., Ekstrom-Jodal, B., and Grimby, G.: Physical activity. Physical fitness and risk of myocardial infarction. *Adv. Cardiol.* 18:217–230, 1976.

Wilkerson, J.E., and Evonuk, E.: Changes in cardiac and skeletal muscle myosin ATPase activities after exercise. *J. Appl. Physiol.* 30:328–330, 1971.

Wood, P.D., Haskell, W., Klein, H., Lewis, S., Stern, M.P., and Farquhar, J.W.: The distributions of plasma lipoproteins in middle aged male runners. *Metabolism* 25:1249–1257, 1976.

Wood, P.D., Haskell, W., Stern, M.P., and Farquhar, J.W.: Plasma lipoprotein distribution in male and female runners. *Ann. N.Y. Acad. Sci.* 301:748–763, 1979.

Wyatt, H.L., and Mitchell, J.H.: Influences of physical training on the heart of dogs. *Circ. Res.* 35:883–888, 1974.

Yenkel, J.T.: Exercise does pay off: Three life insurers lower premiums for the physically fit. *The Minneapolis Star,* Aug. 28, 1979, p. 2D.

Zilvermat, D.B.: Mechanism of cholesterol control in the arterial wall. *Am. J. Cardiol.* 35:559–566, 1975.

CHAPTER 5

Nutrition and the Prevention of Coronary Heart Disease

NORMAN L. LASSER, M.D., PH.D.

Several recent developments have highlighted the pivotal role of nutrition in disease prevention, and no group of diseases better illustrates this than those of the cardiovascular system. The recently published *Surgeon General's Report on Health Promotion and Disease Prevention, Healthy People,* has given a high priority to disease prevention as a key element of national health policy, and a conference, Preventing Disease/Promoting Health, was held in June, 1979, to set objectives for the nation in order to attain progress in several key areas, among them nutrition. The nutritional goals included the attainment of a mean blood cholesterol of 200 mg/dl for adults and 150 mg/dl for children (Preventing Disease, 1979). The dietary goals for the United States issued by the U.S. Senate Select Committee on Nutrition and Human Needs include changes which would help lead to that goal and perhaps surpass it. During the period 1968–1976, there was a dramatic 20.7 percent decline in overall ischemic heart disease mortality in the United States, and some have attributed the decline, at least in part, to the changing American food consumption pattern (Stamler, 1979b; Stern, 1979).

Despite this decline, atherosclerosis and its primary clinical manifestation, the heart attack, remain the leading lethal health hazard and major cause of disability in most affluent societies. Coronary heart disease (CHD) remains the leading cause of death in the United States, being responsible for close to 750,000 deaths per year (Cooper et al., 1978). Whatever the mechanism of the final clinical event, clearly the underlying process is almost always severe coronary atherosclerosis, and the recently published report of the Pooling Project (1978) serves to indicate why prevention is so important for this condition. In the 7,545 men included in this project, 44 percent of the first major coronary events were fatal, but, more important, 70 percent of

134

CHD deaths occurred outside a hospital. For survivors, the likelihood of dying in the subsequent five years was increased fivefold. To paraphrase Professor Jerry Morris of London, "We need to understand precisely why prevention is essential and vital—because for this disease there are no cures."

The implication of this statement is that we now know enough to permit us to develop preventive approaches. Preventive programs will perforce involve changes in lifestyle, for, as pointed out by Virchow more than 100 years ago, the occurrence of an epidemic is almost invariably related to how people live (Ackerknecht, 1953). The etiology of the epidemic of coronary disease which has overtaken industrialized countries in this century includes a confluence of causes related to affluence: a "rich" diet, cigarette smoking, sedentary living habits, and the time-stressed behavior patterns that are common in our current urban competitive industrial society.

A case can be made for assigning a primary role in the prevalence of CHD to our current eating patterns. In terms of total human development, this aspect of our lifestyle is a recent innovation in nutrition. Our contemporary diets are products of a long and complex socioeconomic and cultural development. When man was primarily a hunter-gatherer, his diet consisted of a variety of natural unprocessed foods, with a high ratio of essential nutrients to calories. Once he became a farmer and a herder, making regularly available for the first time many of the foods commonly consumed by most Americans today, this ratio became distorted. As countries have become more economically developed and affluent, people in these countries have consumed less and less grain directly, using it instead more and more as fodder in "corn-hog" and "corn-steer" economies. Figure 5-1 illustrates that as gross national product increases there is a greater and greater intake of saturated (animal) fats, animal proteins, and sugar, with a decrease in the percent calories from vegetable origins (Fejfar, 1974); the long-standing gross protein-calorie malnutrition in developing countries has ceased to be a problem in the economically developed countries, having been replaced by "dysnutrition." When this is added to the other socioeconomically induced changes in lifestyle, such as cigarette smoking, sedentary living, and increased intake of salt, the result is the coronary epidemic plaguing Western industrialized society.

Because the habitual diet of this and other industrialized nations leads to mass hyperlipidemia, only a "public health" approach to this habitual diet will result in a reduction of the hyperlipidemia. This issue of treating the "high risk" individual versus the whole population will be discussed further, but since the best evidence we have for

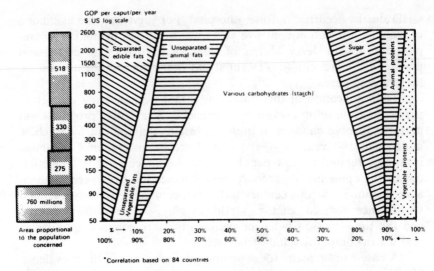

Figure 5-1. Percent calories derived from separated edible fat, unseparated vegetable fats, and unseparated animal fats, high-starch carbohydrates, sugar, animal protein, and vegetable protein according to the income of the countries

Reprinted with permission from Z. Fejfar: "Prevention against ischaemic heart disease: A critical review," *Modern Trends in Cardiology*, edited by M.F. Oliver, Butterworth, London, 1974.

the possibility of prevention is through observation of societies whose members live throughout their lifetime on a lower fat diet, the most productive approach for our society is to provide a better habitual diet to all of us from birth. This approach will also enable high-risk patients to adhere to a new eating style by making it unnecessary for the patient to "swim upstream" against a way of life geared to the production of atherosclerosis.

This chapter, then, will concern itself with the role of nutrition in disease prevention primarily in the cardiovascular system. It will not concern itself with "therapeutic" nutrition, nor will it consider in detail the role of nutrition in preventing other chronic diseases. This chapter focuses on the area which relates to our most pressing problem in chronic disease prevention. Despite the importance, however, of the public health approach alluded to above, this chapter will focus on how the practitioner on the front line of clinical medicine can help his patients change their dietary habits to achieve optimal cardiovascular health. First the evidence relating diet, blood cholesterol, and coronary heart disease will be reviewed, as will the experimental evidence for a cause–effect relationship of these same three factors. Then the arguments will be presented for interpreting this evidence in favor of treatment without unequivocal proof of benefit.

Finally, the practitioner will be provided with a "how to" manual for lowering cardiovascular risk in his patients. This will include a reiteration and, to some degree, expansion of the behavioral tools discussed earlier in this book, for if he is to be successful in preventing disease, the practitioner today must become an effective change agent.

EPIDEMIOLOGIC EVIDENCE ABOUT DIET, LIPIDS, AND CORONARY DISEASE

Epidemiology has provided perhaps the most extensive body of data relating to the question of the causal role of serum cholesterol in atherosclerosis, the ability of diet to modify cholesterol, and, consequently, coronary disease incidence. Indeed it is at the level of population studies, particularly those involving clinical trials, that the clinician must derive the basis for most of his decisions in deciding to treat or not to treat. This is because it is not always possible to wait for the results of experimental studies to indicate precise mechanisms before treating a condition if population-based studies indicate a practical method of treating or preventing disease. The discussion which follows should serve to indicate the persuasiveness of the epidemiological data leading one to conclude that it is prudent to maintain an "optimal" plasma cholesterol to avoid coronary heart disease.

Descriptive-Analytical Studies

Epidemiological studies may be conveniently divided into descriptive, analytical, and experimental. The first two are primarily observational, although analytical studies involve the analysis of relationships among factors studied descriptively. Experimental, or intervention, studies are aimed at perturbing the factors previously studied and observing changes in the incidence of disease or mortality from, in this case, heart disease. Observational studies may conveniently be divided between those relating to individual CHD risk within populations and to comparative CHD risk studies between populations. Stamler (1979b) has divided these studies primarily on the basis of whether they were inter- or intranational, and we shall follow his classification scheme for the framework of this discussion.

Relationships between Nutrition, Plasma Cholesterol, and CHD—International Studies.

1. Analyses of Data on Nutrition and Mortality Patterns among Nations. Analyses of this type are based on Food and Agricultural Organization (FAO) and World Health Organization (WHO) data. It has been possible in at least ten data sets to compare dietary constituents and mortality from CHD by utilizing the national food balance sheets published by the FAO (Stamler, 1979b). The wide range of mortality from coronary heart disease found among various nations is shown in Figure 5-2 for middle-aged men in 18 countries for 1973 (WHO, 1976). This figure serves to illustrate the almost ten-fold dif-

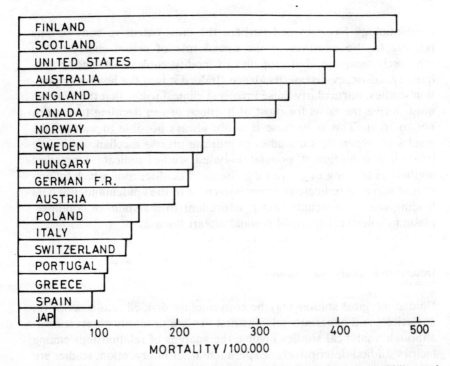

Figure 5-2. Mortality from coronary heart disease (CHD) among middle-aged men in certain countries. WHO = World Health Organization

From: Turpeinen, O.: Effect of cholesterol-lowering diet on mortality from coronary heart disease and other causes. *Circulation* 59:1, 1979. By permission of the American Heart Association, Inc.

ference between the mortality rates in Japan and Finland, with the United States being near the top.

Twenty countries were originally studied by the WHO in regard to cardiovascular mortality. All of the international comparisons of WHO–FAO data show statistically significant associations between dietary constituents and mortality from CHD. Most of these studies have dealt with the nutrient composition of the total diet, with only three considering the relationship of specific foods to mortality (Yudkin, 1957; Armstrong et al., 1975; Stamler, 1978a). Using age-sex-specific and cause-specific mortality data, the more recent studies have found the following dietary variables to be significantly correlated with CHD mortality in univariate analyses: saturated fat, total fat, animal protein, total protein, total calories, meat, eggs, milk, sugar, tea, and coffee (men only). There is also a significant inverse correlation between per capita grain, legume, fruit, and vegetable consumption and CHD mortality rates. Stamler and his group (Byington et al., 1979) have analyzed the combined impact of the three key dietary components shown in metabolic ward studies to influence serum cholesterol (dietary cholesterol, saturated and polyunsaturated fat) and have shown a high-order correlation between the mean Keys-predicted serum cholesterol and the 1973 age-standardized CHD mortality rate in 20 economically developed countries.

These international studies, spanning two decades, have consistently shown associations between nutrients, including saturated fat and cholesterol, and mortality from coronary heart disease. However, there are at least two potential problems with the data: the countries could have been preselected, introducing bias into the conclusions, and since the nutrients and food groups positively related to CHD in these univariate analyses are highly correlated among themselves, it is difficult to determine which of them, if any, are etiologically significant. The consistency of the findings mitigate the first criticism, but it is clear that by themselves these types of data cannot resolve cause-and-effect questions. It does not mean that they are useless, but it does mean that they must be evaluated in the light of other data, simultaneously considered using well-established guidelines to weigh causative relationships.

2. International Autopsy Studies. Initial stuides of this type consisted of observation by pathologists that individuals from countries with infrequent occurrence of severe coronary atherosclerosis had low dietary fat intakes. These observations were followed by large-scale systematic studies, the most comprehensive one of this type being the

International Atherosclerosis Project (IAP) (McGill, 1968). This study quantitated the degree of atherosclerosis of the aorta and coronary arteries at autopsy in over 31,000 individuals ranging in age from 10 to 69, dying in 1960–1965, in 15 cities and countries throughout the world. A strong correlation was found between dietary lipids and the underlying pathologic process, advanced atherosclerosis. Other dietary variables, including sugar consumption, were not significantly related to the severity of disease. The mean level of serum cholesterol of these populations was also correlated with dietary fat, and the cholesterol level with atherosclerosis severity. The IAP also noted findings that indicated hypertension and diabetes to be related to atherosclerosis, particularly in the two industrialized countries studied. This type of study thus confirms previous suggestions of the role of a high-fat diet in establishing the metabolic prerequisite for significant atherosclerosis, and it also highlights the fact that etiology and pathogenesis in this condition is multifactorial.

3. Field Investigations of Population Samples in Different Countries. While in the decade after World War II several studies reported comparisons of living populations among samples from different countries, the International Cooperative Study on the Epidemiology of Cardiovascular Diseases, the "Seven-Country Study," is the most comprehensive investigation of this type so far undertaken (Keys, 1970). This was a prospective international study of 18 population samples in seven countries, and included approximately 12,000 men, originally aged 40 to 59 years. Detailed analyses of the diets consumed, including chemical analyses, demonstrated that the amount and type of lipid habitually eaten, particularly saturated fat and cholesterol, varied markedly among populations. Ten-year mortality data have recently become available (Keys, 1980). If plots are made of the ten-year CHD deaths against median values for total cholesterol taken at baseline in the 1950s and '60s for each of 16 areas in seven countries, a strong correlation is found between median total cholesterol and hard CHD death in ten years ($R = 0.65$), and no clear threshold value of population with respect to CHD risk emerges. It is evident from the data in Table 5-1 that there are marked differences in saturated fat intake, but very little difference in polyunsaturated fat intake among the populations studied. There is quite clearly a correlation between the amount of saturated fat consumed as a percent of calories and the average cholesterol level. The intake of dietary cholesterol among these populations was not measured.

The data from the Seven-Country Study provide a wider range of cholesterol levels than many of the studies conducted in the United

Table 5-1
Dietary Fat, Serum Cholesterol and 10-Year CHD Mortality Rate, Men Originally Aged 40–59, 7-Country Study

Cohort	Total fat % cal	Sat. fat % cal	Poly. fat % cal	2 S-P	Serum cholesterol Median	90th %	10-yr mortality CHD	All
Greece	36	7	3	11	201	258	9	57
Yugoslavia	31	5	5	5	171[a]	219[a]	12[a]	105[a]
Italy	26	9	3	15	198	253	21	126
Rome RR	—	—	—	—	207	260	22	75
U.S. RR	40	18	5	31	236	294	57	115
Finland	37	20	3	37	259	323	65	167
Netherlands	40	18	5	31	230	291	44	125

[a] Excludes Belgrade and Slavonia.

2S-P: S is percentage of calories from dietary saturated fatty acids; P, the percentage of calories from polyunsaturated fatty acids; this expression is, therefore, a measure of the combined impact of these two dietary components on serum cholesterol of the group (45). RR = railroad (from Keys, 1976).

141

States, so that it is worth considering the relationship of the cholesterol level to CHD incidence in some more detail. An analysis of the data from this study shows that all except one of the very low-CHD-incidence areas (0.5 to 1.5 deaths/thousand/year) have cholesterol medians under 200 mg/dl, while all high-CHD incidence areas (3 to 7 cases/thousand/year), have cholesterol medians greater than 235 mg/dl. Table 5-1 illustrates the relationship of the serum cholesterol level at entry to the ten-year CHD death rate. These data, in addition to demonstrating the lack of a threshold as alluded to above, indicates that there is a gradient between 160 and 220 mg/dl, in contrast to the data from the Pooling Project to be discussed below. It is data such as this which gives rise to the recommendations for an "optimal" population mean cholesterol of 190 mg/dl (see below).

    4. International Studies on the Effects of Migration. Studies of the effect of immigration from less-affluent to more-affluent societies provide "natural experiments" for evaluating changes in risk factors. These studies have served to dispel the view that atherosclerosis is an inevitable concomitant of the aging process or that cholesterol levels in different nations represent different genetic backgrounds. Whether the population studied has been Yemenite Jews migrating to Israel, Japanese migrating to Hawaii or the United States, or Italian or Irish who emigrated to the United States, the results are consistent: as groups move from areas with a low incidence of coronary disease to areas with a high incidence, they show a rise in dietary fat intake and a rise in serum cholesterol, taking on the disease incidence of their newly adopted lands (Katz, Stamler, and Pick, 1958).

    Perhaps the most significant of the studies in this area was the major study initiated in 1965 with middle-aged men of Japanese ancestry living in Hiroshima and Nagasaki; in Honolulu; and in the San Francisco Bay area, the so-called "Ni-Hon-San" Study. Baseline nutritional patterns of these populations, assessed by 24-hour dietary recall, indicated that group mean intakes of total fat, saturated fat, and animal protein were much lower in Japanese than in Japanese-American men, while group mean intakes of total carbohydrate, complex carbohydrate, alcohol, and salt were higher in the Japanese. Corresponding to those differences the mean serum cholesterol level in Japanese men was 37 mg/dl lower than that of the Hawaiian men and 47 mg/dl lower than that of the California men (Kagan et al., 1974). Incidence as well as prevalence data on CHD mortality indicate that CHD death rates were consistently and significantly lower for Japanese than for Japanese-American men. Hawaiian men had an incidence of myocardial infarction 2.1 times that of Japanese men, while the California men had a rate 1.5 times that of the Hawaiian and 3.2 times that of the Japanese (Robertson et al, 1977b). Multivariate assessment of the relationship between baseline status for major risk factors and the incidence of CHD for the cohorts studied show that serum cholesterol was significantly and independently related to risk in both populations, as was systolic blood pressure (Robertson et al., 1977a).

Criticisms have been leveled at studies of migrants. For example, they are almost always a selected group, being perhaps more enterprising, or having more problems than those who do not migrate. On the other hand, this type of study provides a unique ability to separate environment from heredity and yields data that is consistent with findings from other studies that demonstrate a correlation of diet with serum cholesterol, which in turn is correlated with CHD mortality rate.

Relationship between Nutrition, Plasma Cholesterol, and CHD— Intranational Studies. Numerous studies of this type have documented the associations indicated by the international studies cited above. Included in these studies have been the evaluation of natural experiments, such as the effects of war, and epidemiological studies of time trends. In addition, analyses have been performed of different regions within a country and of different ethnic and social groups. For example, Sacks et al. (1975) have compared serum lipid values of "pure" vegetarians with omnivores in the United States population, utilizing residents of a Boston commune where a macrobiotic diet was being eaten. Compared to the control group from Framingham, Massachusetts, the vegetarians' mean serum cholesterol as well as their low-density lipoprotein (LDL) cholesterol and very-low-density lipoprotein (VLDL) cholesterol were markedly and significantly lower by 31 to 38 percent. Multivariate analyses showed that avoidance of animal products in general in the preceding week was associated with low levels of serum cholesterol, LDL, and VLDL cholesterol. While high-density lipoprotein cholesterol (HDL-C) was slightly lower in the vegetarians compared to controls, the ratio HDL-C/LDL-C was increased. Studies have confirmed a similar benefit for Seventh Day Adventists compared with the general population (Phillips, Lemon, and Kuzma, 1978).

Of greater significance, however, have been prospective studies relating dietary intake, serum lipids, and other risk factors, and CHD incidence. Data of this type are now available in great quantity from many studies of populations, both in this country and abroad. In the U.S., the Albany, Chicago Gas, Framingham, Tecumseh, and Chicago Western Electric studies have been pooled and analyzed in the National cooperative Pooling Project. The final analyses from this project have recently been published (Pooling Project Group, 1978), and represent results from 8,274 white males originally 40 to 59 years of age, and free of CHD at the initial examination. Table 5-2 represents data from this Pooling Project Report, and shows that population divided into quintiles based on a single measure of cholesterol at entry. The three higher quintiles are compared with quintiles I and II combined, with regard to risk of a first major coronary event. For example, for quintile III, with baseline serum cholesterol ranging from 218 to 240 mg/dl, there was an increase in relative risk of 15 percent, for quintile IV a risk of 64 percent, and for quintile V (cholesterol 268 mg/dl and over) a doubling of risk. Of particular interest, however, is a consideration of the absolute excess risk attributable to having a cholesterol that places one in the upper three quintiles. If again men in quintiles I and II are considered "normal" and cases occurring among quintiles III–V as "excess events," examination of the data in Table 5-2 reveals that almost one-half (44 percent) were due to "moderate" elevations of serum cholesterol in the range of 216–268 mg/dl (quintiles III and IV). This is an important point for the clinician, for any tendency to focus exclusively in the upper 5th percentile of the population, those who are severely hypercholesterolemic, means neglect of most of the patients with hypercholesterolemia and the associated problem of excess risk of coronary disease occurring in almost half the U.S. population. We shall

Table 5-2
Serum Cholesterol and Risk of a First Major Coronary Event between Ages 40 and 64. 8,274 White Men, Pool 5, Pooling Project, Final Report

Quintile of level and level (mg/dl)		No.of events	Risk of an event/1,000	Relative risk	Absolute excess risk/1,000	% of all excess
I + II	≤ 218	166	162.7	1.00	—	—
I	≤ 194	86	172.4	—	—	—
II	194–218	80	153.0	—	—	—
III	218–240	104	186.8	1.15	24.1	8.3%
IV	240–268	167	266.3	1.64	103.6	35.8%
V	> 268	210	324.1	1.99	161.4	55.8%
All		647	222.4	—	—	—

QIII–QV excess events, 3,000 men/all events, 5,000 men = 289.1/1,112.0 = 25.6% of all events are excess events, attributable to hypercholesterilemia.

Reprinted with permission from J. Stamler: "Primary prevention and lifestyles," *Childhood Prevention of Atherosclerosis and Hypertension,* edited by R.M. Lauer and R.B. Shekelle. Copyright © by Raven Press, New York, 1980.

discuss the question of "normal" later in this chapter, but it is important to recognize that apparently trivial elevations of serum cholesterol can, especially when combined with other risk factors, indicate an extremely high risk of coronary disease compared to patients without these risk factors, so that the practitioner should not allow his patients to remain complacent about levels of cholesterol which are "normal" by the usual criteria of clinical laboratories.

The Pooling Project highlights once again the fact that coronary disease is a multifactorial condition. The three major risk factors for coronary heart disease which have emerged from these Pooling Project studies and other studies around the world are: an elevated serum cholesterol, hypertension, and cigarette smoking, each having been proven to be independent and significant factors. This was true for serum cholesterol in the Pooling Project for the age groups including 40 to 55, but not for the 55 to 59 group. Recent reports of the importance of HDL-C help to clarify this situation. It becomes clear when one examines this data (Gordon et al., 1977b) that LDL cholesterol remains positively, independently, and significantly related to risk for both men and women at least into the seventh and eighth decades of life, while HDL cholesterol is inversely related to risk.

It is noteworthy, in light of the criteria for causality, that all Pooling Project studies yielded *consistent* data for the association between cholesterol and risk of CHD, the association being graded and, of course, the hypercholesterolemia preceding the coronary disease. One difficulty, however, which has emerged from studies within single populations has been the inability to correlate cholesterol levels and dietary fat intake in individuals (Gordon, 1970; Nichols et al., 1976). While opponents of the "diet–heart" hypothesis may seize upon such results as important negative evidence relating dietary fat intake to CHD, there are a number of very cogent explanations for this lack of correlation. Recent studies (Liu et al., 1978) indicate that a key factor contributing to the poor correlations reported is the use of dietary survey methods inadequate to distinguish nutritionally among individuals who are members of more or less homogeneous populations. The result is an obscuring of interindividual differences by a large degree of intra-individual variation. It has been calculated by Liu and his colleagues that, to estimate the correlation between dietary lipid intake and serum cholesterol with reasonable precision, nine days of food records are needed under American conditions. Other problems include the fact that present dietary intake may not reflect past habits and both may affect blood lipid levels; and a threshold level of dietary intake may exist above which the relationship between this intake and blood lipid levels are nonlinear or even unrelated. Finally, responsiveness to changes in dietary intake is undoubtedly a genetic trait, adding considerably to interindividual variability. One should thus not discount the large body of diverse other evidence cited above in favor of a relationship between dietary fat intake and CHD when it cannot be shown that this relationship is statistically significant in an individual. In any case, recent within-group observations in both Puerto Rico and Hawaii have shown a relationship between dietary fat, starch, and coronary heart disease (Garcia-Palmieri et al., 1977).

These studies, part of the USPHS International Study, have also demonstrated a gradient relationship between serum cholesterol and CHD incidence, but, interestingly, Framingham CHD rates are higher than can be explained by combined baseline characteristics in the other two populations, indicating that not only can individuals begin at a different *absolute* risk based on genetic traits, but whole populations can begin with a different risk, the explanation for which is not immediately apparent (Gordon et al., 1974).

A large number of other studies have been carried out in other countries. For example, in Tromso, Norway, a two-year prospective case-control study in men aged 20 to 49 years was carried out (Miller et al., 1977), and the Israeli Heart Study (Goldbourt and Medalie, 1979) has provided important information on HDL in a large population with overall CHD rates less than half that of U.S. employee rates.

Criteria for Assessing the Etiologic Significance of Epidemiologic Associations. It is worth reviewing, in light of the associations we have seen to this point, the criteria which help determine whether or not associations of an epidemiologic nature indicate a cause-and-effect relationship between those factors which are associated. The criteria, succinctly presented in the first *Report of the Advisory Committee to the Surgeon General* on smoking and health (1964), in updated form, are as follows:

1. *Strength* of the association
2. *Graded nature* of the association
3. *Temporal sequence,* i.e., does the presumed etiologic factor precede the disease
4. *Consistency* of the findings in multiple studies
5. *Independence* of each of the associations, one from the other
6. *Predictive capacity,* i.e., the ability based on the findings in one or more sets of populations to predict events in other different populations
7. *Coherence* of the findings; i.e., consistency of the epidemiologic

findings with those from other research methods and coherence in the sense that reasonable pathogenetic mechanisms are known whereby the etiologic agents can act to produce the disease.

8. The factor is *susceptible to intervention,* and intervention alters the incidence of disease in humans.

Although we have not discussed the criteria in detail, the first five have clearly been met in the data discussed so far. As to predictive capacity, the Seven-Country Study for the first time assessed the capacity of risk factor findings from an American study to predict CHD rates for European populations. With the use of multiple logistic coefficients from the Framingham Study, a high-order significant correlation was found between the five-year predicted and observed incidence rate for several populations (Keys, 1970). Other analyses of this kind have been carried out (Keys, 1972) and correspondence also found between predicted and observed rates, but the observed rates for the European populations were generally lower than the predicted. While this could mean that additional unidentified risk factors are operating to account for the higher rate in Americans, it is quite likely that a good part of the explanation lies in the problems associated with taking single measurements of risk factors made at one middle-aged point in the life span of the men under study. Also, of course, not all studies took into account other known risk factors. Finally, studies have recently been carried out involving predictive application of multivariate data from one group of Americans to another population in this country, Thus, Section 31 of the Framingham reports has presented data on this matter for five of the Pooling Project studies (McGee and Gordon, 1976), and such data are also considered in the Pooling Project Final Report (1978).

With respect to the biological plausibility of the associations, this will be better assessed after we have looked at some of the animal-experimental data available, but it is by now well known that the majority of the postulated mechanisms for atherosclerosis are consistent with causal roles for most if not all of the known risk factors for CHD. Thus, while it is exceedingly difficult for epidemiological associations to prove cause-and-effect relationships, the data in this area are extremely convincing. The last criterion listed, that of the results of intervention, is the one which has been the most difficult to establish unequivocally, and we shall look at some of the reasons for this later in this chapter, but the effectiveness of intervention on risk factors in middle age remains a source of great controversy. In the final analysis, the practitioner must make his own decision based on the evidence at hand, but we shall look at some of the issues and arguments before discussing how to carry out the intervention.

Studies of Population Cholesterol Levels. On April 11 and 12, 1979, at the American Health Foundation in New York City, a meeting was held entitled "Conference on the Health Effects of Blood Lipids: Optimal Distributions for Populations." The complete report of this conference has recently been published (Wynder et al., 1979) and is a valuable compilation of data on cholesterol levels in populations throughout the world. The conclusion of the conference was that, while an ideal mean for this country might be 160 mg/dl, with a present mean of 210 mg/dl, a feasible mean which would be compatible with a low incidence of CHD would be 190 mg/dl. For children, the comparable values were: ideal mean, 110 mg/dl; present mean, 160 mg/dl; and feasible mean, 140 mg/dl.

There are several sources for recent surveys of the current American mean serum cholesterol. Perhaps the most representative and extensive survey was that conducted by the Prevalence Study of the Lipid Research Clinics Program, the data having been collected between 1971 and 1976. The data have recently been published (Lipid Research Clinics Program Committee, 1979; Heiss et al., 1980) and represent data from ten North American clinics. Although the populations were not selected specifically to be representative of the entire population, the studies were nevertheless prevalence studies and represented lipid determinations in more than 54,000 white participants screened at visit one of the study and over 24,000 participant determinations of lipids and lipoproteins for those attending visit two. The overall mean plasma cholesterol for white middle-aged males was approximately 210 mg/dl. The 45 to 49 year age group had a mean of 212 mg/dl, with a 95th percentile value of 276. The means were 155 mg/dl for the 0 to 4 age group, 160 mg/dl for 5 to 9, and 150 mg/dl for those aged 15 to 19. The 95th percentile remained relatively constant at about 203 mg/dl through age 14, increased to 270 mg/dl for the age group 35 to 39, and then varied between 261 and 277 thereafter. Data is also presented for lipoprotein fractions, and, for example, the LDL cholesterol for age 45 to 49 had a mean of 144 with a 95th percentile of 202. The 95th percentile for LDL cholesterol was 165 for the 25 to 29 age group, remaining 185–189 to age 45, when, as noted, it rose to 202.

In the United States a series of large volunteer populations was recruited for first-generation trials in the 1950s and 1960s and similar populations were recruited in the 1960s and 1970s. In the earlier studies the mean cholesterol was 233.4 ± 45.3 mg/dl compared with 218.8 ± 37.8 in 398,855 men in the later studies. The earlier studies referred to include those collected in the Pooling Project and the Health Examination Survey (HES)(DHEW, 1967), while the later studies included the 1971–1974 Health and Nutrition Examination Survey (HANES)(Abraham et al., 1977), the Multiple Risk Factor Intervention Trial (MRFIT)(Benfari et al., 1975), and the Lipid Research Clinics (LRC). Taken together these studies indicate that there has been an average "spontaneous" cholesterol decrease in the general population mean in the last decade. Perhaps for this reason interventions with a prudent diet in experimental intervention programs now achieve only a 5 percent cholesterol lowering in contrast to the 10 percent lowering in trials of a decade or more ago (Blackburn et al., 1979a). The present adult mean of about 210 mg/dl is about midway between the earlier mean of the 1950s and 1960s (230 mg/dl) and the mean proposed by the American Health Foundation Conference as a feasible target (190 mg/dl). This mean is considered feasible not only because of observations of the group of countries already having such a mean, but because of the probable continued evolution of already existing trends, together with continued and increasing activity in the prevention area, with resulting changes in individual diet and physical activity patterns. The data considered at the conference would seem to indicate that, if there is a threshold, it is at the level of the "ideal" mean of ± 160 mg/dl.

It must be remembered that this discussion has centered around population means, and while suggested means serve as a guideline for the treatment of individual patients, other factors must be taken into account in deciding whether or not a given patient requires aggressive intervention. Some of these will be discussed later in the chapter when treatment is presented.

High-Density Lipoprotein Cholesterol. A brief discussion of the relationship of high-density lipoprotein cholesterol (HDL-C) to CHD is appropriate here, not only because it is one of the more exciting developments in the epidemiology of cardiovascular disease in recent years, but because there are nutritional determinants of this protective fraction, and its relevance must be borne in mind when deciding to intervene with the purpose of lowering total cholesterol or LDL-C. HDL has been "reborn" as an important factor in coronary heart disease, since the first reference to its importance in a paper by Barr, Russ, and Eder in 1951. It was subsequently neglected by the scientific community, but interest reasserted itself following the proposal by Miller and Miller (1975) that it seemed to be an "inverse risk factor." Ten case-control studies have been reported since 1971 and at least two cohort studies. The case-control study of perhaps greatest interest was that of the Cooperative Lipoprotein Phenotyping Study, published in 1977 (Castelli et al., 1977a, 1977b). This was a comparison of HDL-C levels in cases and controls of coronary heart disease in five locations in the continental United States and Hawaii. They demonstrated approximately a twofold gradient of risk, the risk increasing with lower HDL-C levels, but CHD prevalence apparently leveling off at an HDL-C of about 45 mg/dl. In the prospective cohort study from Framingham the original Framingham cohort was studied beginning at the average age of 49 and followed for four years (Gordon et al., 1977a). In this case a sixfold gradient of risk was demonstrated with no leveling off of the risk at any HDL-C level. Multivariate analyses confirmed that, not only was HDL-C a powerful independent predictor of coronary heart disease, but it persisted into the eighth decade and had the highest standardized multivariate coefficient of all the known lipid risk factors. The Israeli Ischemic Heart Disease Study (Goldbourt and Medalie, 1979) confirmed these findings among 6,500 adult males age 50 and over, with no association demonstrable below age 50. All the studies to date seem consistent in demonstrating a negative association between levels of HDL and coronary heart disease.

The Framingham Study has developed "multipliers" by which multivariate risk calculated from the conventional risk factors can be corrected for HDL-C levels. In general, using the risk for a male with a level of 45 mg/dl as standard and that of a female at 55 mg/dl, risk for men is cut about in half for levels above 60 mg/dl and is approximately doubled with levels 30 mg/dl or lower. The corresponding levels for women are 70 and 40 mg/dl, respectively. Galen (1980) has emphasized the use of ratios of total cholesterol or LDL-C to HDL-C in assessing risk. These ratios are summarized in the chart below for men:

Risk	Cholesterol LDL/HDL	Cholesterol Total/HDL
1/2 average	1.00	3.43
average	3.55	4.97
2 × average	6.25	9.55
3 × average	7.99	23.39

These recent findings have stimulated a large volume of laboratory research related to HDL. It has been proposed that the mechanism by which this fraction exerts its protective effect is by its acting as a "scavenger" for cholesterol. Thus HDL acts as a transport mechanism for carrying cholesterol from the peripheral tissues back to the liver in this model. While the details of these mechanisms remain to be worked out, epidemiological studies have demonstrated a number of "determinants" of HDL-C. There are strong positive correlations between alcohol intake and HDL-C levels in a number of studies (Furman, Alaupovic, and Howard, 1967), and there is apparently a positive correlation between exercise, particularly aerobic exercise, and HDL-C levels (Wood and Haskell, 1979). There are also strong inverse relationships between HDL-C and both weight and smoking (Hulley et al., 1979; Garrison et al., 1978). In addition to cross-sectional correlations at a single point in time, several studies have been able to demonstrate a change in HDL-C with a change in particular independent variables such as weight, alcohol, and exercise level (Wilson and Lees, 1972; Huttunen et al., 1979). It has, in addition, been demonstrated that nicotinic acid (Shepherd et al., 1979) and, to some extent, clofibrate are capable of raising HDL-C levels. Undoubtedly the search will continue for pharmacologic agents that will raise HDL-C, particularly if they simultaneously lower LDL and total cholesterol.

These data for HDL reinforce the approaches already advocated for preventing CHD nutritionally, for example, weight loss. Smoking cessation and increased activity levels are also indicated for the prevention of CHD, but the question of alcohol is a difficult one. One must take the findings with relation to alcohol, as indeed is true of all the findings with relation to HDL, with some caution, since these studies are relatively new and have not been extensively duplicated, failing to have the strong positive criteria for establishing etiological relationships as do saturated fat and cholesterol in the diet. Convincing data are available only for populations older than age 50, and it remains possible that some factor other than HDL-C itself is causing the relationship with coronary heart disease. Certainly it is not simply the gross cholesterol content of HDL which is probably responsible for its protective effect, but rather some subfraction. Recent studies suggest that it is the HDL_2 fraction (or some even smaller fraction) which confers protection from coronary heart disease (Anderson, Nichols, and Brewer, 1979).

Finally, the practitioner should be reminded that there is as yet no true standardization program for HDL-C determinations, so that the precision and/or accuracy of a given number provided by a commercial laboratory may be sorely lacking. This, together with the other caveats enumerated above, make it clear that, while HDL-C must be taken into account in the total evaluation of the patient, it is as yet too early to attribute to this fraction the significance given it by some investigators. It would seem wise to treat HDL as being either high, low, or average, and to use this information in modifying one's assessment of the overall risk for CHD in a given patient.

Other Nutritional Factors and the Risk of CHD. It is beyond the scope of this chapter to review in detail all the nutritional factors that may have an influence on serum cholesterol and hence, potentially, on CHD incidence. However, it is essential to consider them at least briefly, since they may have a bearing on the overall nutritional approach taken by the practitioner in instituting a dietary prevention program for cardiovascular disease.

1. Obesity. In studies such as the Framingham Study, increasing weight is associated with increasing incidence of cardiovascular disease, but when multiple regression analyses are done, taking into account all the other known risk factors for coronary disease, weight per se becomes a rather insignificant correlate of disease incidence (Gordon and Kannel, 1976). Despite this, it has been shown in numerous studies that many of the other risk factors are influenced by relative weight (Mann, 1974). For example, data from the Framingham Study indicate that cholesterol, blood pressure, uric acid, and blood glucose all rise as weight rises (Ashley and Kannel, 1974). Recent data from the Multiple Risk Factor Intervention Trial (MRFIT) and other studies (Lasser et al., 1979) clearly demonstrate that weight loss produces a dramatic decrease in VLDL, a smaller but independent and significant decrease in LDL, and a rise in HDL, all potentially beneficial with respect to reducing coronary risk. There appears to be an impact of weight loss on cholesterol-lowering which is not accounted for by adherence to the "prudent" diet lower in saturated fat and cholesterol. Therefore, because of the important relationship of weight loss to the reduction of almost all the other risk factors amenable to dietary intervention, reduction in weight and prevention of obesity is probably the single most important hygienic measure in the nutritional area that one can undertake in preventing CHD.

2. Alcohol. A review of epidemiologic data reveals a U-shaped relationship between alcohol and heart disease. In addition to its well-known effects on the plasma lipoproteins, that is, raising VLDL and HDL, alcohol appears to have some direct protective effect with respect to coronary heart disease. It has been reported from the Honolulu Heart Study that coronary heart disease was less likely to develop in Japanese men in Honolulu who drank alcoholic beverages than in those who abstained and that the more they drank (up to about 60 ml/day of ethanol), the lower the risk (Yano, Rhoads, and Kagan, 1977). In addition, it was the consensus of the data from several large prospective studies in reports presented at a recent Symposium on

Alcohol and Cardiovascular Disease (1980) that moderate alcohol intake, up to approximately 2 drinks per day, was associated either with no increased risk of cardiovascular disease or with a slight decreased risk. A recent geographic analysis has been done of alcohol consumption and coronary heart disease, and such an analysis of 20 countries in 1972 suggested that moderate alcohol consumption appeared to be negatively related to rates of heart disease mortality. A temporal analysis in the U.S. indicated that changes in alcohol consumption, particularly beer, were highly negatively related to changes in CHD mortality from 1950 to 1975 (LaPorte, Cresanta, and Kuller, 1980). However, all of these studies demonstrated that, as alcohol intake increased, particularly when it exceeded six to eight drinks per day, risk from cardiovascular disease rose precipitously, as did other problems associated with alcohol. The same relationship has been shown to relate alcohol consumption to blood pressure; that is, a moderate alcohol intake may be associated with a slight drop in blood pressure, while more excessive alcohol intake is associated with increasing blood pressure (Klatsky et al., 1977). Recent work in nonhuman primates has also indicated a protective effect for alcohol. In *Macaca nemestrina* it has been shown that, when young adult males are fed alcohol as 36 percent of calories, whether the diet was low or high in cholesterol, the index of coronary atherosclerosis was lower in animals given alcohol (Leathers, Bond, and Rudel, 1978). It appears that there is an effect on the size of the LDL, in the direction of producing smaller molecules, but with an increased total concentration of both LDL and HDL. On the other hand, the Honolulu Heart Study (Blackwelder et al., 1980) has recently reported that, while it is true that Japanese men in Honolulu who drank had a lower risk for coronary heart disease, the reverse is true for risk of death from cancer and from stroke. In this study, men who drank were more likely to die from these causes than those who abstained, and the more they drank the greater was the risk of death. In addition, there are the well-known adverse effects of alcohol, which produces fatty liver and ultimately cirrhosis, as well as producing a direct toxic effect on the myocardium resulting in alcoholic cardiomyopathy. Therefore, particularly in light of the fairly short history of alcohol effects on HDL and of the effects of HDL itself, prudence should be exercised in advising patients to drink. The risk of alcoholism itself is sufficiently high that encouraging patients to drink probably has an adverse risk/benefit ratio. Thus, the risk of excess intake must temper any advice that the physician gives his patients with regard to alcohol intake, but in view of the possible beneficial effects of moderate intake, the wisest course is probably to inform the patient of the facts and let him make his own decision with regard to this controversial subject.

3. Hyperglycemia. Although hyperglycemia itself is not amenable to dietary treatment except through weight loss, it is worthwhile noting its relationship to CHD in evaluating the total risk profile of the patient. While it is clear that in industrialized countries diabetics are more likely to suffer or die from coronary heart disease than are non-diabetics (Jarrett and Keen, 1975), the data with regard to impaired glucose tolerance is less clear. Studies in 15 populations have recently been reported in a symposium issue of the *Journal of Chronic Diseases* (Stamler and Stamler, 1979) and subsequently further commented upon in *Lancet* (Editorial, 1980). Most studies showed higher rates of ECG abnormalities in the highest quintile of blood glucose distribution at baseline examinations. Eleven of the studies reported data on long-term mortality. While by univariate analysis six studies showed a relative risk of 1.4 or more when the highest quintile of blood glucose distribution was compared to the lowest, multivariate analyses led to significant association of CHD death rate with glucose levels in only one study, that of the Chicago People's Gas Company. It appears, however, that there may be a threshold effect so that, for example, the Whitehall study (Fuller et al., 1979) showed that, above the 98th percentile of blood glucose distribution (106 mg/dl) the relative risk of CHD mortality was doubled even when corrected for other risk indices. Impaired glucose tolerance carries a definite, although small, risk of progress to overt diabetes. As indicated above, it may also confer some increased risk of coronary heart disease but, in any case, it has not been shown that measures which lower the blood sugar and improve glucose tolerance will reduce the risk of CHD, so that the importance of treating an abnormal glucose remains unclear. However, since measures such as weight loss which will improve glucose levels are usually advisable in the general prevention of coronary disease, it is probably wise to consider impaired glucose tolerance at least a mild additional risk factor in the assessment of the individual patient.

4. Long-chain Polyunsaturated Fatty Acids. Recent enthusiasm has been expressed for the importance of the qualitative content of the polyunsaturated fatty acids which are ingested in potentially preventing platelet aggregation, and hence, overt coronary heart disease. In a series of papers, Dyerberg and Bang have investigated the role of the intake of ω-3 polyunsaturated fatty acids [such as cis 5,8,11,14,17-eicosapentenoic acid (C 20:5)] in the low death rate from cardiovascular disease reported among Eskimos (Dyerberg, Bang, and Hjorne, 1975; Dyerberg and Bang, 1979). They have shown that the intake of the fatty acids is reflected in the blood platelet lipids, there being a shift in Eskimos from polyunsaturated fatty acids belonging to ω-6 group (18:2 and 20:4) to those of ω-3 group (18:3, 20:5, 22:5, and 22:6). The ratio of ω-3 polyunsaturated fatty acids to ω-6 acids was 1.38 and 0.10 for Eskimos and Danish controls, respectively. The investigation demonstrated that, in the Eskimos, there is substantially decreased platelet aggregation, and it is proposed that the mechanism of this decreased aggregation is through competitive inhibition of formation of pro-aggregatory arachidonate (C 20:4) metabolites and through conversion of eicosapentenoic acid (EPA) to a prostacyclin (PGI) of the 3 series, with biological properties similar to those of PGI_2. In brief, these results indicate that by some mechanism, probably related to prostaglandin metabolism, intake of EPA may exert a beneficial effect on cardiovascular events. In addition to the evidence just noted, a study carried out comparing characteristics of the populations of Stockholm and Edinburgh, where CHD mortality rates are markedly different despite similar risk factors in every other respect, demonstrated that the one difference in the risk profile of these populations was in their intake of long-chain fatty acids of the ω-3 series, for example, eicosapentanoic acid (Oliver, 1979). While it is too early to suggest prescription of eicosapentenoic acid through such devices as the high mackerel diet as recently reported (Siess et al., 1980), this is an exciting new area which holds promise for the future.

5. Fiber. It has been suggested that the low-fiber diet of Western societies may be a factor in atherogenesis (Roth and Mehlman, 1978), by possibly permitting increased cholesterol absorption. The data in this field are rather confusing, in part because fiber is a complex chemical mixture requiring better definition than is presently available. Wheat fiber does not lower cholesterol (Kay and Truswell, 1977b), but pectin does (Kay and Truswell, 1977a) and so does the pulp of two apples taken three times a day (Cannella, Golinelli, and Melli, 1962). It cannot even be said, however, that all whole-grain cereals lack a hypocholesterolemic effect because oatmeal may lower plasma cholesterol (De Groot, Luyken, and Pikaar, 1963). Despite the lack of convincing proof of benefit, it would seem prudent, however, to maintain a reasonable level of fiber in the diet, since this produces other potentially beneficial effects.

6. Dietary Carbohydrate. International epidemiological studies have demonstrated that populations with low CHD mortality consume a high proportion of calories in the form of complex carbohydrate, and a high sucrose intake has been claimed to play a causal role in CHD. However, a review of the descriptive-analytical studies relating diet

and CHD indicates that sucrose, in multivariate analyses, does not remain a significant independent correlate of CHD (Armstrong et al., 1975). In addition, the epidemiologic data, in contrast to those for dietary cholesterol and fat, are not supplemented by the large body of additional evidence from other fields relating dietary carbohydrate to atherogenesis and CHD. While increased ingestion of carbohydrate may, at least temporarily, raise the levels of VLDL, this lipoprotein in itself is not an independent risk factor for CHD. Moreover, in one series of isocaloric experiments, exchange of sucrose for starches at 23 percent of dietary energy had no effect on plasma total cholesterol (Mann and Truswell, 1972). It therefore must be concluded at present that ingestion of carbohydrate poses no threat for increasing risk of CHD. Indeed, the ingestion of increased levels of carbohydrate, particularly complex carbohydrate, is an inherent accompaniment of the "Phase 3" diet which many are advocating and which we shall discuss later.

   7. Dietary Protein. There is considerable evidence, in both animals and humans, that dietary proteins of animal and plant sources do not exert equivalent effects on plasma cholesterol. Much of this evidence has been summarized recently by Carroll (1978). It is reported that proteins derived from animals, especially casein, exert a hypercholesterolemic effect, while plant proteins, particularly soy protein, exert a cholesterol-lowering effect. Carroll and associates (1978) reported that replacement of meat and dairy protein by soy protein/isolate resulted in a 10–15 mg/dl decrease in plasma cholesterol from an initial average level of 175 mg/dl. It has also been reported (Sirtori et al., 1977) that substitution of soy protein for animal protein led to a 31 percent reduction in plasma cholesterol in Type II patients even with the addition of 500 mg/day in the form of egg powder. However, there were many differences between the experimental and control diets. For example, the soybean preparation ("Temptein") was a concentrate with only 80 percent protein and 15 to 20 percent indigestible polysaccharides (Hems, 1977). A repetition of this experiment using a pure soybean product has not confirmed these earlier results (Holmes, Rubel, and Hood, 1980).

   The mechanisms of the sterol-lowering effect of plant protein, if they are real, are unclear. The data reported by Carroll suggest that a plasma decrease of 8 mg/dl might be expected if the current American dietary plant protein content of 30 percent were increased to 50 percent. The data concerning the effects of protein in humans, however, are still too preliminary to make firm recommendations with respect to dietary management of hypercholesterolemia.

8. Trace Elements. While some epidemiologic studies have suggested a relationship between soft water and increased CHD incidence, the validity and reason for this relationship remain unclear. It is perhaps yet too early to make a specific recommendation in this area. While it has been reported that 2 gm/day of calcium lowers plasma cholesterol (Bierenbaum, Fleischman, and Raichelson, 1972), these results have not been widely confirmed. The roles attributed to vitamin C, vitamin E, lecithin, zinc/copper ratios, and other trace elements in preventing heart disease remain unconvincing. The reader is referred to recent reviews of dietary effects of plasma lipids for further information in this interesting area (Truswell, 1978; Merz, 1979).

9. Coffee. While a positive correlation between CHD and coffee drinking has been claimed in some studies, multivariate analyses, particularly taking into account the association between coffee drinking and cigarette smoking, fail to confirm an independent relationship between coffee drinking and heart attacks. While coffee-drinking may raise plasma triglycerides, it does not raise cholesterol and is no longer considered an independent risk factor for CHD (Shank, 1979).

Experimental (Intervention) Studies

Despite the extensive and impressive observational data linking dietary fat and cholesterol, plasma cholesterol levels, and coronary heart disease incidence, it remains to be unequivocally proven that the lowering of plasma cholesterol through dietary change, drugs, or surgical procedures reduces cardiovascular disease mortality. While it appears clear from descriptive studies that dietary changes at the community and national levels should ultimately result in a lower incidence of CHD, it is not immediately obvious that similar changes in the middle-aged individual will be beneficial. The explanation for this is at least twofold. First, epidemiological studies in themselves have not, and probably cannot, prove a causal relationship between diet and serum cholesterol on the one hand and atherosclerosis and coronary heart disease on the other hand, although numerous animal and other experimental studies indicate such a relationship. Second, it is not clear that the process of atherosclerosis is indeed reversible, and, if it is reversible, at what stage of life it might cease to be so. In order to test the question of whether lowering the serum cholesterol will result in a reduction in coronary heart disease morbidity and mortality, a number of intervention studies have been carried out in which interventions on lipid levels were made in a medical center model and in the community health setting as well. Most of the previous studies have been flawed so that their results cannot be interpreted unequivocally, but a "second generation" of clinical trials is currently underway which may produce more definitive results. Nevertheless, the results from the earlier trials of the 1950s and 1960s have led the Intersociety Commission and numerous other advisory groups throughout the world to recommend to the population at large that it modify its eating pattern in a direction which would lower serum cholesterol: a decreased intake of cholesterol and saturated fat, with modest substitution of polyunsaturated fat (Report of Inter-Society Commission, 1970).

An extensive discussion of all these experimental studies is beyond the scope of this chapter, but they have been reviewed extensively elsewhere (Stamler, 1978a, 1979b; Blackburn, 1979a; Davis and Havlik, 1977). They will be relatively briefly reviewed here in order to enable the reader to evaluate their results as they bear on the decision-making process involved in the treatment of hyperlipidemia. The studies may conveniently be divided into the earlier, "first generation" studies of the 1950s and 1960s and the more recent "second generation" studies of the 1970s.

Earlier Studies. Intervention studies of cholesterol-lowering can be divided into those carried out in patients with (secondary prevention) or without (primary prevention) existing coronary heart disease; within these categories studies have been done using both free-living and institutionalized populations, utilizing both dietary and drug interventions. Of most relevance for this chapter are those most often quoted studies of dietary intervention. Two of the earlier ones involve subjects with and without clinically evident CHD at baseline. Dayton and coworkers carried out a randomized double-blind trial of diet in a Veterans Administration domicile (Dayton et al., 1969). The diets contained 40 percent of calories as fat, the experimental diet having a polyunsaturated to saturated fat (P:S) ratio of 1.7 and a daily cholesterol intake of about 365 mg. The study was carried out in 846 subjects approximately equally divided between the control and treated group, with a eight-year follow-up period. A 20 percent lowering of cholesterol was obtained in the experimental group, with a 7 percent reduction in the control group. Both groups had a baseline cholesterol averaging about 234 mg/dl. Utilizing sudden death or death from definite myocardial infarction as primary endpoints, the study produced a difference between the two groups (event rate of 15.4 percent in controls and 12.3 percent in experimental patients) which was favorable but not statistically significant. Only when these events were pooled with cerebral infarction, ruptured aneurysm, and amputation was the difference between the two groups statistically significant. There was no difference between the two groups in total mortality. Several reasons are cited for the lack of conclusive results in this study: the sample size was too small and the adherence rate too low; about one-half the population was over 65 or had preexisting complications, and these subgroups were associated with less significant results when compared with young, asymptomatic men. Of additional potential significance was a reported increased cancer death rate in the treatment group, although this observation has not been confirmed in a review of four other similar studies (Ederer et al., 1971).

A second noteworthy dietary study was carried out in two Finnish mental hospitals (Turpeinen, 1979), Hospital K and Hospital N, a crossover design being utilized. A cholesterol-lowering diet was administered from 1959 to 1965 in Hospital K, while N was on the control diet, and from 1966 to 1971 the diets were reversed. The experimental diet achieved a P:S ratio of 1.4–1.8, with a ratio of 0.2–0.3 on the usual hospital diet. Cholesterol was reduced 12–18 percent when each hospital was used as its own control, comparing levels before and after institution of the diet. For analysis the results for the two hospitals were pooled and event rates were compared for the periods on and off the special diet. These analyses show that the death rate in the diet period was about half that during the control periods. This study has been the subject of several criticisms (Halperin, Cornfeld, and Mitchell, 1973). Because of population turnover during the 12-year duration of the trial, the population had only a small proportion which was constant for both periods. Of course a patient's death precluded his or her participation in the other phase of the study. There were no population comparisons for other potential coronary risk factors, or baseline coronary status. However, differences in age distribution were adjusted for and cholesterol levels were determined. But there may have been a major discrepancy between the baseline pretreatment cholesterol level and subsequent control level in at least one hospital. That is, the mean cholesterol level was substantially higher during the control period than at the start of the dietary period; this could account for a higher mortality rate during the control period. These criticisms, together with the fact that the reduction in total mortality rate, while sizable, did not reach statistical significance, greatly weakened the suggestive positive results with respect to coronary event rates.

Of the greatest potential significance was the U.S. Diet-Heart Study. The then National Heart Institute initiated this study in 1962; it was designed to determine the feasibility of conducting a definitive dietary trial of the lipid hypothesis in free-living populations free of disease initially. The trial was double-blind in design, the food being provided to the experimental and control groups in special commissaries. Approximately a 10 percent cholesterol reduction was achieved through this design, and in the final report the investigators concluded that such a study could be conducted (National Diet-Heart Study, 1968). Had this study been carried out in its full scale, it would have been the most appropriate test of the diet-heart question, being a large-scale single-factor primary prevention trial. Unfortunately, following the completion of the feasibility study and years of discussion, the Task Force on Arteriosclerosis of the National Heart and Lung Institute in 1970–1971 recommended that it not be undertaken (1971). There were major concerns about the resources of money and manpower needed to conduct such a study, since estimates of the sample size indicated that it would require 50,000–100,000 subjects (men age 40 to 59) and would cost almost one billion dollars at that time. There was also concern that such a study would inevitably be confounded by the modification of other risk factors by the subjects. The result was that the Task Force recommended, and the National Heart, Lung, and Blood Institute (NHLBI) subsequently implemented, several new intervention trials, utilizing the device of choosing high-risk subjects in order to reduce the necessary sample size. Another approach recommended was to study individuals with several risk factors, including elevated cholesterol level, smoking, and high blood pressure. These recommendations led directly to some of the currently ongoing trials, which will be discussed below.

The Oslo Diet-Heart Study (Leren, 1966) was a secondary prevention trial utilizing dietary lowering of cholesterol. It was carried out in 412 men aged 30 to 64 who had had a documented myocardial infarction during the years 1956–1958. The patients were randomly placed on a cholesterol-lowering diet with a P:S ratio of about 1.8, achieving a 17.6 percent cholesterol reduction over five years, with a net difference of 13.9 percent as compared with controls. The incidence of fatal events alone, as well as fatal and nonfatal events combined, was significantly decreased in the treated group, but sudden deaths were kept separate from the above events and showed no difference between the two treatment groups. However, based on the experience of the Coronary Drug Project (see below), a 14 percent reduction in cholesterol should have theoretically resulted in about a 14 percent reduction in CHD. The excessive reduction in event rate in the Oslo study (about 35 percent) suggests other interventions occurring simultaneously, or perhaps some other bias operating. The lack of double-blinding makes such bias more likely. An 11-year follow-up report of this study has also been published (Leren, 1970), but there was a change in endpoint definitions from the original papers in order to reach a significant reduction in CHD mortality. If total CHD mortality is considered, including both fatal infarctions and all sudden deaths combined, the results are not statistically significant. Thus these results, too, must be considered encouraging but not conclusive.

It should be noted that several other studies demonstrated the capability to achieve sizable cholesterol reductions through dietary intervention, including the New York Anti-Coronary Club Study (Rinzler, 1968) and the Chicago Coronary Prevention Evaluation Program (Stamler, 1971), the latter a multifactor study without, however, a control group. These will not be considered in detail here, but before proceeding to a consideration of current trials, three *secondary prevention drug trials* should be discussed, since they, too, bear on the lipid hypothesis. The largest of these, and the immediate predecessor of the current large multicenter trials, was the Coronary Drug Project. This was a randomized, double-blind trial of the efficacy of drug treatment for cholesterol-lowering in patients who had sustained at least one prior myocardial infarction. The first patients were enrolled in March 1966 and a total of 8,341 men was randomized. Two of the original four drugs tried, estrogen and D-thyroxin, were discontinued during the course of the trial because of the suggestion of increased toxicity in the groups receiving these drugs. The Project was completed in January 1975 with the publication of final results from the groups on clofibrate, 1.8 gm/day, and nicotinic acid, 3.00 gm/day. Neither drug caused a significant lowering in total or CHD mortality. Clofibrate was associated with significant excessess of angina, pulmonary embolism, and intermittent claudication without any reduction in the myocardial infarction rate, but in the case of nicotinic acid, there was a statistically significant lower incidence of definite nonfatal myocardial infarction (Coronary Drug Project Research Group, 1975).

What is the significance of the CDP results for clinical practice (Coronary Drug Study Project Research Group, 1977)? First, the failure of the drugs to produce a demonstrable improvement of life expectancy in these subjects indicates that these agents are probably of little or no utility for widespread general use in such patients, but does not necessarily mean that they are of no value if the risk of subsequent infarction is sufficiently high. On the other hand, these negative results did not indicate that all efforts to reduce serum cholesterol levels post-myocardial infarction are useless. For example, the study says nothing about the efficacy of reducing serum cholesterol by dietary means and does indicate that hypercholesterolemia (and smoking) are definite risk factors in people who have had a myocardial infarction. More important, the lipid hypothesis was probably not well tested in the Coronary Drug Project. The natural history experience of the placebo group in this study suggested that the effect of cholesterol-lowering would not be so potent in subjects who have had a coronary event as compared to subjects without such a history (Coronary Drug Project Research Group, 1978). The data suggest that to achieve a 25 percent reduction in mortality, a constant 25 percent lowering of cholesterol levels would have to have been maintained, and no group within the trial attained a lowering even close to this. Moreover, since subjects did not come into the study on the basis of any lipid criterion, they were not representative of the types of patients who might be subjected to cholesterol-lowering by a practicing clinician. In other words, a practitioner might choose patients with a more definitely favorable risk-benefit ratio for such treatment. When one adds to the weakness of cholesterol as a risk factor in secondary prevention the results of selection biases which brought in a younger and less diseased group of participants than anticipated, the inevitable conclusion is that the trial simply did not have enough subjects to produce a positive result even if cholesterol-lowering by these drugs was indeed beneficial.

Predating the final report of the Coronary Drug Project were the results of two other secondary prevention trials of clofibrate in Great Britain (Group of Physicians, Newcastle Upon Tyne, 1971; Research Committee, Scottish Society of Physicians, 1971). Both these studies, one in the Newcastle region and one in Scotland, reported beneficial effects in subgroups. The Newcastle study concluded that clofibrate gave protection against death in infarction among patients with a history of angina, with or without a previous myocardial infarction, while it failed to do so in patients whose background was solely one of previous infarction. The Scottish trial also concluded that clofibrate was beneficial in patients with angina, but had no apparent effect in subjects who entered the study with a history of myocardial infarction without angina. Both studies concluded that the beneficial effects occurred independent of the serum lipid effects. The Coronary Drug Project Final Report presented a statistical comparison of the three studies, but, in any case, since the benefits in the British trials were independent of lipid levels and lipid lowering, they showed negative results with respect to the lipid hypothesis.

Current Studies. Of the "current studies," only two are primary prevention trials devoted solely to lowering cholesterol, and one, a drug study, has already been reported (Committee of Principal Investigators, 1978). This was a study sponsored by the World Health Organization and utilized clofibrate. This trial included subjects, male, 39 to 50 years of age, free of known CHD, and with a cholesterol level in the upper one-third of the cholesterol distribution. About 15,000 subjects were included in this study, which also included a control group in the upper third of cholesterol distribution and a low cholesterol control group. The study achieved a 6–9 percent fall in cholesterol level and reported a 25 percent reduction in the rate of nonfatal myocardial infarction which was not, however, accompanied by benefits in rates of fatal myocardial infarction or angina. There was, however, unfortunately an increased noncardiovascular mortality rate in the clofibrate-treated group, with signs of systemic toxicity as well. Thus, while there was a significant reduction in nonfatal myocardial infarctions, total mortality was greater in the treated than nontreated group. Although the study was well designed, including large numbers, adequate follow-up, and double-blind randomization technique, its follow-up procedures have been criticized, especially with respect to nonfatal coronary events. Thus this trial, too, yields results which are not sufficiently conclusive to make possible specific recommendations for positive action with respect to cholesterol. However, the positive results which were obtained indicate that, in patients with sufficiently high risk, the benefit of using the drug could exceed the risk, which is a real one, as indicated by this trial. Again, utilization of drug therapy to test the hypothesis is fraught with the danger of an adverse risk/benefit ratio because of drug toxicity.

Another drug, cholestyramine, is being utilized in the other primary cholesterol-lowering trial, coronary Primary Prevention Trial of the Lipid Research Clinics (Central Patient Registry, 1972). Subjects for this trial, still underway, are male, 35 to 59 years at entry, free of known CHD, and with an LDL cholesterol in the estimated upper 5 percent of the population LDL distribution. For this purpose an initial level of 190 mg/dl was chosen as the cut-off point for LDL cholesterol, and a final recruitment yielded 3,800 subjects, who were randomized. A potential 28–30 percent reduction in cholesterol should be possible in this trial through the combined use of diet and cholestyramine. The control group receives a placebo and an identical diet, producing a 3–5 percent lowering of cholesterol. The trial is scheduled to end in 1983 and provides a strong potential for definitive results. The same can be said of the study using ileal bypass surgery for cholesterol reduction being carried out by Buchwald and his colleagues, if sufficient numbers of subjects can be recruited and the study successfully completed.

The remainder of the trials currently underway which involve reduction of serum cholesterol are multifactor trials which include this as at least one of their modalities. Some such studies enroll and treat subjects individually, while the remainder of the trials intervene on whole populations. Among the former, one trial, the randomized Smoking–Lipid Trial of the Oslo study, has recently reported its results (Hjermann, 1977, 1979). For this trial 1,232 healthy men with high coronary risk, aged 40 to 49, were randomized into an intervention and a control group. The mean cholesterol at entry was 330 mg/dl, and 80 percent of the men were smokers. A P:S ratio of 1 was achieved for the treatment group with a ratio of 0.39 in the control group. There was a 15 percent reduction of cholesterol in the treated group, with a 50 percent decrease in smoking in this group. This study was not designed to test total mortality, since the total population of the study was not large enough, but the results did show a significant and sizable reduction in coronary events. These results are encouraging for the other multifactor trials currently underway.

The other study treating multiple risk factors in individuals is the Multiple Risk Factor Intervention Trial (MRFIT) being carried out in the United States (Benfari, 1979; Multiple Risk Factor Intervention Trial, 1976). This is a multicenter trial being carried out in 12,866 men, originally aged 35 to 57 and in the upper tenth percentile of multivariate risk. Cholesterol is being lowered by dietary means alone, while blood pressure is being treated to some degree with weight loss, but primarily through a stepped-care drug regimen. Smoking cessation, of course, is being accomplished through hygienic means. The control group for this study consists of a "usual care" group being sent to their usual source of medical care for treatment and followed annually at the 22 MRFIT clinical centers. This study is scheduled to end in February of 1982 and is using as its endpoints fatal and nonfatal coronary mortality, as well as mortality from all causes. The difficulty with this trial, as is the case for all multifactor trials, is that it is changing several risk factors simultaneously, so that a positive result may not provide unequivocal evidence validating the lipid hypothesis. The nutrition modality within this study is, however, demonstrating the utility of a new multidisciplinary medical center model in achieving results. The use of behavioral scientists and a behavioral medicine approach in this trial has set the stage for the future importance of behavioral science in any risk-reduction programs conducted in the future, whether at an individual or a community level.

The remainder of the multicenter trials, being carried out in Europe, involve intervention on groups of people. While such studies do not provide a model for the utilization of the clinician in treating individual patients, they do serve as an appropriate model for generalizing these studies for the public health approach. The North Karelia Project has attempted, with some success, to change the cardiovascular risk in an entire community. The Project consists of a systematic, comprehensive community program to control CHD in the county of North Karelia, Finland. At the end of the first five-year period, good feasiblility of the project has been reported (Puska et al., 1980). Follow-up data showed that there was a continuous trend among the whole population in North Karelia toward the desired direction in their health behavior. Smoking among males, for example, was reduced from 54 to 43 percent. The number of registered hypertensives increased, approaching 9 percent of the total population by the end of the study period. There were considerable changes in dietary habits, with a decrease in the average serum cholesterol in North Karelia by 10 mg/dl. The preliminary results from the five-year data analysis indicates a decrease of 20–30 percent in coronary event rates, both fatal and nonfatal.

The World Health Organization (WHO) European Collaborative Trial (ECT) is a multicenter trial utilizing both face-to-face and mass media techniques in achieving intervention. It is being carried out in an industrial population with random allocation of factories to experimental and control groups (WHO European Collaborative Group, 1974). The preventive program is aimed at male subjects from 40 to 59 years of age. The changes in the coronary risk profile two years after the baseline examination has recently been reported for the Belgian Heart Disease Prevention Project, a part of the WHO Trial (Kornitzer et al., 1980). In the high-risk intervention group, multivariate risk showed a decrease of 20 percent after two years, and there was a drop of risk of 2.26 percent in a random sample of the total intervention group, with an increase in risk of 25 percent found in the control group. These initial results indicate, as have results from the Stanford Three-Community Study (Farquhar et al., 1977), that risk reduction can take place through the successful use of mass media.

It should be noted that the Stanford Study has now been extended to include five new communities, and surveillance techniques will be used to gain an estimate of impact on CHD mortality. A similar approach will be used in a community study to be carried out in Minnesota under the direction of Henry Blackburn and his colleagues at the Laboratory of Physiological Hygiene. These studies hold the promise of more encouraging results with regard to the community approach to risk reduction. However, it is the medical center model of the treatment of individuals which has the most relevance for the clinical practitioner, and all clinical trials in this area have problems which limit their contribution to decisions for individual patients.

ANIMAL-EXPERIMENTAL AND CLINICAL STUDIES

The criterion of coherence as a measure of etiologic significance of epidemiological associations is more than amply met by the vast array of animal-experimental and clinical findings in atherosclerosis research in recent years. The highlights of these findings will be briefly reviewed here and have been more extensively reviewed in several recent publications (Stamler, 1979a; Lauer and Shekelle, 1980; Steinberg, 1979; Wissler, 1979). A discussion of protein metabolism is not included here, but will be found in the section below on "Preventive Care."

Effects of Dietary Lipid Composition on Serum Cholesterol Levels

Since the publication by Ahrens and his colleagues (1957) 25 years ago of the first clear proof that plasma lipids can be predictably altered by changes in the quality of dietary fat, a large number of outpatient and metabolic ward studies have amply confirmed and extended this landmark work. Intensively studied have been the effect of the degree of saturation or unsaturation of ingested triglyceride and the effect of dietary cholesterol on plasma lipids and lipoproteins. Of particular importance were a series of metabolic ward studies carried out in the 1960s showing that the plasma cholesterol concentration rises as the proportion of calories derived from saturated dietary fat is increased and falls as the proportion of polyunsaturated fat is increased. In addition to the 63 experiments carried out by Keys, Anderson, and Grande (1965), 36 were carried out by Hegsted and his colleagues (1965), and several by Mattson, Ericson, and Kligman (1972) and Connor, Stone, and Hodges (1964). These workers have also studied in depth the relationship of dietary cholesterol to changes in serum cholesterol. Keys, Hegsted, and Mattson and their colleagues have derived empirically expressions for relating changes in the percentage composition of dietary fats and cholesterol to changes in serum levels. The Keys equation is as follows:

$$\Delta \text{ cholesterol} = 1.35 \ (2 \ \Delta s - \Delta p) + 1.5 \ \Delta z$$

where s is the percentage of total calories provided by saturated fatty acids and p is that provided by polyunsaturated fat; z is the square root of the dietary cholesterol in milligrams per 1,000 kCal. of diet. It is evident from this formula and that of Hegsted that saturated and poly-unsaturated fats have opposing actions, and that the cholesterol-lowering effect of removing one gram of saturated fat is approximately equal to that of adding two grams of polyunsaturated fat. Monounsaturated fat, as shown in experiments with oleic and erucic acids (Keys, Anderson, and Grande, 1958) do not significantly influence plasma cholesterol levels. The general relationships demonstrated by these metabolic ward studies have been corroborated by the National Diet–Heart Feasibility Study (1968) and a number of outpatient studies have demonstrated these effects as well as the importance of the percent of calories from carbohydrate, protein, and fat; the total number of calories ingested; and the intake of alcohol and concentrated sweets. Eighteen of these outpatient studies have been summarized recently by Gotto, Foreyt, and Scott (1980).

Connor and associates (1964) have shown with the use of diets of mixed ordinary foods that dietary cholesterol from eggs and beef considerably influences serum cholesterol, irrespective of neutral fat composition of the diet, and Hegsted and co-workers (1965) confirmed that the effect of dietary cholesterol is independent of the degree of saturation of dietary fat. Some outpatient studies have failed to demonstrate a consistent relationship between dietary cholesterol and serum levels, but the cause of the continuing controversy concerning dietary cholesterol may lie partly in confusion stemming from the extreme heterogeneity of the response to this factor (McGill, 1979), so that group data may mask a true effect. Moreover, metabolic studies in man have shown that a further increase in cholesterol intake above 500–600 mg/day does not usually further substantially increase plasma cholesterol concentrations. Because of this threshold, studies done in subjects who already have a high basal diet of cholesterol will not likely demonstrate an increase in serum levels with an increase in dietary intake. The groups headed by Connor and Mattson have demonstrated that dietary cholesterol has a decisive effect on plasma cholesterol concentration from approximately 0 cholesterol per day to 300–600 mg/day.

It has also been demonstrated that a high polyunsaturated fat diet can lower VLDL, and that cholesterol feeding can increase the concentration of HDL_1, a fraction at the lower end of HDL density which is also found in animals fed cholesterol (Mahley et al., 1978). Of course, diets low in saturated fat and cholesterol, with moderate substitution of polyunsaturated fat, will lower the concentration of LDL, probably the most atherogenic of the lipoprotein fractions.

**Atherosclerosis and Its Relationship
to Serum Lipids**

A number of clinicopathologic studies have been carried out by assessing coronary artery atherosclerosis by X-ray examination and by autopsy. Both methods show that the severity of atherosclerosis is greatest in people with higher levels of LDL and also with lower levels of HDL, with no apparent threshold levels of LDL below which atherosclerosis becomes inapparent. One of the first to report this were Heinle and associates (1969), who showed that the majority (54 percent) of patients with angiographic evidence of coronary atherosclerosis had either Type II or Type IV plasma lipoprotein phenotype (see below). With multivariate analysis, an atherosclerosis score has been shown to be independently correlated with age and with the plasma total cholesterol concentration, being inversely correlated with HDL-cholesterol concentration and not related to VLDL-triglyceride concentration. Patients with angiographically proven peripheral vascular disease also tend to have elevated LDL and reduced HDL concentrations, as well as elevated VLDL.

Experimental pathology provides a large body of evidence supporting the importance of lipid and cholesterol in the progression of atherosclerosis. Anitschkow first showed more than 50 years ago that by feeding small amounts of animal products to rabbits, low-order hypercholesterolemia could be induced, with subsequent development of atherosclerosis (Anitschkow, 1933). Since then it has been shown that advanced atheromatous lesions can be induced in a wide variety of animals with dietary manipulations resulting in sustained elevations of serum cholesterol, and that the reaction to arterial endothelial injury is greatly augmented toward severe atherosclerosis by dietarily induced hypercholesterolemia (Ross and Harker, 1976). In general, the severity of atherosclerosis in these experimental situations is related to the average serum cholesterol (LDL) elevation. Of particular interest is the recent extensive research on diet-induced atherosclerosis in nonhuman primates. The lesions produced in monkeys have been shown to be relatively easy to induce with a high-fat, high-cholesterol diet, are progressive, and resemble in most respects the spectrum of lesions seen in human subjects. Wissler and Vesselinovitch (1975) have been able to induce atherosclerosis in Rhesus monkeys by feeding the customary American diet. When a "prudent" diet, lower in saturated fat, cholesterol, and calories, was fed, hypercholesterolemia and atherogenesis were less marked. These experimental models in primates have been able to produce massive infarction, gangrene of lower extremities, aneurysms, and severe cerebral atherosclerosis. Work in the primate model has also demonstrated the interplay between multiple other factors and the nutritional cause once it is operating. For example, the work of Pick, Johnson, and Glick (1974) has shown the aggravating effects of hypertension in cholesterol-fat-fed monkeys, and the benefits of discontinuation of the atherogenic diet for the hypertensive animal. Results of many of these primate studies are found in a monograph edited by J. Strong entitled *Atherosclerosis in Primates* (1976).

At the cellular level, evidence from *cell pathobiology* continues to implicate cholesterol and LDL as possible primary factors in atherogenesis. The most prevalent theory of atherogenesis involves an initiating event of some type of injury, and Ross and Harker (1976) have indicated in recent reports that sustained hypercholesterolemia itself can be an important factor in producing endothelial cell damage. The proliferation of smooth muscle cells, which is characteristic of atherosclerosis, has been shown in tissue culture to be stimulated by elevated LDL concentrations in serum (Fischer-Dzega, Frazer, and Wissler, 1976). It has also previously been shown that the B protein of LDL can be identified in atheromatous plaques.

The work of Ross and his colleagues (1974) has been instrumental in demonstrating the importance of platelets in atherogenesis. He has shown that, in response to injured endothelium, platelets release a "mitogenic" factor which stimulates smooth muscle cells in the artery wall to proliferate. Indeed, platelet adherence at the artery wall in general may be an important factor in the response which causes atherosclerosis following endothelial injury. The platelets release factors which influence further aggregation of platelets. A prostaglandin derivative, thromboxane A_2, formed by the platelet from a cycloperoxide of arachidonic acid, is a powerful stimulant to platelet aggregation as well as a potent vasoconstrictor. However, the same cycloperoxide can be converted by another pathway in endothelial cells to prostacyclin (PGI_2), which inhibits platelet aggregation and favors vasodilatation. It has recently been reported that prostacyclin generation in arterial walls from rabbits on atherogenic diets was severely depressed. These studies were confirmed in atherosclerotic human arteries, which also generated smaller amounts of PGI_2 than morphologically unaltered control arteries (Sinzinger et al., 1979).

Regression Studies

One of the most important consequences of the ability to produce experimental atherosclerosis in nonhuman primates has been the resulting *regression studies* which have been carried out in the last few years. *Regression of atherosclerotic lesions* has been repeatedly demonstrated in monkeys by a number of groups: Armstrong, Warner, and Connor (1970), Wissler and Vesselinovitch (1975), Wagner and Clarkson (1975), and others. All of the regression studies record morphological evidence of substantial removal of cholesterol, cholesterol esters, and triglycerides from lesions. In addition, there is evidence that simply lowering serum cholesterol to very low levels also results in a substantial decrease in lesion concentrations of collagen and elastin in the rate of cell proliferation and possibly in the quantity of calcium deposited (Armstrong, 1977). That is, essentially complete healing has been shown to occur in animals first fed an atherogenic diet and then fed a regression diet leading to low cholesterol levels. Cholestyramine has also been effective in producing regression (Vesselinovitch et al., 1976).

Attempts have also been made to study the *regression of atheromata in man* through serial angiographic studies. A number of such studies have been carried out utilizing the femoral artery in patients with symptoms of peripheral vascular disease (Blankenhorn, 1978). Those studies, which were purely observational, demonstrated that, without treatment, the majority of lesions progressed when examined a second time after several years. Therefore, subsequent studies have interpreted lack of progression as a positive treatment effect. A series of such studies has been published. Buchwald and his colleagues, utilizing partial ileal bypass as the therapy, has shown lesion size decrease with sequential arteriography (Knight et al., 1972). Nikkila, Viikinkoski, and Valle (1978) reported a study of 30 patients with primary hyperlipoproteinemia with moderate or severe coronary atherosclerosis, who responded to lipid-lowering treatment, with 15 patients showing stable lesions and the remaining 15 showing progression. Eleven of 15 patients with a greater-than-median reduction in cholesterol level showed stable lesions, while 11 of the 15 with a less-than-median reduction in serum cholesterol showed progressive lesions. Thompson and co-workers (1978) recently reported eight familial Type II patients who were treated with plasma exchange to produce a major reduction of lipid level. Aortic valve and coronary artery lesions observed by angiography showed partial regression in two homozygotes and one heterozygote still receiving treatment at the end of the study. Kuo and associates (1979) reported that, over a three to four year follow-up, repeat coronary angiography demonstrated stable lesions in eight out of twelve patients.

There are several problems with these types of studies. The current nature of arteriography makes a control group impossible; selection of patients who have had two angiograms for study may bias the outcome in advance, since repeat angiography is usually performed only when a patient has new symptoms. Moreover, the longer the interval between angiograms, the more convincing the evidence for benefit, but long-term follow-up has its own problems. Change in X-ray equipment may become a problem, for example. Of course, a major problem lies in the technical area of carrying out good angiograms and of consistent and accurate interpretation. The technical problems have in part been overcome by Blankenhorn and his colleagues, utilizing a procedure which measures the severity of atherosclerosis from the density profile of edges of a contrast-medium shadow: computer-estimated atherosclerosis (CEA). They obtained a continuous variable by measuring CEA/age and CEA percentage change per month. In their recently published studies (Barndt et al., 1977; Blankenhorn et al., 1978), 15 of the 25 patients were in the "latent" stage of atherosclerosis because they had no signs or symptoms. They were being treated primarily for hyperlipoproteinemia, and the results of the studies over a 13-month average follow-up period indicated that blood cholesterol level and blood triglyceride level were significant correlates with the rate of atherosclerotic change. Nine of the 25 patients showed lesion regression, and the average cholesterol reduction in this group was much greater than it was in the group showing lesion progression. These arteriograms were all carried out in the femoral artery, and the technique offers much promise, but it too has problems which weaken its conclusions. First, to date, the number of patients has been small, and the patients were selected. Second, the estimate of risk factor status during a control period of atherosclerosis development was limited. Additionally, the atherosclerosis measurement used is not expressed in quantitative terms relative to the amount of preexisting atherosclerosis. Finally, the improvement observed was in lesions at relatively early stages of development. Nevertheless, developments in this area are encouraging, in that they offer at least tentative evidence that the same stability and even regression of lesions can occur in humans, as has been demonstrated in animals, and it is hoped that developments in noninvasive techniques will make possible adequately controlled experiments in the future in which actual regression can be demonstrated in humans.

RESEARCH QUESTIONS, OPEN ISSUES, AND PUBLIC POLICY: TO TREAT OR NOT TO TREAT

The position taken in this book is that prevention is possible, and the position taken in this chapter is that the weight of evidence suggests that elevated serum lipids, particularly cholesterol and LDL, should be lowered to optimal levels in the practice of preventive medicine. There remains, however, lively controversy concerning the advisability of treating either individual patients or the public at large for hyperlipidemia. Reports continue to appear which urge action now on the basis of our best current evidence (Stamler, 1980a, 1980b), while others appear urging caution since the benefit of changing diet or otherwise lowering serum lipids has yet to be conclusively proven (Ahrens, 1976). Blackburn (1979b) has perhaps most aptly described these several points of view as (1) the clinical view, concerned with the individual; (2) the academic view, preoccupied with basic mechanisms at the molecular and cell levels; and (3) the public health view. The clinical view is concerned primarily with the diagnosis and treatment of an individual patient, which may make the decision about a "high-risk" patient easier, but leaves unanswered the question concerning the "borderline" patient. The academician is concerned about prescribing preventive measures until specific mechanisms are understood, so that the preventive measures can be tailored to specific groups. In the public health view, testing hypotheses as it does with epidemiological methods, "proof" is rarely established. The mass metabolic disorder reflected by our mass hyperlipidemia reflects, in part, sociocultural determinants, which therefore provide the potential for mass prevention. Thus, decisions cannot wait for final proof.

Does Lowering Cholesterol Reduce The Risk of Coronary Heart Disease?

It must be said, as it has been above, that epidemiological studies have not proven conclusively evidence of benefit from lowering cholesterol, even though many of these studies have yielded suggestive data. On the other hand, none of these studies has proven conclusively that the risk of CHD is *not* reduced by lowering cholesterol. The problems with studies to date have been summarized (Cornfeld and Mitchell, 1969):

1. The numbers of subjects in the studies were to small to yield statisically significant results.
2. The intervention was introduced too late in the stage of the disease to be of benefit.
3. Follow-up time was too short.
4. Serum cholesterol reduction was by too small a degree.
5. Randomization and/or double-blind procedures were not employed, or experimental and control groups were not comparable.
6. Statistical aproaches used in analysis were flawed.

There are indeed many reasons to think that clinical trials will never give unequivocal answers to the question "to treat or not to treat." First, because of the practical requirements stemming from cost in time, human effort, and money, it has been, and probably will continue to be, necessary to begin such trials so late in the "latent" period of atherosclerosis that the best one is hoping to accomplish is to delay the end of the latent period. Since the process of atherosclerosis is probably more reversible in its early stages, we may be beginning too late in the process to achieve our goals. The ideal study would be one beginning in the late teenage years and proceeding throughout the lifetime of the subjects, testing the single hypothesis that changing one's diet prevents the clinical manifestations of CHD. Such a trial obviously will never be carried out. Indeed, in a sense, the results of all these trials are separate from the issue of primary CHD prevention at the community level because they are based on the medical center care model rather than multiple community health strategies, and the results of intervention on a single risk characteristic late in the stage of disease may be irrelevant to the potential effects of achieving lower lipid levels throughout the younger and older population through a change in the whole community.

Kuller (1980) has summarized the problems with current clinical trials. The cost and practicality of blinding nutrition and intervention trials has essentially ruled them out as susceptible to a double-blind design. We do not know how large a reduction in the risk factors is necessary to observe a decrease in heart attacks, but the results in the health education phases of the Belgium and Stanford Three-Community Studies have been disappointing, and it may be difficult to attain the necessary lowering of risk to achieve the desired results. The measurement of outcome is critical in these studies, but requires individualized trials such as MRFIT to maximize the chance of demonstrating the difference between the groups. Some of the current studies, such as MRFIT have an additional problem in that there is no true control group, so that the "usual care" group may be receiving advice and thus decreasing the differences between it and the experimental group. All of these studies are confounded by the uncertainty of the interval between risk factor change and the expected reduction in risk of disease. If the population is not followed long enough to include both the lag period and the effects of initial selection of those with advanced clinical disease, an erroneous interpretation of the study results is possible, if not likely. Intermediate "soft" endpoints might help, but would probably not be accepted, so that we may, after the trials are over, be left facing the same question we are now, that of accepting lifestyle changes as good preventive medicine without solid scientific proof.

The Arguments against Action

Ahrens (1979) has recently given a thoughtful review of the argument that the time is not yet ripe for drawing up national guidelines and dietary recommendations for the general public. He was chairman of a panel assembled in 1978 by the American Society for Clinical Nutrition to weigh the quality of all published scientific evidence relating to six dietary issues—fat, cholesterol, carbohydrates, alcohol, excess calories, and salt. The nine panelists measured the cohesiveness of their views on each of the issues; they found less agreement concerning recommendations regarding saturated fat and dietary cholesterol than for most other factors. The panel felt it could not guarantee that lipid-lowering by dietary means would necessarily lead to a reduced incidence of new events of CHD.

Ahrens lists the following four reasons for resisting the advocacy of a low-fat national diet:

1. There has been no previous test of the "prudent" diet. He points out that the basis of current advocacy is suggestive evidence obtained from tests of a *different* kind of diet.
2. The "prudent" diet will have only a small effect on plasma lipid levels. He feels that a mean decrease in plasma cholesterol of 6 percent is what will be attained by 50 percent compliance with the current recommendations—a decrease from 220 to 207 mg/dl.
3. Any one diet produces different results in different people. The point here is that it is unwise to recommend a single diet for the entire population.
4. Crucial questions remain to be resolved. In essence, this is the

academic view noted above, that the "success" of prevention depends upon the thoroughness of our understanding of the root causes of disease. He feels we may be in danger of "launching an all-out war against the wrong foe."

Other arguments against the advocacy of lowering dietary fat intake in order to prevent CHD have been enumerated by Mann (1977) and McMichael (1979), as well as others. The reader is referred to these publications for a more extended discussion of this side of the problem.

The Activist "Public Health" View

This view has been eloquently stated in many places by Blackburn (1979a), Stamler (1978b), Kristein, Arnold, and Wynder, (1977), and a host of others. Before summarizing these views, I should like to present a response to the objections enumerated above. With regard to the first one, there probably will never be a test of the "prudent" diet. The National Diet–Heart Feasibility Study was the closest to that test we have had, and no recommendation for carrying out a full-scale study was forthcoming. In view of the expenditure for large clinical trials like MRFIT and the increasing difficulties of carrying out such a trial because of currently changing lifestyles, no tests of this diet will ever be possible, so that if it is recommended, it must be done without final proof. The potentially small decrease in plasma cholesterol, even if it is only 6 percent, is an extremely important change. On a mass scale, it would correspond approximately to the average "spontaneous" 5 percent cholesterol decrease in the general population mean in the last decade. This decrease may have been a major factor in the 20 percent decrease in CHD mortality we have seen in this period. That is, as pointed out by the report of the Inter-Society Commission (1970), a small change in the mass cholesterol leads to a tremendous potential saving of lives. In any case, it must be remembered that, in those 50 percent who do comply with the recommendation, a 12 percent or greater decrease in cholesterol will probably occur, from the mean of 220 mg/dl to 194 mg/dl, the very decrease which has been recommended in the American Health Foundation's conference on optimal cholesterol (Wynder, 1979).

The other two objections cited above are best answered by a general discussion of the public health approach, but it should be pointed out that, instead of the recommended dietary change, Ahrens suggests that the incidence of CHD may decrease as the population adopts a lifestyle characterized by reduced cigarette-smoking and reduced body weight, but he fails to recognize that these two changes have not been conclusively proven to reduce the purported results either. Neither have the benefits of increased exercise attributed to it by Mann (1977).

The counterarguments to those favoring a delay in recommendations center around a consideration of risk versus benefit. The nature of atherosclerosis, with its long latent period, its high rate of sudden coronary death outside the hospital, and its very magnitude as a problem necessitates a preventive strategy. Decisions on the public's health often may require that a position be taken, based on the best evidence available, which may have the greatest potential benefit for the public. It is amply documented that there are a large number of susceptible individuals in our population who are adversely affected with regard to their serum lipids, their blood pressure, and the effect of cigarette smoking by our current lifestyle. There is also ample evidence that changes in lifestyle have the potential for altering mass hyperlipidemia. It is quite clear to anyone who has attempted intervention in this area that changing eating patterns will ultimately require, even for the individual, practical changes in food supply availability and acceptability in order to permit long-term adherence to a desirable pattern. Ultimately these things can come about only through a national plan, policy, and administrative structure, not currently complete in American society. Of course the clinician should individualize the diet for his patients, but public health recommendations cannot be made for individuals; they can be made only for the public at large, and the diet recommended is one which attempts to counter the current pattern, which has been shown to be deleterious.

Certainly the presumptive evidence is sufficiently strong to indicate the desirability of lowering serum cholesterol. Many therapeutic maneuvers undertaken by the clinician are based on much less conclusive evidence than is available concerning the diet–heart question. Those who tell us to wait are making the assumption that today's diet in the United States is satisfactory and optimal. This optimal diet has led to a high prevalence rate of obesity in childhood and youth, increases in serum cholesterol and blood pressure levels of the population as it evolves from childhood into adulthood, and so on. Moreover, life expectancy for males at birth is greater for Italians and Japanese than for Americans and remains true through age 55, despite our greater wealth and per capita expenditure on medical services. The dietary changes recommended are clearly feasible, palatable, and safe (Stamler, 1980a; 1980b). The potential benefit is tremendous, and the risk vanishingly small. The issue of increased cancer incidence in those with very low cholesterol levels has recently been shown probably to be due to preexisting disease in study populations when baseline cholesterol values were obtained (Rose and Shipley, 1980). We have no reason to think that the adherence to a diet lower in fat and cholesterol will have anything but a beneficial effect.

Based on these arguments and others, at least 16 expert committees on dietary fat and coronary heart disease have made recommendations for changes such as those we have been discussing. They have been summarized by Blackburn (1979b). The last one he lists is the recommendation of the Senate Select Committee on Nutrition (U.S. Senate Select Committee on Nutrition and Human Needs, 1977); this is summarized here in Figure 5-3. Included in the recommendations are also the avoidance of overweight, reduction of cholesterol consumption to about 300 mg/day, and limitation of salt intake to about 5 gm/day. The implementation of the new recommendations for the individual patient is the subject of the next section.

PREVENTIVE CARE

The basic principles and some of the details of the dietary management of hyperlipoproteinemia will be presented in this section. It is assumed that the physician wishes to lower the cholesterol and LDL levels in his patients to optimal ones and that he will supplement his own counseling by working with allied professional personnel, especially nutritionists, in gaining the patient's adherence to the new eating style. We shall begin with a discussion of the fundamental aspects of lipid transport in man as a background for diagnosis and treatment.

Lipoprotein Metabolism

All three of the major classes of serum lipids—cholesterol, triglycerides, and phospholipids—are carried as part of a complex macromolecule, the lipoprotein. Lipoproteins are distinguished from all other plasma proteins by having a density less than 1.210 gm/ml. Based on physical separation methods, the plasma lipoproteins have been classified into four major families, depending on their rate of flotation in salt solutions in the ultracentrifuge or on their migration in electrophoretic systems. At the native density of serum, 1.006 gm/ml, two groups

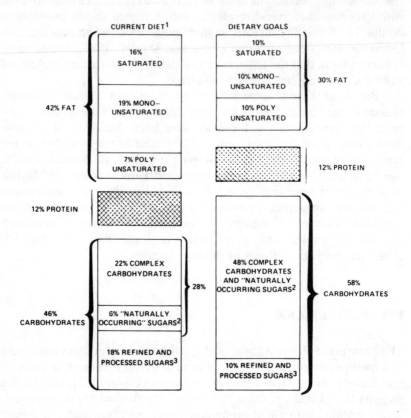

Figure 5-3. Dietary Goals for the United States. U.S. Senate Select Committee on Nutrition and Human Needs, 1977.

[1]These percentages are based on calories from food and nonalcoholic beverages. Alcohol adds approximately another 210 calories per day to the average diet of drinking age Americans.

[2]"Naturally occurring" sugars which are indigenous to a food, as opposed to refined (cane and beet) and processed (corn sugar, syrups, molasses, and honey) sugars which may be added to a food product.

[3]In many ways alcoholic beverages affect the diet in the same way as refined and other processed sugars. Both add calories (energy) to the total diet but contribute few or no vitamins or minerals.

178

of proteins will float in the ultracentrifuge: the chylomicrons and the very-low-density lipoproteins (VLDL). The largest and the least dense are the chylomicrons, which are the form in which fat is absorbed from the intestine, being found in the blood following a fatty meal. The next higher density lipoprotein, VLDL, is found in normal subjects even after a 12-hour fast. The next higher density class, the low-density lipoprotein (LDL) floats between the densities of 1.006 and 1.063 gm/ml, the highest density class, the high-density lipoprotein (HDL), floating between 1.063 and 1.21 gm/ml. HDL can be subdivided into two, and possibly three, subclasses (Anderson et al., 1979): HDL_2, density 1.063–1.125 gm/ml; and HDL_3, density 1.125–1.21 gm/ml. Proteins of density greater than 1.21 gm/ml are not classified as lipoproteins, although free fatty acids and other lipids are carried in this density range. Each of the density classes has a characteristic mobility in electrophoresis. In commonly used electrophoresis media, such as paper or agarose, chylomicrons remain at the origin, VLDL migrates in the pre-beta position, the LDL as beta-globulin, and the HDL as $alpha_1$. The composition of the plasma lipoproteins is summarized in Table 5-3. All lipoprotein clases have the same chemical composition, consisting of different proportions of the three lipid classes (cholesterol, triglyceride, and phospholipid) and protein. The chylomicrons, at the lower end of the density scale, are the largest and carry the most triglyceride and the least protein, while the lipoprotein at the other end of the density scale, the HDL, has approximately 50 percent by weight of protein and very little triglyceride. While there is cholesterol in all the fractions, most of it, approximately two-thirds, is carried in the LDL, which consists of 50 percent by weight of cholesterol. The size of chylomicrons and pre-beta lipoproteins causes them to scatter light, so that their presence in excess results in a turbid appearance of the serum. Because of their content of triglycerides, turbidity is synonymous with hypertriglyceridemia. Since the lipids and the proteins in lipoproteins are not bound covalently, proteins may be isolated by delipidation of the whole lipoprotein. It has been found through studies of these apoprotein components that VLDL and HDL contain multiple nonidentical peptides, Apo-1 A-I and A-II in HDL, Apo-C-I, C-II, C-III, D, and E in both. LDL contains a single peptide, Apo B, also found in VLDL. In recent years, great progress has been made in the study of the detailed structure of these apoproteins and the understanding of the binding of lipid to protein. Methods have become available, primarily immunological, for quantitating the levels of the various apoproteins, leading to a better understanding of their role in normal and pathological situations.

Table 5-3
Composition and Properties of Human Plasma Lipoproteins

Properties	Chylomicrons	VLDL	IDL	LDL	HDL
Density (g/ml)	< 0.95	0.95–1.006	1.006–1.019	1.019–1.063	1.063–1.210
Molecular weight	$> 0.4 \times 10^9$	5–10×10^6	3–5×10^6	2.7–4.8×10^6	1.8–3.6×10^5
Major apoproteins	ApoB ApoC-I ApoC-II ApoC-III	ApoB ApoC-I ApoC-II ApoC-III ApoE	ApoB	ApoB	ApoA-I ApoA-II
Minor apoproteins	ApoA-I ApoA-II	ApoA-I ApoA-II ApoD	ApoC ApoE		ApoC-I ApoC-II ApoC-III ApoD ApoE
Major lipids	Dietary triglyceride	Endogenous triglyceride	Cholesteryl esters Triglyceride	Cholesteryl esters Phospholipids	Phospholipids Cholesteryl esters
Minor lipids	Phospholipids	Phospholipids Cholesteryl esters	Free cholesterol Phospholipids	Free cholesterol Triglyceride	Free cholesterol

VLDL = Very low density lipoproteins. IDL = Intermediate density lipoproteins. LDL = Low density lipoproteins. HDL = High density lipoproteins.

Reprinted with permission from A. Gotto et al.: "Hyperlipidemia and nutrition: Ongoing work," *Atherosclerosis Reviews*, Vol. 7, edited by Ruth Hegyeli, M.D. Copyright © by Raven Press, New York, 1980.

The two major sources of lipoproteins circulating in the plasma are the liver, the source of endogenously derived lipoproteins, and the gut, secreting exogenously derived fat but also an important source of increasingly proven lipoprotein synthesis. VLDL is primarily synthesized in the liver. Newly secreted VLDL is acted upon by lipoprotein lipase bound to the capillary endothelium, the triglyceride breakdown products being taken up in peripheral tissues. Most of the apoproteins other than Apo B, and much of the phospholipid and cholesterol, are lost in the process, resulting in a smaller, triglyceride-poor lipoprotein of intermediate density (IDL), which is finally converted to LDL. Most LDL is derived as an end product of this VLDL breakdown, but LDL can also be secreted by the liver directly, especially in patients with familial hypercholesterolemia. The catabolic pathways of lipoproteins are also becoming increasingly clear. The catabolism of chylomicrons is known to occur in two stages, a remnant being produced by the action of lipoprotein lipase; the remnant, which must be further metabolized by the liver, apparently requires a normal component of Apo E for recognition by the liver, and it is the absence of one of the subclasses of Apo E which is thought to be the lesion responsible for dysbetalipoproteinemia, Type III. The site of HDL degradation is uncertain, but some evidence indicates that HDL apoproteins may be degraded peripherally as well by the liver. One of the most important recent advances has been the elucidation of LDL–cell interaction, indicating that LDL catabolism occurs primarily in the periphery. Studies carried out by Goldstein and Brown (1977), as well as others, have provided evidence that, in cultured cells, catabolism of LDL occurs through a specific LDL receptor found in the plasma membrane. The best evidence for these receptors has come from studies of cells from patients with familial hypercholesterolemia, cells that lack the high-affinity receptor. One mechanism proposed for the protective effect of HDL has been its role in "reverse cholesterol transport," that is, transport of cholesterol from peripheral tissue back to the liver. According to this scheme, nascent HDL may pick up cholesterol at the plasma membrane of peripheral cells, thereby transporting it away from these tissues.

Our knowledge of the mechanisms of hyperlipoproteinemia has increased a great deal in the last few years. Thus we can now, in at least five categories of hyperlipoproteinemia, identify the protein deficiency involved. In addition, we can now draw schemes to account for forms of secondary hyperlipoproteinemia within the context of known lipoprotein physiology.

For more extensive discussions of the fundamental aspects of lipoprotein structure and metabolism, the reader is referred to several recent reviews (Wissler, 1979; Jackson, Morrisett, and Gotto, 1976, 1977; Schaefer, Eisenberg, and Levy, 1978; Gotto et al., 1980; New York Academy of sciences, 1980).

Diagnosis

Laboratory Diagnosis of Hyperlipidemia. Hyperlipidemia means "too much fat in the blood." The appropriate diagnostic workup for a patient with suspected hyperlipidemia is as follows:

1. Samples, two or three approximately one week apart, of serum or plasma for determination of cholesterol and triglyceride levels after a 12-hour fast
2. Observation of the plasma or serum sample after an overnight stand in the refrigerator, for chylomicrons
3. HDL cholesterol level determined at least once initially
4. A search for causes of secondary hyperlipidemia
5. A thorough and detailed family history with special attention to known hyperlipidemia, history of xanthomata, and history of premature heart disease

Samples are obtained after an overnight fast in order to measure triglycerides under standardized conditions, since a nonfasting state may lead to spurious chylomicronemia. The value of cholesterol is essentially unaffected by nonfasting. The value is affected, however, by several *technical factors*. Plasma values may run 3–5 percent lower than serum values, depending on the anticoagulant used for the plasma. Factors causing hemoconcentration or prolonged increased venous pressure will tend to increase cholesterol values. Included are venous occlusion by the tourniquet for more than one minute, which raises the cholesterol value, and the effect of position, the value becoming higher as one goes from recumbent to sitting to upright. For this reason the patient should be seated for at least ten minutes before the blood is drawn. Repeated samples are needed simply because of laboratory and biological variability, in order to establish a more accurate mean baseline value, particularly at the beginning of therapy. The value is, of course, affected by the accuracy of the method used in the laboratory. The most important factor determining accuracy is the availability of a reference standard which has been measured by a highly accurate specific method, such as the semi-automated Abell-

Kendall method utilized at the Lipid Standardization Laboratory at the Center for Disease Control (CDC) in Atlanta. Standardization at the CDC is desirable, either directly or indirectly, for the laboratory chosen by the physician for his determinations. One of the most common methods in use today, the automated cholesterol oxidase method, will tend to give low values unless it is carefully standardized.

Chylomicrons will manifest themselves as a cream layer after an overnight stand in the refrigerator, indicating hyperchylomicronemia or a nonfasting sample. VLDL will not form a cream layer, but will remain dispersed throughout the serum, giving rise to a lactescent or turbid sample. The combined use of the lipid values and observation of this type makes electrophoresis unnecessary by today's standards.

Causes of secondary hyperlipidemia include the following conditions or medications:

Estrogens or contraceptives	Diabetes
Steroids	Obstructive jaundice
Diuretics	Porphyria
Hypothyroidism	Dysproteinemia
Renal disease: nephrotic	Pregnancy
syndrome or chronic failure	Alcohol

Treatment of secondary hyperlipidemia should, of course, be directed at the primary disease which is causing it. *Family history* and *family screening* are important not only to determine whether the condition is familial or sporadic, but to detect other family members who may be at high risk of CHD, since hyperlipidemia is often an inherited metabolic disorder. Of course measurement of other risk factors, such as blood pressure, should be carried out as part of the overall evaluation.

The question of *normality* has been discussed earlier. Because of the environmental component of the otherwise genetically determined cholesterol level, it is clearly inappropriate to speak of a "normal" range for cholesterol, but rather an optimal one. A value of 190 mg/dl or lower is a feasible goal for the average American and should be the goal for most patients, male or female, except for those with familial hyperlipoproteinemia (HLP), especially of the familial hypercholesterolemia type. In the case of the latter, the goal is as low as possible, approaching 200 as closely as possible. Of course, what is optimal for an individual patient will also be influenced by family history, presence of other risk factors, and age.

Included in this list of other risk factors is HDL-cholesterol. One method of utilizing the HDL-C value is to use it as an independent risk factor which modifies your assessment of the patient's overall risk based on the three major risk factors: cholesterol level, blood pressure level, and smoking habit. Thus, if a male patient's HDL-C is approximately 45–50 mg/dl, he can be treated as at average risk with respect to his HDL-C, and his risk is not modified by this value. If he has a value around 60, his risk is approximately half what it would otherwise be, and he is at above-average risk if his HDL-C approximates 35, the multiplier in this case being approximately 2. The comparable values for women are 10 mg/dl higher than for men. Castelli (Galen, 1980) prefers to use the ratio of total cholesterol/HDL-C or LDL-C/HDL-C as a measure of relative risk, and the relationship of risk to these ratios has been presented under "Epidemiologic Evidence" above.

A normal triglyceride level is difficult to establish, partly because there is such a wide range between mean values and 95th percentile values. Thus, for a middle-aged American male, the mean is 150 mg/dl, while the 95th percentile value is 300 mg/dl. More important, except for postmenopausal women, neither serum triglyceride nor VLDL-cholesterol has been shown to be an independent risk factor for CHD when other known risk factors are taken into account (Gordon et al., 1977b). Therefore it should not usually be taken into account in making a decision to embark on treatment. Of course, when triglyceride values exceed approximately 500 mg/dl, chylomicrons begin accumulating, as do lipoprotein particles with densities between those of chylomicrons and VLDL and that of LDL, so that treatment on the basis of cholesterol in these intermediate density particles may be indicated. In addition, extremely high values of triglycerides, even with relatively normal cholesterol levels, may be associated with eruptive xanthomata and/or abdominal pain, requiring treatment of the hypertriglyceridemia per se.

A final word about desirable levels. The ideal cholesterol level of 160 mg/dl should ordinarily be associated with an LDL-cholesterol level of 100 mg/dl, and this is a goal which should be striven for. As an approximation, LDL-cholesterol may be calculated from the following formula:

LDL-cholesterol = plasma cholesterol − [(triglyceride/5) + HDL-C]

Triglyceride divided by 5 is used to approximate the value for VLDL cholesterol (Friedewald, Levy, and Fredrickson, 1972).

Classifications of Hyperlipidemia. Fredrickson, Levy, and Lees (1967) have classified hyperlipidemias into five types, based primarily on which lipoprotein fraction(s) is elevated. The characteristics of these five types of hyperlipoproteinemia were recently reviewed by Gotto and co-workers (1979) and will be discussed only briefly here, since "dietary management" in this chapter is not based on this classification, which attempts to translate hyperlipidemia into hyperlipoproteinemia. Thus, Type I represents elevation of chylomicrons; Type II, hyperbetalipoproteinemia; Type III, accumulation of IDL (see above); Type IV, increased VLDL; and Type V, increases in chylomicrons and VLDL. It was for a time believed that these types might each represent a homogeneous genetically determined metabolic disorder, but this is not the case. Based on an extensive genetic study of myocardial infarction survivors in Seattle, Goldstein and his colleagues (1973) determined that there were three major monogenetic types of hyperlipidemia: familial hypertriglyceridemia, familial hypercholesterolemia, and familial combined hyperlipidemia. Correlations between this classification and the phenotypic one of Fredrickson demonstrated that the phenotypes are not genetically homogeneous. Some of them are probably also not phenotypically homogeneous, so that, while this classification into five types serves a useful purpose for empirically characterizing a patient and as a shorthand descriptive jargon, it need not form the basis for a diagnostic workup or for therapy. It is nevertheless desirable to be aware of which lipoprotein fraction is responsible for a particular cholesterol elevation, since future progress in this area may be lipoprotein and apoprotein based.

Other Clinical Findings. Other findings may characterize patients with hyperlipidemia (HLP), particularly of the familial type, and these are conveniently described according to the Fredrickson classification. Skin lesions, or xanthomata, associated with HLP include tendon xanthomata in Type II, and tuberous xanthomata in this type and Type III, where planar xanthomata are also found. Eruptive xanthomata, generalized pruritic lesions, are characteristically found with extremely high values of triglycerides in Types I and V. Hepatosplenomegaly with or without abdominal pain also characterizes patients with extremely high triglyceride values. Types I and II commonly manifest themselves in early childhood, while the other types usually first appear clinically in adulthood.

Dietary Management of Hyperlipidemia

1. General Principles of Dietary Management—the Unitary Diet. It should be emphasized that the majority of patients seen by most physicians will not be of the exotic familial hyperlipidemic type with extremely elevated serum lipids, but will be the patient with a serum cholesterol value which to some might seem trivially elevated. It is

precisely these patients with cholesterol values between 200 and 250 mg/dl, in the middle quintiles of the cholesterol distribution, who account for almost half of the excess risk attributable to cholesterol, as noted in the discussion of Pooling Project data above. For these patients, dietary management alone will usually be sufficient to bring the cholesterol level near an optimal one, and even in patients who ultimately will need drug therapy, diet should be the mainstay of therapy and should initiate any therapeutic regimen. When drugs are begun, dietary management should continue, since its effects are additive to the effects of the medication.

In view of the metabolic effects of dietary manipulations and the heterogeneity of the phenotypes described by Fredrickson, a single diet concept has become the basis for most dietary regimens advocated for the treatment of hyperlipidemia aimed at reducing CHD risk. This "unitary" diet is the one which is in the process of being implemented by the American Heart Association through its Nutrition Committee. Of course any dietary plan should be individualized, but all plans aimed at lowering serum lipids will have the following elements:

A decrease in total fat intake
A decrease in the percentage of calories from saturated fat
A substitution of polyunsaturated fat for some of the saturated fat
A decrease in dietary cholesterol intake
A reduced calorie intake to achieve ideal body weight, if necessary

While much work has been done isocalorically studying the effects of compositional changes in dietary fat on serum cholesterol, it is very difficult to separate the effects of a change in dietary fat intake and the effect of weight loss. It has been stated by the proponents of the phenotypic classification described above that the treatment of choice for Type II patients involves primarily the first three elements in the diet changes listed above and that for Types III, IV, and V, those with elevated serum triglycerides, reduction to ideal body weight should be the first approach taken. However, there is evidence from MRFIT and other studies (Lasser et al., 1979) that there is an effect of weight loss in lowering cholesterol and LDL concentrations which exceeds that expected on the basis of adherence to compositional change alone, even in Type II patients. In addition, there is evidence that patients on a prudent lower-fat diet will also lower their triglycerides. There seems little doubt that VLDL is particularly sensitive to decreases in alcohol intake and to weight loss, but all serum lipids are lowered considerably through loss of weight.

The Nutrition Committee of the American Heart Association recommends the development of a progressive type of eating plan for the dietary treatment of hyperlipidemia. The levels which will be used by physicians and nutritionists as guidelines will be as follows:

Phase I: 30–35 percent calories from fat, 300 mg cholesterol
Phase II: 30 percent calories from fat, 200–250 mg cholesterol
Phase III: 20–25 percent calories from fat, 100 mg cholesterol

This stepwise approach seems particularly appropriate from a behavioral point of view and has become a favored approach by a number of workers. Thus, Connor and Connor (1977) have described a stepwise approach toward an "alternative" American diet. MRFIT, in its second phase of nutrition intervention, has instituted a "Progressive Eating Plan" in order to help its participants move in the direction of the alternative American diet. Phase I of the American Heart Association Diet corresponds approximately to what has been described as the "prudent" diet, in which the fat calories are approximately equally divided between saturated fatty acids, polyunsaturated fat, and monounsaturated fat, and this was essentially the diet advocated at the beginning of MRFIT. Phase III of the AHA dietary plan corresponds approximately to Connor's Phase III diet. He proposes that progress through the three phases may take years, and, for some patients this may be the case. It should be noted that, in Phase III, meat, fish, and poultry are used as "condiments." The meat dish no longer occupies the center of the table, but will supplement vegetable-, grain-, or legume-based dishes. The use of special low-cholesterol cheeses is also an important component of Phase III.

Table 5-4 lists the food sources of nutrients that are to be modified. In general the following changes will have to be made by most patients:

Reduction in Saturated Fat

Reduction in red meat intake, with substitution of chicken (minus the skin) and fish. This should include the choice of lean cuts of red meat when it is eaten, trimming of all visible fat, and the use of cooking methods (e.g., broiling) which help remove fat.

Table 5-4
Food Sources of Fat and Cholesterol

FAT COMPONENT	ANIMAL	VEGETABLE
Polyunsaturated fatty acids	Fish, oil and fat	Walnuts Salad Oils Oils - Safflower, Sunflower, Corn Soybean, Sesame Cottonseed Certain margarines (soft type) Commercial mayonnaise
Monounsaturated fatty acids	Poultry skin Egg yolk fat	Peanuts Oils - Olive, Peanut Olives Hydrogenated soybean oil Some margarines
Saturated fatty acids	Animal fat, lard, visible fat incl. cold cuts, frankfurters, bacon sausage, whole milk and whole milk products, butter	Coconut oils, cocoa butter Palm and palm kernel oil Chocolate Hydrogenated shortening (may also contain sat. animal fats)
Cholesterol	Organ meats - including liver, kidney, brains, sweetbreads Egg yolk Meats, poultry, fish Butter fat	None

Reduction of any type of meat to 6 oz. per day (Phase I).

Discontinuation of use of *whole milk dairy products* with the substitution of skim milk products. This means the use only of specialized cheeses such as low fat cottage cheese.

In the case of *visible fats*, the use of polyunsaturated oils for cooking whenever possible and the substitution of soft margarines made with polyunsaturataed oil for butter.

Discontinuation of the use of *commercial baked goods*, with the substitution of baked goods using modified recipes (for example, from the *American Heart Association Cookbook*).

Reduction in Cholesterol Intake

Reduction in egg yolk intake to no more than two per week and discontinuation of use of organ meats such as liver or brains. Sparing use of sardines and shrimp, but other shellfish are not restricted.

Note that all animal products contain cholesterol, so that even meats low in fat will contain significant amounts of cholesterol, as illustrated in Table 5-5. For this reason a Phase III diet takes on many of the characteristics of a vegetarian approach to eating. The foods listed above relating specifically to cholesterol intake are those foods which contain little or no fat as such, but are extremely high in cholesterol. The fatty acid composition of selected foods is also presented, in Table 5-6, to enable the reader to assess the relative merits of some specific foods in dietary plans and to make clear the quantitative aspects of the tables which follow.

2. Implementation of the Modified Fat Diet

a. Overall approach. What will be described in the section which follows is the approach used in the Heart Attack Prevention Program at the New Jersey Medical School in Newark. This is a multidisciplinary program aimed at multiple risk factor reduction, with particular emphasis on treatment of hyperlipidemia. While every practitioner cannot utilize such a specialized approach, he can follow the broad outlines described here and certainly employ many of the general principles which we feel are optimal in such a program. For example, even if a physician does not have a nutritionist working within his own office, he can and should identify one to whom he can refer patients and with whom he can form an effective team.

It should be emphasized that in any case the physician cannot simply hand a patient a printed diet from a file drawer and expect that any real change, even temporary, will ensue. Instead, he should act as a patient educator and counselor. He should be particularly attentive to the patient's belief system, while assessing major problem areas and potential difficulties in changing the dietary patterns. The team approach, including a minimum of a physician, a nutritionist, and possibly a behavioral scientist is most productive. The physician plays a key role in the team. If the nutritionist and the patient have identified problem areas and have agreed upon specific limited goals, the physician can, if kept informed about these goals, reinforce the plans agreed upon. The physician brings additional "clout" to the patient with regard to these agreed-upon changes. The nutritionist provides specific dietary expertise as well as more in-depth analysis of the patient's

Table 5-5
Cholesterol Content of Common Measures of Selected Foods (in ascending order)

Food	Amount	Cholesterol (mg)
Milk, skim, fluid, or reconstituted dry	1 cup	5
Cottage cheese, uncreamed	½ cup	7
Lard	1 tablespoon	12
Cream, light table	1 fluid ounce	20
Cottage cheese, creamed	½ cup	24
Cream, half and half	¼ cup	26
Ice cream, regular, approximately 10% fat	½ cup	27
Cheese, cheddar	1 ounce	28
Milk, whole	1 cup	34
Butter	1 tablespoon	35
Oysters, salmon	3 ounces, cooked	40
Clams, halibut, tuna	3 ounces, cooked	55
Chicken, turkey, light meat	3 ounces, cooked	67
Beef, pork, lobster, chicken, turkey, dark meat	3 ounces, cooked	75
Lamb, veal, crab	3 ounces, cooked	85
Shrimp, sardines	3 ounces, cooked	130
Heart, beef	3 ounces, cooked	230
Egg	1 yolk or 1 egg	250
Liver, beef, calf, hog, lamb	3 ounces, cooked	370
Kidney	3 ounces, cooked	680
Brains	3 ounces, raw	more than 1700

Excerpted with permission from Feeley, R. M., Criner, P. E., and Watt, B. K. Cholesterol Content of Foods. *Journal of the American Dietetic Association*, Vol. 61:134, 1972.

habits. It is in any case imperative, in light of today's knowledge, that the team members be grounded in the rudiments of behavioral and counseling techniques.

It should also be emphasized that the treatment of hyperlipidemia should be done in the context of a multiple risk factor approach, since

Table 5-6
Fatty Acid Composition of Selected Foods

Foods	Total Fat (gms)	Sat. Fat (gms)	Unsaturated Fat (gms)	
			Oleic	Linoleic
8 oz. whole (3.5%) milk	9	5	3	-
8 oz. skim milk	trace	-	-	-
1 cubic inch cheddar cheese	6	3	2	trace
½ cup cottage cheese (creamed)	5	3	1.5	trace
½ cup cottage cheese (uncreamed)	1	trace	trace	trace
1 cup ice cream (10%) fat	14	8	5	trace
1 cup ice milk	7	4	2	trace
3 oz. regular hamburger*	17	8	8	trace
3 oz. lean round*	4	2	2	trace
3 oz. pork*	26	9	11	2
3 oz. veal cutlet*	9	5	4	trace
3 oz. canned salmon	5	1	1	trace
3 oz. tuna (in oil, drained)	5	2	1	1
2 pork sausage links*	11	4	5	1
1 T. butter	12	6	4	trace
1 T. soft margarine	11	2	4	4
1 T. safflower oil	14	1	2	10
1 T. corn oil	14	1	4	7
1 T. soybean oil	14	2	3	7
1 T. peanut Oil	14	3	7	4
1 T. olive oil	14	2	11	1
1 T. peanut butter	8	2	4	2
¼ cup walnuts	19	1	6.5	9

*Cooked
From Nutritive Value of Foods, *Home and Garden Bulletin* No. 72, U.S.D.A.

the primary aim of cholesterol-lowering is the reduction of overall risk for CHD. Thus, the physician must not only take risk factors into account in deciding whether to initiate therapy and whether to progress to drugs, but must help the patient in setting priorities. For example, when the patient is simultaneously trying to correct hyperlipidemia and hypertension, weight loss, since it benefits both conditions, should be a priority over sodium restriction, although the latter can be carried out to a moderate degree. Further, if smoking is a problem, it may be beneficial to begin with weight loss which will not only help the patient's hyperlipidemia, but will also prepare him for the avoidance of weight gain when he stops smoking. As a final example, the physician should strive as far as possible to achieve therapy for hypertension with nonpharmacologic treatment in a patient with hyperlipidemia, since the diuretics usually constituting step one in anti-hypertensive therapy are known to raise serum cholesterol (Ames and Hill, 1976).

Prior to his initial visit the patient should if possible have had some initial laboratory work, and, possibly, a blood pressure measurement and electrocardiogram. Initial cholesterol, triglycerides, and HDL-cholesterol should be determined prior to the initial visit. Some type of self-adminstered history form can also be mailed prior to the visit, or filled out at the visit if preferred. The patient should be informed as to the overall content of the initial vist, including the potential duration of the visit. Ideally, if appropriate patient education material and assessment are included, the visit may last two to three hours.

b. Initial visit. At the initial visit both medical and nutritional assessment are carried out and the patient is given a message both about the rationale for his treatment and about the content of the new dietary pattern, as well as an orientation to the planned approch. If it has not already been filled out, a self-administered medical history form is completed and the patient is oriented concerning the content of the day's visit. Following this, the patient may be exposed to a variety of audiovisual materials, depending on his known problem. For example, he can be shown a slide/tape concerning risk factors in general in prevention of CHD; material introducing him to the new dietary pattern; material describing hypertension; and specific information concerning food preparation. Other media, of course, may include motion pictures, videotape, cartridge movies, etc. Weight and blood pressure should be determined at every visit, including the first one. An additional determination of serum lipids should be carried out so that the baseline consists of at least two measurements; and a battery of screening chemistries obtained as well, including tests of hepatic, renal, and thyroid function, in order to rule out causes of secondary hyperlipidemia. The usual medical history should be obtained, with an in-depth analysis of the family history as it pertains to cardiovascular disease. The inheritance of known risk factors should be assessed as far as possible.

A physical examination should also be carried out if indicated, but time should be allowed to include an explanation of risk factors and of the "state of the art" with respect to the degree to which risk reduction is or is not proven to be effective in prevention. The appraisal of what can be expected should be realistic, but the physician should maintain a positive enthusiastic attitude about the new way of life he is asking his patient to embark on. The gradient nature of risk factors, including cholesterol, should be explained so that the patient understands that there is really no "normal" value, but rather an optimal one to aim at. Realistic goals should be set both for weight and cholesterol, as well as a goal of less than 90 mm Hg for blood pressure. It should be made clear that the goal weight, while it may approximate that found in a table, should be that weight which is required to obtain optimal cholesterol and blood pressure measurements. Finally, the broad outlines of the approach to be used should be provided, including the behavioral principles indicated below. Thus, positive aspects of the program should be highlighted and the long-term nature of follow-up emphasized. The patient should understand that he is not expected to change a lifetime's habits overnight, but that a gradual, stepwise approach will be most successful, with some expected backsliding.

The initial visit with a nutritionist should follow the physician visit, but can also precede it in the interest of flexibility of patient flow. A good dietary history should be taken and should include not only the usual record of the daily eating pattern and its nutrient content but also an assessment of daily activity, location and circumstances of eating, cooking facilities, shopping pattern, history of weight and the patient's assessment of his own ideal weight, previous diets, and ascertainment of who does the cooking. An attempt should be made to assess the patient's current lifestyle and his/her food preferences as a starting point for suggesting changes. The visit should include an initial exposition of the overall content of the new style of eating as discussed above. Specific initial goals for changes should be set, and, of course, a follow-up nutrition visit scheduled.

The *food and nutrient content of the recommended dietary plan* are shown in Tables 5-7 and 5-8. Table 5-7 presents the nutrient content of the current American and two alternate diet plans—the prudent diet and a Phase III diet. Note that in Phase III, there has been essentially a reversal of the proportions of protein from vegetable and animal sources as compared to the current American diet, and that there has been a concomitant increase in complex carbohydrate (starch) as a source of carbohydrate calories. In addition there is a considerable increase in the amount of fiber and potassium taken in with this type of a diet compared to the current American one. As one progresses from the current American diet through these several phases, meat intake decreases from up to 16 oz. per day currently to no more than 6 oz.

Table 5-7
Nutrient Content of Current American and Two Alternate Diets

	Current American Diet	AHA Diet (Prudent)	Final Phase Diet (Step III)
Cholesterol (mg/day)	750	300	100
Fat (percent total calories)	40	30	20
Saturated fat (percent calories)	15	10	5
Monounsaturated fat (percent calories)	16	10	8
Polyunsaturated fat (percent calories)	6	10	7
Protein (percent total calories)	15	15	15
Vegetable protein (percent protein)	32	31	56
Animal protein (percent protein)	68	69	44
Carbohydrate (percent total calories)	45	44	65
Starch (percent calories)	22	26	40
Sucrose: added to food (percent calories)	15	4	10
Naturally occurring dietary sugars (percent calories)	8	14	15
Crude fiber (g.)	2-3		12-15
Sodium (mEq.)	200-300		*50-75
Potassium (mEq.)	30-70		120-150

*Should sodium restriction be necessary.

194

Table 5-8
Food Group Content of Current American and Two Alternate Diets

	Current American Diet	AHA Prudent Diet	Final Phase Diet (Step III)
Lean meat, poultry, fish	11 oz.	6 oz. or less/day	3 oz. or less/day
Meatless meals	rarely	As often as possible	At least one meatless meal/day (Emphasis on well complemented veg. protein intake (breakfast presumed meatless)
Eggs (yolk)	1 daily	2 or less/week	None
Margarines and oils	4 Tb. daily	2-4 Tb./day	2-3 Tb./day (1/3 can come from mayo or mayo-type dressings)
Dairy products (skim milk, low fat cheese)	2½ servings (not low fat)	2 servings (1% fat)	2 servings (skim only)
Breads, cereals, grains	10 servings	4 servings or more	5 servings or more
Fruits and vegetables	3-4 servings	4 servings or more	5 servings or more
Alcohol	3-4 servings	Limited (for weight control)	Limited (for weight control)
Sugar	Unlimited	Limited (for weight control)	Limited (for weight control)

per day in the prudent diet, and finally to 3 oz. or less per day in the Phase III diet. There is an emphasis on meatless meals, including at least two per day, and, if possible, several meatless days per week.

Table 5-9 lists suggested foods and foods to avoid when choosing the day's menu. They are grouped according to the meal at which they are usually eaten, and, although a given food is listed only once, it may obviously be chosen for whichever meal is desired. Foods from the "suggested" list should be chosen in the context of the quantitative and qualitative patterns suggested in Table 5-8. Table 5-10 illustrates some sample menus based on these three dietary patterns, and Table 5-9, while not exhaustive, should provide a starting point for preparing other menus. The patient should be given specific menu plans, as well as recipes, to facilitate implementation of the proposed changes in dietary habit. These sample menus illustrate that all of these diets can be palatable, and, indeed, a Phase III diet can be an exciting, innovative new way of eating if it is viewed positively.

While the dietary approach suggested is not phenotype-specific, the qualitative content of the diet should take into account the patient's lipoprotein pattern. For example, a very low total fat intake (less than 10 percent of calories) is appropriate for a Type I patient, since the patient cannot handle chylomicrons. Some therapists prohibit alcohol consumption in Type IV and Type V patients. While alcohol consumption in certain susceptible individuals may cause a marked increase in VLDL, for most patients it is the caloric content and the liberalizaion of other eating habits resulting from alcohol intake that are the major problems, so that this intake should at least be moderated to permit appropriate weight loss when that is the goal. The Phase III diet previously described is high in carbohydrate, and emphasis has been placed on lowering this in Type IV patients in the past, but it is the opinion of most workers in this field that weight loss is the single most important maneuver which will help reduce VLDL levels in the Type IV patient, rather than carbohydrate restriction.

These diets are in general *nutritionally adequate* (Connor and Connor, 1977), although it remains to be absolutely proven that no trace minerals are deficient in a Phase III-type diet. It is important in this regard that the patient by taught the concept of "complementary protein" for consuming a vegetarian-type diet. That is, in order to obtain essential amino acids in the appropriate proportions in the absence of animal protein, one must usually consume two different vegetable sources of protein at the same time. For quality protein, therefore, one should choose a food from Column I in combination with a food from Column II in the chart below:

	COLUMN I	COLUMN II
Legumes		Low-fat dairy. products
	Beans: aduki, black, cranberry, fava, kidney, limas, pinto, marrow, mung, navy, pea, soy (tofo)(sprouts)	
		Grains
		Nuts & Seeds
Grains		
	Whole grains: barley, corn (corn bread)(grits); oats rice; rye: wheat (bulgur, wheat germ)(sprouts)	Low-fat dairy products
		Legumes
Nuts & seeds		
	Nuts: almonds, beechnuts, brazil, cashews, filberts, pecans, pine (Pignolia), walnuts	Low-fat dairy products
	Seeds: pumpkin, sunflower	Legumes

From: *American Heart Association Cookbook,* 3rd ed. New York: American Heart Association, Inc. Copyright 1979 by David McKay Co. Reprinted with permission.

c. Follow-up. Long-term follow-up should be an integral part of a program aimed at reducing serum cholesterol. Generally it is necessary for visits to be more frequent at the beginning of a change program than after the rate of change has reached a plateau. It is the practice in our own program to see the patient at the end of approximately one month for a complete visit, that is, to both the physician and the nutritionist. It is also the practice, however, to have the patient see the nutritionist more frequently as needed. If weight loss is a part of the program, weekly visits are in order if they are possible, telephone contact being a reasonable substitute when this is not possible. At the initial visit, the patient is given a seven-day food record to keep, and this is repeated as often as is necessary to assess the patient's habits and to establish appropriate goals for future visits. A balance must be struck between the value of documenting a patient's food habits and the "nag effect" of keeping a record for some patients.

After the initial several follow-up visits at monthly intervals, patients may be seen at two-month intervals until the desired goal is reached, after which increasingly infrequent visits are in order. However, the patient should be seen regularly at least every four months until changes have remained permanent for several years, after which

Table 5-9
Food Choices for a Modified Fat Diet

Suggested Foods*	Foods to Avoid
A. Breakfast	

Suggested Foods*	Foods to Avoid
Fruit and fruit juices	Whole eggs, egg yolks
Egg whites, egg substitutes	Commercial home fried potatoes
Homemade fried potatoes	Commercial donuts, Danish,
Bagel, english muffin	coffee cake, sweet rolls,
Homemade modified pancakes,	waffles, muffins, pancakes,
waffles, muffins	mixes
Cooked or dried cerals except	Bacon, sausage
granola with coconut or	
coconut oil	
Canadian bacon	
Meat substitutes: soybean	
products	

Suggested Foods*	Foods to Avoid
B. Lunch	

Suggested Foods*	Foods to Avoid
Pastas, macaroni	Vegetables in butter or cream sauce
Peanut butter	Commercial french fried or hash
Beans, dry; all types w/o pork	brown potatoes
All plain breads, including rye,	Whole milk yogurt
whole wheat, raisin, white	Natural and processed cheese, cheese
pumpernickel, French, Italian,	spreads
hard rolls	Commercial cream type, meat or
Vegetables: all, plain, coleslaw	fish soups
Low fat yogurt, all flavors	Frankfurters
Cheese: farmer's cottage, 1% fat,	Commercial hamburger, cheeseburger
plain uncreamed cottage cheese	Luncheon meats: bologna, pastrami,
Broth and vegetable-type soups	corned beef, salami, and canned
Canned or dried fish	types
Frozen or smoked fish	
Boiled ham, deli-type	
Luncheon meats: lean, pressed ham,	
turkey, beef; ground round,	
chicken loaf	*Continued*

*Animal products listed here should be consumed in limited quantities and some (red meat) only occasionally.

Table 5-9 *continued*

Suggested Foods	Foods to Avoid
C. Dinner	
Chicken and turkey without skin	Commercial egg roll
Fish, shellfish; all except	Chow mein noodles
shrimp and sardines	Beef: corned brisket, chuck,
Beef: round, rump, sirloin,	ground beef, rib, club chuck,
flank, tenderloin, all	porterhouse, T-bone
trimmed	Breaded, pre-fried fish and
Lamb: leg, sirloin, shanks,	shellfish
rib	Herring in sour cream
Pork: loin, sirloin, tender-	Commercial meatloaf
loin, ham, fresh, smoked	Organ meats, including tongue
Veal: all cuts except breast	Pork: picnic shoulder, butt,
Homemade gravy, with soft mar-	spare ribs, head cheese, salt
garine or vegetable oil and	pork
fat-free drippings	Commercial sauces containing meat,
Homemade white sauce, modified	sauce mixes, gravy made with
Cheese: part skim mozzarella	meat or poultry fat
and ricotta, parmesan	Frozen dinners and main dishes
Homemade popovers, modified	Commercial pot pies
D. Miscellaneous Foods	
a. Beverages	
All carbonated, "diet," chocolate	Whole milk
flavored drinks, shakes made	Cream: heavy, light (sweet), sour
with skim milk	cream
Tea, coffee, Postum	Powder and liquid non-dairy creamers
	Ice cream, frozen custard
b. Dairy	
Low fat cheeses (certain brands)	Butter, stick margarine
Skim milk, 1% fat milk	Shortening
Skimmed buttermilk	Coconut and palm kernel oil
Polyunsaturated non-diary	Baking chocolate
creamer	Coconut
Ice milk (certain brands)	Salad dressings: creamy and cheese
Frozen yogurt	types
Frozen dietary desserts	Lard
c. Fats and Oils	
Soft margarines	
Polyunsaturated oils: sunflower,	
safflower, corn, cottonseed,	
sesame, soybean	
Mayonnaise	

Continued

Table 5-9 *continued*

Suggested Foods	Foods to Avoid
Miscellaneous Foods (cont'd.)	

Cocoa
Salad dressings: clear types
  and mayo-types
Walnuts, other nuts (except macadamia)

d. Desserts and Snacks

Suggested Foods	Foods to Avoid
Hard candy, jellies, mints, glazed fruit	Commercial or mix-type cakes, cookies, pie crusts, frostings, pizza, crackers
Sherbert, fruit ices	
Fig bars, graham crackers, ginger snaps, commercial or homemade	Chocolate, carmel, cream or nut candy
Angel food cake	Potato chips (unless made with polyunsaturated oil)
Homemade modified recipes for cakes, pastries, pies, cookies, pizza, frostings	Buttered popcorn
Pretzels	
Crackers: Oyster, matzoh, saltines, soda, flat bread, rye crisp	
Popcorn (dry)	

biannual or annual visits are sufficient. Prior to each visit, blood is drawn for a follow-up determination of serum lipids and for other tests which are appropriate, so that the values are available at the time of the visit. The patient should be kept informed of his cholesterol level, since this provides the feedback necessary in the behavioral approach suggested below. The physician, while playing the usual medical role, can also play the role suggested above as part of a team including himself and the nutritionist.

Follow-up visits, particularly those conducted by the nutritionist, should have a "trouble shooting" and goal-setting format, with the patient being given specific skills to help him deal with problems he is likely to encounter. For example, the patient must be given practice with *coping mechanisms for special situations,* such as restaurant eating and eating in other people's homes. Actual practice with restaurant menus is useful, and, even in Phase III, Oriental, Mexican, Italian, and Middle Eastern restaurants have palatable foods to choose from which are compatible with the diet. The patient can be taught to choose only acceptable foods and when the food choices are minimal,

Table 5-10
Sample Menus for Current American and the Two Alternate Diets

	Current American Diet	Prudent Diet (AHA)	Final Phase Diet
BREAKFAST:	Orange juice	4 oz. orange juice	4 oz. fruit or vegetable juice
	Soft-cooked egg	corn flakes with banana	2 slices raisin toast with
	2 slices toast with butter	and skim milk	2 tsp. polyunsaturated tub
	Coffee with non-dairy creamer	½ English muffin with	margarine
		2 tsp. polyunsaturated	8 oz. skim milk
		margarine	black coffee
		Coffee	
		2 oz. skim milk	
SNACK:	Coffee with non-dairy creamer	1 cup coffee	Coffee, black
	Danish pastry	2 oz. skim milk	1 piece fresh fruit
		1 graham cracker	
LUNCH:	Cheesburger	2 oz. chicken loaf in a	1 cup navy bean soup
	French fries	sandwich, with mayonaise	green salad with 1 Tb. oil and
	Coke	1 carrot	vinegar dressing
	Vanilla ice cream	6 oz. apple juice	1 slice whole wheat bread
		1 pear	1 piece fresh fruit
SNACK	Coffee with non-dairy creamer		
	2 cookies		

201

take only small amounts of animal or high-fat foods. This type of rehearsal of situations is, of course, an intimate part of the behavioral approach outlined below. Other special topics discussed should include food for lunch bags; shopping, including label reading; and snacking.

It is important that the patient be given something positive to replace those things which are taken away from the diet, to minimize the feeling of sacrifice on his part. Important in this respect are *recipes* for the new eating style and the technique of *recipe modification*. Thus, for example, it is important for patients to learn specifics, such as the substitution of 3 or 4 tablespoons of cocoa plus 1½ teaspoons of margarine for 1 oz. of chocolate. In order for modifications of favorite recipes to take place, the patient must know, for instance, that for 1 cup of shortening, butter, or margarine in baking, he can substitute ¾ cup polyunsaturated oil. Yogurt or blended low-fat cottage cheese can be substituted for sour cream, egg substitutes can be substituted for eggs, low-fat mozzarella for hardened cheeses, and so on.

Finally, when *weight reduction* is the primary goal of the dietary management plan, the specific paradigms of behavior modification may be useful in helping the patient achieve the weight loss desired. Thus the approach and priorities are different when weight loss is the primary goal. The importance of *activity* must also be stressed in encouraging weight loss, to aid in achieving a negative caloric balance. A walking program is the single most effective activity which will both potentially reduce coronary risk and help in calorie consumption. In many preventive programs, of course, more strenuous aerobic activity, such as jogging, is recommended, and this has, at the least, the advantage of being more conservative of the patient's time for the number of calories burned and may appeal to him for its own sake.

Liberal use should be made of patient education materials in follow-up visits. Particularly useful publications are the *American Heart Association Cookbook* (1979), *"Cooking Without Your Salt Shaker"*(1978), and *"The Heart Saver Eating Style"* (1977). In general your local Heart Association is a good source of information about materials available and other local resources, such as nutrition counseling services.

Behavioral Aspects of Dietary Management. It is important to remember that ultimately the prescription of dietary change will be successful only if the patient actually makes the changes. Rarely, if the changes are made, will the serum lipids not respond to some degree to this manipulation. It should be possible in most patients to lower the lipids as much as 30 percent through dietary approaches alone. A 15–20 percent reduction should be fairly readily attainable in most patients. For this to occur, however, it is important to remember that what is being asked of patients is a change in lifestyle, and this then becomes a problem in behavior change. The importance of behavioral science in clinical preventive programs has been emphasized earlier in this chapter and in Chapter 2 as well, and it is beyond the scope of this chapter to present a detailed history and background of the principles of behavioral medicine. This chapter would not be complete, however, without a few words concerning the application of behavioral principles to dietary change specifically, especially as they concern the role of the physician in achieving a change in lifestyle.

In order for the physician to be a successful change agent, he should abandon the conventially held model of the authoritarian figure who prescribes treatment for the patient, following which the patient *complies* with his direction. This approach implies a militaristic psychology which will produce a "yes" in the office but in fact will usually not result in any change in the long term. Rather the physician, and indeed any counselor, should consider that he or she is entering into a "therapeutic alliance" with the patient in which they are both trying to achieve the same end, an improvement in the patient's serum cholesterol, and, hopefully, a decrease in his risk of CHD. The implications of this approach include the assumption by the patient of an important role for his own care and long-term systematic follow-up by the physician—characteristics, as we shall note, of any good change program.

1. Theoretical Background. It would not be appropriate here to present an extensive theoretical background, but it should be noted that principles of behavior therapy or behavior modification have played an increasingly important role in weight loss programs and other dietary programs aimed at lifestyle change (Foreyt and Gotto, 1979; Foreyt et al., 1979; Leventhal and Cleary, 1979). It is important to realize, however, that neither the physician nor the patient should expect a miracle from this approach, and that, whatever the approach used, it will require a great deal of time and effort on the part of both therapist and patient to achieve permanent success. Behavior modification makes the assumption that eating, and indeed all habits, are learned behaviors, and that changing them involves a learning process in which new behaviors are practiced. Behavior modification derives from the classical conditioning experiments of Pavlov and has in the past placed great emphasis on stimulus control and control of the environment in general in controlling an undesirable act or response. The earlier models of self-control or behavioral self-management programs have emphasized a three-stage approach, consisting of self-observation, self-evaluation, and self-reinforcement. Within the "oper-

ant" perspective of behavior modification, environmental control of behavior occurs primarily through differential consequences. The self-control model referred to retains this perspective, but does not encompass the full complexity of interdependent, cognitive, and environmental processes influencing behaviors.

More recently the cognitive side of behavior has had a resurgence as an important factor in determining outcome. Thus, the patient's belief system, it is now assumed, does play some role in whether or not he can achieve a change, and the Health Belief Model conceptualizes some aspect of this belief system as it is relevant to health behavior (Becker and Maiman, 1975). Going a step further, Coates and Perry (1980) have proposed a "reciprocal interaction model" of behavior, displayed in outline form in Figure 5-4. The model presents a framework designed to return to center stage the reciprocal influence of external and internal factors. This interactive system thus includes the *person*, the physical and social *environment*, and the person's *behaviors*. One important consequence of this model, derived from social learning theory, is that the behaviors themselves may influence the subject's belief system. This opens as one avenue for behavior change

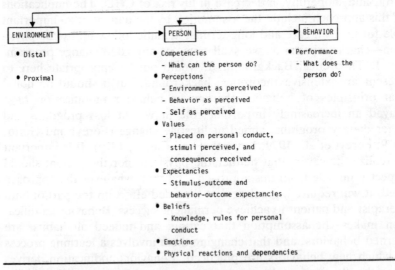

Figure 5-4. A social learning/reciprocal interaction model

Reprinted with permission from T.J. Coates and C. Perry, "Multifactor risk reduction with children and adolescents: Taking care of the heart in behavioral group therapy," *Behavioral Group Therapy, 1980: An Annual Review,* edited by D. Upper and S.M. Ross, Research Press Co., Champaign, Ill., 1980.

the possibility of convincing a patient to help carry out a particular activity whether he thinks he will like it or not, in the hope that the act of carrying it out may change his belief about it.

The reciprocal-influence model suggests that an effective intervention for patients should (1) use behavioral rehearsal with corrective feedback as a major method for teaching skills; (2) teach a variety of personal-influence skills so that individuals know how to respond to a variety of problem situations; and (3) structure the environment so that skills may be used consistently and persistently outside treatment sessions and the person may experience positive feedback.

It is hoped that this model and others presented elsewhere will form a useful framework within which to place the generalizations which follow.

2. Characteristics of a Successful Change Program. Despite the vast array of models and theoretical background material which has developed in the last few years in this area, the characteristics of a successful change program which involves the physician can be summarized by listing a few cogent points. The goal inherent in this list, and the objective of this behavioral approach, is to maximize success and minimize failure. The following characteristics are an attempt to fulfill that goal:

a. The patient should be made responsible for his/her own health. The patient must understand that he/she is not making the change to make the physician happy or for approval, but must take the responsibility when away from the therapist/counselor to make the right decisions for his/her own health improvement.

b. Health beliefs should be taken into account. It should be ascertained whether the patient believes that he/she is susceptible to disease and that what he/she is doing will not only help him/her but is worth whatever sacrifice is involved. It is sometimes worthwhile simply to stop and discuss with him/her what the patient believes.

c. Positive changes should be emphasized. Positive reinforcement should be utilized, with negative aspects of the patient's behavior played down.

d. The program should be specific. Suggested changes the patient is asked to make should be spelled out in detail, and he/she should leave the office with specific goals to be achieved before the next visit. For example, it is not sufficient to suggest that the patient be "more active." A specific program, such as 30 minutes a day of walking, should be agreed upon, including agreeing on what time of day it should occur and under what circumstances.

e. Changes should be gradual. This is perhaps the most important characteristic of a successful change program. Most patients will not be willing or able to change a lifetime's habits in a few weeks or even a few months. Therefore, long-term follow-up should be provided and a "step by step" approach should be taken except for the rare case in which the patient appears to be able to make large changes. Even when the patient insists on making these changes, it is wise to discourage this, because in the long run it will be deleterious to the overall program.

f. "Backsliding" should be built in. Part of the gradual approach should be the expectation that the patient's progress will not always be in the right direction, and that it is human to "backslide." In any case, confrontation concerning the lack of achievement of goals should be avoided, the positive being emphasized as noted above.

g. Realistic goals should be set. By doing this, success is maximized and situations avoided which will guarantee failure. Thus, a patient who wants to lose ten pounds in one week should be discouraged from doing so because he is likely to fail and this will have a negative effect on his ability to carry out a change program in the future.

h. Self-monitoring should be included in the program. The patient should be asked to keep records. This is informative both to the patient and to the physician or nutritionist and in itself will act as a tool in effecting change.

Other Aspects of Dietary Counseling. Zifferblatt and Wilbur (1977a, 1977b) and Wilbur and colleagues (1980) have provided some guidelines for counseling aimed primarily at nutritionists, but the physician would be wise to avail himself of as many of these tools as he can in working effectively with a nutritionist, or, if necessary, by himself. The reader is referred to the literature cited for a full discussion of these counseling principles.

Pharmacologic Therapy

There is as yet no perfect drug for the treatment of hyperlipidemia. It must be borne in mind that the certainty of a desirable benefit to risk ratio has not been demonstrated for the reduction of serum lipids, so that the use of medication, which always carries with it some risk, should be undertaken only when dietary therapy is not successful after a reasonable trial or when the lipids in any case cannot be brought below 240 mg/dl. An elevation of serum triglyceride should be treated with medication probably only when it is considerably over 500 mg/dl unless there is a sufficient elevation of accompanying cholesterol to justify the lowering of both together, since it is the cholesterol which undoubtedly carries with it the greatest increased risk of premature coronary disease. As stated above, particularly if the decision to use drugs has already been made, a desirable cholesterol is one that is well below 200 mg/dl, so that the average cholesterol over a period of time will remain below 200 mg/dl. A variety of drugs are approved for use in the treatment of hyperlipidemia. The drug of choice for patients without a triglyceride elevation is the bile acid-sequestering anion exchange resin cholestyramine (Questran®, Mead Johnson). Another similar resin has recently been marketed by the Upjohn Company under the trade name Colestid® (generic name: colestipol). The only serious side effect from the use of these drugs is constipation, and this can usually be handled through the administration of stool softeners. Compliance is sometimes a problem because the medication does not dissolve and often remains in the mouth after the liquid suspension has been swallowed. A positive approach by the physician will be beneficial in this case. One other side effect of this medication is a temporary increase in triglyceride level, but this usually can be expected to return to its pretreatment level. This side effect does, however, prevent the drug from being useful in patients with elevated triglycerides. But if the triglyceride can be lowered through weight loss, it is still desirable to use a resin, since it is not absorbed and systemic side effects are unlikely. This drug is the drug of choice for familial Type II patients, and the best second drug, when it is tolerated, is nicotinic acid, although adverse effects often make it very difficult to administer the latter. Treatment is usually more successful if it is started at low levels and the dosage gradually increased, taken at mealtimes when necessary. It is very successful at lowering almost every serum lipid fraction. It must, however, be used in doses up to 6 gm/day in order to accomplish the desired changes. Clofibrate (Atromid S®, Ayerst) is one of the most commonly used hypolipidemic agents. It is also sometimes used in combination with a resin when treating some Type II patients, and the same patients may respond to Atromid S alone, although usually not to any great degree. Clofibrate may be useful in the treatment of patients with elevated triglycerides, particularly Type III patients. Patients may be resistant to the effects of this drug, however, if they have not first lost weight. It can be administered at 2.0 gm/day in two doses. Side effects are usually minimal, and include transient elevations of SGOT. It can also, however, cause rather severe myositis and has even been reported to cause cardiac arrhythmias. It must be particularly cautiously used in patients with low serum proteins and/or decreased renal function, since it is excreted in the urine. It also has been shown to be associated with an increased incidence of gallstones (Coronary Drug Research Group, 1975). In view of the results of the WHO Clofibrate Study (Committee of Principal Investigators, 1978), care should be exercised to use clofibrate only when the risk of hyperlipidemia clearly exceeds that of the drug. Other drugs used in treating hyperlipidemia include D-thyroxine (Choloxin®), neomycin, and plant sterols (β-sitosterol).

Although we now know much more than previously about methods of lowering serum lipids both by dietary and by pharmacologic means, there are still many patients, particularly familial Type II patients, who are extremely resistant to treatment. It must constantly be borne in mind by the physician that an adverse benefit/risk ratio is a possibility in these situations, since the treatment of symptomless disorders such as those described is predicated on the yet unproved "lipid hypothesis" that lowering lipid levels will decrease morbidity and mortality from premature atherosclerosis. While there is yet debate about what advice should be given to the public at large, there is little debate about the advisability of treating high-risk individuals. Therefore, an evaluation of every patient with regard to risk factors, including serum lipids, should be carried out and appropriate measures instituted for high-risk patients. Evaluation should also be carried out in children in which a family history for premature coronary disease may in fact be an inherited risk factor. Certainly, whenever a proband of any family is found who seems to have familial hyperlipidemia, all family members should be screened so that high-risk patients in that family do not go undetected. While immediately following a myocardial infarction is the worst time to measure a patient's cholesterol, since it often falls precipitously, it is often a very good time to screen the rest of the family, since they are usually all at the hospital.

In treating patients with these disorders, the total patient should always be taken into account. Thus, not only should the total serum lipid values be a factor in deciding to begin treatment, but also the HDL cholesterol, the presence of other risk factors, family history, and a variety of other factors. The decision to treat cannot be made lightly, since we are, when treating these disorders, treating patients who are asymptomatic, treating them for the rest of their lives in many cases, and at times with drugs which have potentially serious side effects. It is hoped that studies currently underway will give us more definitive answers concerning the value of treatment and that more specific approaches to therapy may become available in the future.

CONCLUSION

Even though there are those who do not believe that there is now any justification for considering a change in the U.S. dietary pattern and those who believe that the diet–heart hypothesis has some validity but are troubled by the gaps in our understanding, leading to a "wait and see" attitude, there are those who argue that the evidence presently available is sufficient to justify embarking on the measures which could reduce population blood cholesterol levels. They argue that the fat-modified diet is both acceptable and safe. A study of the changes in the American diet which have occurred in the last two decades give clear evidence that, while the experts are arguing, Americans are making these suggested changes on their own. Secular trends in diet are most easily measured by reviewing "food disappearance" estimates prepared by the U.S. Department of Agriculture annually (Board of Agriculture and Renewable Resources, 1976). Between 1909 and 1973, vegetable fat consumption tripled, and animal fat consumption declined modestly. These changes were due in part to reduced consumption of whole milk and increased consumption of lower-fat milks, an increased consumption of salad and cooking oil, and the virtual replacement of butter and lard in the American diet by margarine and shortening since the Second World War. Egg consumption, rising sharply after the war, has fallen sharply to prewar levels; beef consumption, after declining, began an irregular rise that accelerated after the war; and poultry consumption has risen substantially since the war. Saturated fat consumption peaked in the period 1957–1959 at 15.7 percent of calories consumed, declining to 15.0 percent in 1974. Comparing the same two periods, linoleic acid consumption rose from 4.8 percent of calories to 6.5 percent of calories and cholesterol consumption declined from 184 mg/kCal to 164 mg/kCal (Gortner, 1975).

The more educated the stratum of the population the more changes in the direction of a fat-modified diet is taking place. This is illustrated in Table 5-11 by the data on the health-conscious men entering MRFIT in the mid-1970s compared to men entering the studies of the 1960s. As one progresses toward the later study, total fat intake becomes lower, saturated fat and dietary cholesterol are down even more, while polyunsaturated fat is somewhat higher (Stamler, 1980a, 1980b).

The changes in consumption that have occurred would be predicted by the Keys and Hegsted equations to produce a 4–6 mg/dl reduction in serum cholesterol, and a comparison of the cholesterol

Table 5-11
Baseline Nutrient Intake[a]

Nutrient	MRFIT (6,298 men)	Framingham (864 men)	ND-HS (1,196 men)
Calories (per day)	2,473	2,608	2,565
Protein (% of cal)	16.2	15.8	15.6
Carbohydrate (% of cal)	37.9	38.6	40.7
Alcohol (% of cal)	7.4	6.7	4.1
Total fat (% of cal)	38.4	39.0	40.4
Saturated fatty acids (% of cal)	13.9	15.0	15.6
Monounsaturated fatty acids (% of cal)	14.8	15.5	17.6
Polyunsaturated fatty acids (% of cal)	6.6	5.4	3.9
Cholesterol (mg/day)	450	530	533

[a]Men in the Framingham and National Diet-Heart Studies (ND-HS)(early 1960s), and men in the MRFIT (mid-1970s).

Reprinted with permission from J. Stamler, "The fat-modified diet: Its nature, effectiveness, and safety," *Childhood Prevention of Atherosclerosis and Hypertension,* edited by R.M. Lauer and R.B. Shekelle. Copyright © by Raven Press, New York, 1980.

levels found in National Health Examination Survey of 1960–1962 and that found in the HANES Survey of 1971–1974 shows that serum cholesterol concentrations declined by 1.9–5.9 mg/dl in men (Abraham et al., 1977). An even larger decrease in cholesterol is reflected by the data from epidemiological studies when one compares the Pooling Project mean cholesterol level (1950s) of 235 with the mean value of 210 obtained in population studies of the mid-1970s. If one assumes an average 10 mg/dl decline in serum cholesterol over the past decade, the predicted decline in coronary heart disease mortality for men aged 45 to 74 is 13.7 percent (Stern, 1979).

Age-adjusted overall ischemic heart disease mortality declined by 20.7 percent in the United States between 1968 and 1976. There have been numerous conferences in which the reasons for this decline have been discussed (Havlik and Feinlieb, 1979). The reasons remain unclear, and an advisory panel at the NIH has recommended that more surveillance be undertaken to provide a data base for monitoring the causes of the decline in mortality, but utilizing the multivariate risk model, it can be shown that 40 percent of the predicted CHD mortality change is accounted for by the 25 mg/dl decrease in mean cholesterol noted above and almost all of the CHD change is predicted if blood pressure and smoking changes are also taken into account (Blackburn, 1979b; Beaglehole et al., 1979). It thus appears that the American people have "gotten the message" about the adverse health effects of the recent American diet and are doing something about it. They are increasing activities at the community and governmental level in line with and encouraging these trends. Thus, the American Heart Association is increasingly active in the area of nutrition programming, and there is an Office of Prevention, Education, and Control attached to the National Heart, Lung, and Blood Institute. The accelerating pace of these activities should increase the rate at which current trends continue.

It is clear that the educated consumer simply will not wait while the academician continues to search for conclusive proof of benefit. The National Heart, Lung, and Blood Institute has recently initiated a Preventive Cardiology Academic Award, given to faculty members at U.S. medical schools for developing curricula in Preventive Cardiology. It is to be hoped that the educated physician can lead the way in this trend, since there are multiple popular sources of misinformation for the patient. It would be a happy occurrence if the practitioner interested in disease prevention could provide the patient with the advice he is so urgently seeking.

REFERENCES

Abraham, S., Johnson, C.L., and Carroll, M.D.: A comparison of levels of serum cholesterol of adults, 18–74 years of age in the United States in 1960–62 and 1971–74, in: Advance Data from Vital and Health Statistics of the National Center for Health Statistics, No. 6. Washington, D.C.: DHEW, 1977.

Ackerknecht, E.H.: *Rudolph Virchow—Doctor, Statesman, Anthropologist.* Madison, Wis.: University of Wisconsin Press, 1953.

Ahrens, E.H., Jr., Insull, W., Blomstrand, R., Hirsch, J., Tsaltas, T.T., and Peterson, M.L.: The influence of dietary fats on serum-lipid levels in man. *Lancet* 1:943–953, 1957.

Ahrens, E.H., Jr.: The management of hyperlipidemia: Whether, rather than how. *Ann. Intern. Med.* 85:87–93, 1976.

Ahrens, E.H., Jr.: Dietary fats and coronary heart disease: unfinished business. *Lancet* 2:1345–1348, 1979.

American Heart Association Cookbook. New York: David McKay, 1979.

Ames, R.P., and Hill, P.: Elevation of serum lipid levels during diuretic therapy of hypertension. *Am. J. Med.* 61:748–757, 1976.

Anitschkow, N.: Experimental arteriosclerosis in animals, in E.V. Cowdry, editor, *Arteriosclerosis.* New York: Macmillan, 1933, p. 271.

Armstrong, B.K., Mann, J.I., Adelstein, A.M., and Eskin, F.: Commodity consumption and ischemic heart disease mortality, with special references to dietary practices. *J. Chron. Dis.* 28:455–469, 1975.

Armstrong, M.L., Warner, E.D., and Connor, W.E.: Regression of coronary atheromatosis in rhesus monkeys. *Circ. Res.* 27:59–67, 1970.

Armstrong, M.L.: Connective tissue changes in regression, in G. Schettler, Y. Goto, Y. Hata, and G. Klose, editors, *Atherosclerosis IV* (Proc. 4th Int. Symp.). Berlin: Springer-Verlag, 1977, p. 405–413.

Anderson, D.W., Nichols, A.V., and Brewer, H.B.: Ultracentrifugal characterization of the human high density lipoprotein distribution, in K. Lippel, editor, in Report of the High Density Lipoprotein Methodology Workshop, NIH Publication No. 79-1661, 1979.

Ashley, F.W., and Kannel, W.B.: Relation of weight changes to changes in atherogenic traits. The Framingham Study. *J. Chron. Dis.* 27:103–114, 1974.

Barndt, R., Jr., Blankenhorn, D.H., Crawford, D.W., and Brooks, S.H.: Regression and progression of early femoral atherosclerosis in treated hyperlipoproteinemic patients. *Ann. Intern. Med.* 86:139–146, 1977.

Barr, D.P., Russ, E.M., and Eder, H.A.: Protein-lipid relationships in human plasma. II. In atherosclerosis and related conditions. *Am. J. Med.* 11:480–493, 1951.

Beaglehole, R., LaRosa, J., Heiss, G., Davis, C.E., Williams, O.D., Tyroler, H.A. and Rifkind, B.M.: Serum cholesterol, diet and the decline in coronary heart disease mortality. *Prev. Med.* 8:538–547, 1979.

Becker, M.H., and Maiman, L.A.: Sociobehavioral determinants of compliance with health and medical care recommendations. *Med. Care* 13:10–24, 1975.

Benfari, R.C., for the MRFIT Research Group: Lifestyle alteration and the primary prevention of CHD: The Multiple Risk Factor Intervention Trial (MRFIT), in M.L. Pollock and D.N. Schmidt, editors, *Heart Disease and Rehabilitation.* Boston: Houghton Mifflin, 1979, p. 341.

Bierenbaum, M.L., Fleischman, A.I., and Raichelson, R.I.: Long term human studies on the lipid effects of oral calcium. *Lipids* 7:202, 1972.

Blackburn, H., Chairman: Epidemiological Section, Conference on the Health Effects of Blood Lipids. *Prev. Med.* 8:612–678, 1979a.

Blackburn, H.: Diet and mass hyperlipidemia: A public health view, in R.I. Levy, B. Rifkind, B. Dennis, and N. Ernst, editors, *Nutrition, Lipids, and Coronary Heart Disease.* New York: Raven Press, 1979b.

Blackwelder, W.C., Yano, K., Rhoads, G.G., Kagan, A., Gordon, T., and Palesch, Y.: Alcohol and mortality: The Honolulu Heart Study. *Am. J. Med.* 68:164–169, 1980.

Blankenhorn, D., Brooks, S.H., Selzer, R.H., and Barndt, R., Jr.: The rate of atherosclerosis change during treatment of hyperlipoproteinemia. *Circulation* 57: 355–361, 1978.

Blankenhorn, D.H.: Reversibility of latent atherosclerosis. Studies by femoral angiography in humans. *Mod. Concepts Cardiovasc. Dis.* XLVII:79, 1978.

Board of Agriculture and Renewable Resources. Commission on Natural Resources and Food and Nutrition Board, Assembly of Life Sciences: Fat Content and Composition of Animal Products. Washington, D.C.: National Academy of Sciences, 1976.

Byington, R., Dyer, A.R., Garside, D., Liu, K., Moss, D., Stamler, J., and Tsong, Y.: Recent trends of major coronary risk factors and CHD mortality in the United States and other industrialized countries, in Proceedings of the Conference on the Decline in Coronary Heart Disease Mortality. Washington, D.C.: DHEW, Public Health Service, Publ. No (NIH) 79-1610, 1979.

Cannella, C., Golinelli A., and Melli, A.: Influenza sui valori colesterolemici della polpa di mela aggiunta alla normale alimentazione. *Arcispedale S. Anna de Ferrara* 15:803, 1962.

Carroll, K.K.: Dietary protein in relation to plasma cholesterol levels and atherosclerosis. *Nutr. Rev.* 36:1, 1978.

Castelli, W.P., Doyle, J.T., Gordon, T., Hames, C.G., Hjortland, M.C., Hulley, S.B., Kagau, A., and Zukel, W.J.: HDL cholesterol and other lipids in coronary heart disease. The Cooperative Lipoprotein Phenotyping Study. *Circulation* 55:767–772, 1977a.

Castelli, W.P., Gordon, T., Hjortland, M.C., Kagan, A., Doyle, J.T., Hames, C.G., Hulley, S.B., and Zukel, W.J.: Alcohol and blood lipids. The Cooperative Lipoprotein Phenotyping Study. *Lancet* II:153–155, 1977b.

Central Patient Registry and Coordinating Center for the Lipid Research Clinics: *Protocol for the Lipid Research Clinics Type II Primary Prevention Trial,* Vol. 1 Dept. of Biostatistics, Univ. of North Carolina, Chapel Hill, 1972.

Coates, T.J., and Perry, C.: Multifactor risk reduction with children and adolescents: Taking care of the heart in behavioral group therapy, in D. Upper and S.M. Ross, editors, *Behavioral Group Therapy, 1980: An Annual Review.* Champaign, Ill.: Research Press Company, 1980.

Committee of Principal Investigators: A cooperative trial in the primary prevention of ischemic heart disease using clofibrate. *Br. Heart J.* 40:1069–1118, 1978.

Connor, W.E., Stone, D.B., and Hodges, R.E.: The inter-related effects of dietary cholesterol and fat upon human serum lipid levels. *J. Clin. Invest.* 43:1691–1696, 1964.

Connor, W.E., and Connor, S.L.: Dietary treatment of hyperlipidemia, in B.M. Rifkind and R.I. Levy, editors, *Hyperlipidemia, Diagnosis and Therapy.* New York: Grune and Stratton, 1977, p. 281–326.

Cooking Without Your Salt Shaker. American Heart Association Publication, No. 53-002-A, Dallas, Tex., 1978.

Cooper, R., Stamler, J., Dyer, A., et al.: The decline in mortality from coronary heart disease; U.S.A., 1968–1975. *J. Chron. Dis.* 31:709–720, 1978.

Cornfeld, J., and Mitchell, S., Selected risk factors in coronary disease. Possible intervention effects. *Arch. Environ. Health* 19:382–394, 1969.

Coronary Drug Project Research Group: Clofibrate and niacin in coronary heart disease. *JAMA* 231:360–381, 1975.

Coronary Drug Study Project Research Group: The Coronary Drug Project: Implications for primary care. *Primary Care* 4:247, 1977.

Coronary Drug Project Research Group: The natural history of myocardial infarction in the Coronary Drug Project: Long-term prognostic importance of serum lipid levels. *Am. J. Cardiol.* 42:489, 1978.

Davis, C.E., and Havlik, R.J.: Clinical trials of lipid lowering and coronary artery disease prevention, in B.M. Rifkind and R.I. Levy, editors, *Hyperlipidemia—Diagnosis and Therapy*. New York: Grune and Stratton, 1977.

Dayton, S., Pearce, M.L., Hashimoto, H., et al.: A controlled clinical trial of a diet high in unsaturated fat in preventing complications of atherosclerosis. *Circulation* 40 (Suppl. II):1–63, 1969.

De Groot, A.P., Luyken, R., and Pikaar, N.A.: Cholesterol-lowering effect of rolled oats. *Lancet* 2:303, 1963.

Department of Health, Education, and Welfare: Serum cholesterol levels of adults, United States, 1960–62, in National Health Survey, National Center for Health Statistics, Series 11, No. 22. Washington, D.C.: DHEW, 1967.

Dyerberg, J., and Bang, H.O.: Hemostatic function and platelet polyunsaturated fatty acids in Eskimos. *Lancet* II:433–435, 1979.

Dyerberg, J., Bang, H.O., and Hjorne, N.: Fatty acid composition of the plasma lipids in Greenland Eskimos. *Am. J. Clin. Nutr.* 28:958–966, 1975.

Ederer, F., Leren, P., Turpeinen, O., et al.: Cancer among men on cholesterol lowering diets. *Lancet* 2:203–206, 1971.

Editorial. Diabetes, hyperglycemia, and coronary heart diease. *Lancet* 1:345–346, 1980.

Farquhar, J.W., Wood, P.D., Breitrose, H., Haskell, W.L., Meyer, A.J., Maccoby, N., Alexander, J.K., Brown, B.J., McAlister, A.L., Nash, J.D., and Stern, M.P.: Community education for cardiovascular health. *Lancet* 1:1192, 1977.

Feeley, R.M., Criner, P.E., and Watt, B.K.: Cholesterol content of foods. *J. Am. Dietetic Assoc.* 61:134, 1972.

Fejfar, Z.: Prevention against ischemic heart disease; a critical review, in M.D. Oliver, editor, *Modern Trends in Cardiology*, Vol. 3. London: Butterworth, 1974, pp. 465–499.

Fischer-Dzega, K., Fraser, R., and Wissler, R.W.: Stimulation of proliferation in stationary primary cultures of monkey and rabbit aortic smooth muscle cells. I. Effects of lipoprotein fractions of hyperlipemic serum and lymph. *Exp. Mol. Pathol.* 24:346–359, 1976.

Foreyt, J.P., and Gotto, A.M.: Behavioral treatment of obesity, in A.M. Gotto and R. Paoletti, *Atherosclerosis Reviews*, No. 6. New York: Raven Press, 1979, p. 179–201.

Foreyt, J.P., Scott, L.W., Mitchell, R.E., and Gotto, A.M.: Plasma lipid changes in the normal population following behavioral treatment. *J. Consult. Clin. Psychol.* 47:440–452, 1979.

Fredrickson, D.S., Levy, R.I., and Lees, R.S.: Fat transport in lipoproteins—an integrated approach to mechanisms and disorders. *N. Engl. J. Med.* 276:34–44, 94–103, 148–156, 215–255, 273–281, 1967.

Friedewald, W.T., Levy, R.I., and Fredrickson, D.S.: Estimation of the concentration of low-density lipoprotein cholesterol in plasma, without use of the preparative ultracentrifuge. *Clin. Chem.* 18:499, 1972.

Fuller, J.H., McCartney, P., Jarrett, R.J., et al.: Hyperglycemia and coronary heart disease: The Whitehall Study. *J. Chron. Dis.* 32:721–728, 1979.

Furman, R.H., Alaupovic, P., and Howard, R.P.: Effects of androgens and estrogens on serum lipids and the composition and concentration of serum lipoproteins in normolipemic and hyperlipidemic states. *Prog. Biochem. Pharmacol.* 2:215, 1967.

Galen, R.S.: HDL cholesterol: How should we use it? *Diagnostic Med.* 3:61, 1980.

Garcia-Palmieri, M.R., Tillotson, J., Cordero, E., et al.: Nutrient intake and serum lipids in urban and rural Puerto Rican men. *Am. J. Clin. Nutr.* 30:2092–2100, 1977.

Garrison, R.J., Kannel, W.B., Feinleib, M., Castelli, W.B., McNamara, P.M., and Padgett, S.J.: Cigarette smoking and HDL cholesterol. The Framingham Offspring Study. *Atherosclerosis* 30:17, 1978.

Goldbourt, U., and Medalie, J.H.: High density lipoprotein cholesterol and the incidence of coronary heart disease—the Israeli Heart Disease Study. *Am. J. Epidemiol.* 109:296–308, 1979.

Goldstein, J.L., Schrott, H.G., Hazzard, W.R., Bierman, E.L., and Motulsky, A.G.: Hyperlipidemia in coronary heart disease. *J. Clin. Invest.* 52:1544–1568, 1973.

Goldstein, J.L., and Brown, M.S.: Atherosclerosis: The low density lipoprotein receptor hypothesis. *Metabolism* 26:1257–1275, 1977.

Gordon, T.: The Framingham Diet Study, diet and the regulation of serum cholesterol, in The Framingham Study—An Epidemiological Investigation of Cardiovascular Diseases. Washington, D.C.: DHEW, Section 24, 1970.

Gordon, T., and Kannel, W.B.: Obesity and cardiovascular disease: The Framingham Study. *Clin. Endocrinol. Metab.* 5:367–376, 1976.

Gordon, T., Garcia-Palmieri, M.R., Kagan, A., Kannel, W.B., and Schiffman, J.: Differences in coronary heart disease in Framingham, Honolulu, and Puerto Rico. *J. Chron. Dis.* 27:329–344, 1974.

Gordon, T., Castelli, W.P., Hjortland, M.C., Kannel, W.B., and Dawber, T.R.: High density lipoprotein as a protective factor against coronary heart disease. *Am. J. Med.* 62:707–714, 1977a.

Gordon, T., Castelli, W.P., Hjortland, M.C., Kannel, W.B., and Dawber, T.R.: Predicting coronary heart disease in middle-aged and older persons. *JAMA* 238:497–499, 1977b.

Gortner, W.A.: Nutrition in the United States. 1900 to 1974. *Cancer Res.* 35:3246–3253, 1975.

Gotto, A.M., Shepherd, J., Scott, L.W., and Manis, E.: Primary hyperlipoproteinemia and dietary management, in R.I. Levy, B. Rifkind, B. Dennis, and N. Ernst, editors, *Nutrition, Lipids and Coronary Disease.* New York: Raven Press, 1979.

Gotto, A.M., Foreyt, J.P., and Scott, L.W.: Hyperlipidemia and nutrition: Ongoing work, in Ruth Hegyeli, editor, *Atherosclerosis Reviews,* Vol. 7. New York: Raven Press, 1980, p. 169.

Group of Physicians of the Newcastle Upon Tyne Region: Trial of clofibrate in the treatment of ischemic heart disease. *Br. Med. J.* 4:767–775, 1971.

Havlik, R.J., and Feinleib, M., editors: Proceedings of the Conference on the Decline in Coronary Heart Disease Mortality, Washington, D.C.: DHEW, Public Health Service, Publ. No. (NIH) 79-1610, 1979.

Halperin, M., Cornfeld, J., and Mitchell, S.C.: Effect of diet on coronary heart disease mortality. *Lancet* 2:438–439, 1973.

Heart Saver Eating Style, Chicago Heart Association, no. 99-7051B, 1977.

Hegsted, D.M., McGandy, R.B., Myers, M.L., and Stare, F.J.: Quantitative effects of dietary fat on serum cholesterol in man. *Am. J. Clin. Nutr.* 17:281–295, 1965.

Heinle, R.A., Levy, R.I., Fredrickson, D.S., and Gorlin, R.: Lipid and carbohydrate abnormalities in patients with angiographically documented coronary artery disease. *Am. J. Cardiol.* 24:178–186, 1969.

Hems, P.: Soybean-protein diet and plasma cholesterol. *Lancet* 1:805, 1977.

Hjermann, I.: Current objectives in prevention. Panel on diet, in A.T. Hansen, P. Schnohr, and G. Rose, editors, *Ischemic Heart Disease—The Strategy of Postponement.* Copenhagen: FADL Publishing, 1977, p. 162.

Hjermann, I.: The randomized "Smoking-Lipid Trial" of the Oslo Study. Presented at the Fifth International Symposium on Atherosclerosis, Nov. 6–9, 1979, Houston, Tex.

Huttunen, J.K., Lansimies, E., Vontilainen, E., Ehnholm, C., Hietanen, E., Penttila, I., Siitonen, O., and Raurammaa, R.: Effect of moderate physical exercise on serum lipoproteins. *Circulation* 60:1220–1229, 1979.

Hulley, S., Ashman, P., Kuller, L., Lasser, N., and Sherwin, R., for the MRFIT Research Group: HDL Cholesterol levels in the Multiple Risk Factor Intervention Trial (MRFIT). *Lipids* 14:119–125, 1979.

Jackson, R.L., Morrisett, J.D., and Gotto, A.M.: Lipoprotein structure and metabolism. *Physiol. Rev.* 56:259–316, 1976.

Jackson, R.L., Morrisett, J.D., and Gotto, A.M.: Lipoproteins and lipid transport: Structural and functional concepts, in B.M. Rifkind and R.I. Levy, editors, *Hyperlipidemia, Diagnosis and Therapy.* New York: Grune and Stratton, 1977, p. 1–16.

Kagan, A., Harris, B.R., Winkelstein, W., Jr., Johnson, K.G., Kato, H., Syme, S.L., Rhoads, G.G., Gay, M.L., Nichaman, M.Z., Hamilton, H.B., and Tillotson, J.: Epidemiologic studies of coronary heart disease and stroke in Japanese men living in Japan, Hawaii, and California; demographic, physical, dietary, and biochemical characteristics. *J. Chron. Dis.* 27:345–364, 1974.

Katz, L.N., Stamler, J., and Pick, R.: *Nutrition and Atherosclerosis.* Philadelphia: Lea and Febiger, 1958.

Kay, R.M., and Truswell, A.S.: Effect of citrus pectin on blood lipids and fecal steroid excretion in man. *Am. J. Clin. Nutr.* 30:171, 1977a.

Kay, R.M., and Truswell, A.S.: The effect of wheat fiber on plasma lipids and fecal steroid excretion in man. *Br. J. Nutr.* 37:227, 1977b.

Keys, A., editor: Coronary heart disease in seven countries. *Circulation* 41:Suppl. 1, 1970.

Keys, A.: Predicting coronary heart disease, in G. Tibblin, A. Keys, and L. Werko, editors, *Preventive Cardiology.* Stockholm: Almqvist and Wiksell, 1972, p. 21.

Keys, A.: Mortality and coronary heart disease in Mediterranean area, in *Proceedings of the II International Congress on the Biological Value of Olive Oil, Torremolinos, Spain.* Organizaction de Exposiciones y Congresos, S.A., Madrid, 1976, pp. 281–286.

Keys, A., editor: *Seven Countries: Death and Coronary Heart Disease.* Cambridge, Mass.: Harvard University Press, 1980.

Keys, A., Anderson, J.T., and Grande, F.: Effect on serum cholesterol in man of mono-ene fatty acid (oleic acid) in the diet. *Proc. Soc. Exp. Biol. Med.* 98:387, 1958.

Keys, A., Anderson, J.T., and Grande, F.: Serum cholesterol response to changes in the diet. Part I. Iodine value of dietary fat vs. 2 S-P; Part II. The effect of cholesterol in the diet; Part III. Differences among individuals; Part IV. Particular saturated fatty acids in the diet. *Metabolism* 14:747–787, 1965.

Klatsky, A.L., Friedman, G.D., Siegelaub, A.B., et al.: Alcohol consumption and blood pressure, Kaiser-Permanente Multiphasic Health Examination Data. *N. Engl. J. Med.* 296:1194, 1977.

Knight, L., Schebel, R., Ampatz, K., Varco, R.L., and Buchwald, H.: Radiographic appraisal of the Minnesota partial ileal bypass study. *Surg. Forum* 23:141–142. 1972.

Kornitzer, M., DeBacker, G., Dramaix, M., and Thilly, C.: The Belgian Heart Disease Prevention Project. Modification of the coronary risk profile in an industrial population. *Circulation* 61:18–25, 1980.

Kristein, M.M., Arnold, C.B., and Wynder, E.L.: Health economics and preventive care. *Science* 195:457–462, 1977.

Kuller, L.: Prevention of cardiovascular disease and risk-factor intervention trials. *Criculation* 61:26–28, 1980.

Kuo, P.T., Hayase, K., Kostis, J.B., and Moreyra, A.E.: The use of combined diet and Colestipol in long-term (7–7 ½ years) treatment of patients with Type II hyperlipoproteinemia. *Circulation* 59:199–211, 1979.

Lasser, N.L., et al.; for the MRFIT Group: Contribution of weight loss to changes in lipoprotein cholesterol levels in the Multiple Risk Factor Intervention Trial (MRFIT). *J. Oil Chem. Soc.* 59:204a, 1979.

La Porte, R.E., Cresanta, J.L., and Kuller, L.H.: The relationship of alcohol consumption to atherosclerotic heart disease. *Prev. Med.* 9:22–40, 1980.

Lauer, R.M., and Shekelle, R.B., editors: *Childhood Prevention of Atherosclerosis and Hypertension.* New York: Raven Press, 1980, p. 41–74.

Leathers, C.W., Bond, M.G., and Rudel, L.L.: Effects of ethanol on dyslipoproteinemia and coronary artery atherosclerosis in non-human primates. *Circulation* 58(II):77, 1978.

Leren, P.: The effect of plasma cholesterol-lowering diet in male survivors of myocardial infarction. *Acta Med. Scand.* (Suppl.) 466:1–89, 1966.

Leren, P.: The Oslo diet heart study. *Circulation* 42:937–942, 1970.

Leventhal, H., and Cleary, P.D.: Behavioral modification of risk factors: technology or science? in M.L. Pollock and D.H. Schmidt, editors, *Heart Disease and Rehabilitation.* Boston: Houghton Mifflin, 1979, p. 297–313.

Liu, K., Stamler, J., Dyer, A., McKeever, J., and McKeever, P.: Statistical methods to asess and minimize the role of intra-individual variability in obscuring the relationship between dietary lipids and serum cholesterol. *J. Chron. Dis* 31:399–418, 1978.

Mahley, R.W., Weisgraber, K.H., Bersof, T.P., and Innerarity, T.L.: Effects of cholesterol feeding on human and animal high density lipoproteins, in A.M. Gotto, N.E. Miller, and M.F. Oliver, editors, *High Density Lipoproteins and Atherosclerosis.* Amsterdam: Elsevier-North Holland, 1978, pp. 149–176.

Mann, J.I., and Truswell, A.S.: Effects of isocaloric exchange of dietary sucrose and starch on fasting serum lipids, postprandial insulin secretion and alimentary lipemia in human subjects. *Br. J. Nutr.* 27:395, 1972.

Mann, G.V.: The influence of obesity on health. *N. Engl. J. Med.* 291:178–185, 226–232, 1974.

Mann, G.: Current concepts. Diet-heart: End of an era. *N. Engl. J. Med.* 297:644–650, 1977.

Mattson, F.H., Erickson, B.A., and Kligman, A.M.: Effect of dietary cholesterol on serum cholesterol in man. *Am. J. Clin. Nutr.* 25:589–594, 1972.

Merz, W.: Effect of dietary components on lipids and lipoproteins—mineral elements, in R.I. Levy, B.M. Rifkind, B.H. Dennis, and N. Ernst, editors, *Nutrition, Lipids, and Coronary Heart Disease.* New York: Raven Press, 1979, p. 175.

Miller, G.J., and Miller, N.E.: Plasma high-density lipoprotein concentration and development of ischemic heart disease. *Lancet* 1:16, 1975.

Miller, N.E., Forde, O.H., Thelle, D.S., and Mjos, O.D.: The Tromso Heart Study. *Lancet* 1:965–968, 1977.

McGee, D., and Gordon, T.: The Framingham Study—an epidemiological investigation of cardiovascular disease. Section 31. The results of the Framingham Study applied to four other U.S.-based epidemiologic studies of cardiovascular disease. Washington, D.C.: DHEW, Publication No. (NIH), 76-1083, 1976.

McGill, H.C. Jr., editor: *Geographic Pathology of Atherosclerosis,* Baltimore: Williams and Wilkins, 1968.

McGill, H.: The relationship of dietary cholesterol to serum cholestrol concentration and to atherosclerosis in man. *Am. J. Clin. Nutr.* 32:2664, 1979.

McMichael, J.: Fats and atheroma: an inquest. *Br. Med. J.* 1(6151):173–175, 1979.

Multiple Risk Factor Intervention Trial (MRFIT): A national study of primary prevention of coronary heart disease. *JAMA* 235:825, 1976.

National Diet–Heart Study Final Report, National Diet Heart Study Research Group. *Circulation* 37 (Suppl. I):1–419, 1968.

New York Academy of Sciences: Lipoprotein structure. *Ann. N.Y. Acad. Sci.* (in press), 1980.

Nichols, A.B., Ravenscroft, C., Lamphiear, D.E., and Ostrander, L.D.: Independence of serum lipid levels and dietary habits. The Tecumseh Study. *JAMA* 236:1948–1953, 1976.

Nikkila, E.A., Viikinkoski, P., and Valle, M.: Effect of lipid lowering treatment on progression of coronary atherosclerosis assessed by angiography (abstr.). *Circulation* 58:11–50, 1978.

Oliver, M.: Coronary heart disease in Edinburgh and Stockholm. Presented at Fifth International Symposium on Atherosclerosis, Nov. 6–9, 1979, Houston, Tex.

Phillips, R., Lemon, F., and Kuzma, J.: Coronary heart disease mortality among Seventh-Day Adventists with differing dietary habits—a preliminary report. *Am. J. Clin. Nutr.* 31(Suppl.):S191–S198, 1978.

Pick, R., Johnson, P.J., and Glick, G.: Deleterious effects of hypertension on the development of aortic and coronary atherosclerosis in stumptail macaques (Macaca Irus) on the atherogenic diet. *Circ. Res.* 35:472, 1974.

Pooling Project Research Group: Relationship of blood pressure, serum cholesterol, smoking habit, relative weight and ECG abnormalities to incidence of major coronary events. *J. Chron. Dis.* 31:201–206, 1978.

Preventing Disease/Promoting Health: Drafts of working papers by participants in a public conference held in Atlanta, Ga., June 13–14, 1979. DHEW. U.S. Government Printing Office: 1979-644-770, p. 95.

Puska, P., Tuomilehto, J., Nissinen, A., Salonen, J., Maki, J., and Pallonen, U.: Changing the cardiovascular risk in an entire community: The North Karelia Project, in *Childhood Prevention of Atherosclerosis and Hypertension.* New York: Raven Press, 1980, p. 441.

Report of the Advisory Committee to the Surgeon General of the Public Health Service: Smoking and Health. Washington, D.C.: DHEW, Public Health Service Publ. No. 1103, 1964.

Report of Inter-Society Commission for Heart Disease Resources: Primary prevention of the atherosclerotic diseases. *Circulation* 42:A55, 1970.

Research Committee of the Scottish Society of Physicians: Ischemic heart disease: A secondary prevention trial using clofibrate. *Br. Med. J.* 4:775–784, 1971.

Rinzler, S.H.: Primary prevention of coronary heart disease by diet. *Bull. N.Y. Acad. Med.* 44:936, 1968.

Robertson, T.L., Kato, H., Rhoads, G.G., Kagan, A., Marmot, M., Syme, S.L., Gordon, T., Worth, R.M., Belsky, J.L., Dock, D.S., Myanishi, M., and Kawamoto, S.: Incidence of myocardial infarction and death from coronary heart disease. *Am. J. Cardiol.* 39:239–243, 1977a.

Robertson, T.L., Kato, H., Gordon, T., Kagan, A., Rhoads, G.G., Land, C.E., Worth, R.M., Belsky, J.L., Dock, D.S., Myanishi, M., and Kawamoto, S.: Epidemiologic studies of coronary heart disease and stroke in Japanese men living in Japan, Hawaii, and California. Coronary heart disease risk factors in Japan and Hawaii. *Am. J. Cardiol.* 39:244–249, 1977b.

Rose, G., and Shipley, M.J.: Plasma lipids and mortality: A source of error. *Lancet* 1:523–526, 1980.

Ross, R., Glomset, J., Kariya, B., et al.: A platelet-dependent serum factor that stimulates the proliferation of arterial smooth muscle cells in vitro. *Proc. Natl. Acad. Sci.* 71:1207–1210, 1974.

Ross, R., and Harker, L.: Hyperlipidemia and atherosclerosis. *Science* 193:1094–1100, 1976.

Roth, H.P., and Mehlman, M.A., editors: Proceedings of the symposium on Role of Dietary Fiber in Health. *Am. J. Clin. Nutr.* 31 (10 Suppl.):S1–S291, 1978.

Sacks, F.M., Castelli, W.P., Donner, A., and Kass, E.H.: Plasma lipids and lipoproteins in vegetarians and controls. *N. Engl. J. Med.* 292:1148–1151, 1975.

Schaefer, E.J., Eisenberg, S., and Levy, R.I.: Lipoprotein apoprotein metabolism. *J. Lipid Res.* 19:667–687, 1978.

Shank, R.E.: Nutrition in relation to other aspects of cardiovascular disease, in R.I. Levy, B., Rifkind, B. Dennis, and N. Ernst, editors, *Nutrition, Lipids, and Coronary Heart Disease.* New York: Raven Press, 1979, pp. 523–553.

Shepherd, J., Packard, C.J., Patsch, J.R., Gotto, A.M., and Taunton, O.D.: Effects of nicotinic acid therapy on plasma high density lipoprotein subfraction distribution and composition and on apolipoprotein A metabolism. *J. Clin. Invest.* 63:858–867, 1979.

Siess, W., Scherer, B., Bohlig, B., Roth, P., Kurzmann, I., and Weber, P.C.: Platelet-membrane fatty acids, platelet aggregation, and thromboxane formation during a mackerel diet. *Lancet* I:441–444, 1980.

Sinzinger, H., Clopath, P., Silberbauer, K., and Auerswald, W.: Prostacyclin synthesis in human and experimental atherosclerosis. *Atherosclerosis* 34:345–347, 1979.

Sirtori, C.R., Agradi, E., Conti, F., Mantero, O., and Gatti, E.: Soybean protein diet in the treatment of type II hyperlipoproteinemia. *Lancet* 1:275–278, 1977.

Stamler, J.: Acute myocardial infarction—progress in primary prevention. *Br. Heart J.* 33 (Suppl.):145–164, 1971.

Stamler, J.: Lifestyles, major risk factors, proof and public policy. *Circulation* 58:1–19, 1976a.

Stamler, J.: Introduction to risk factors in coronary artery disease, in H.D. McIntosh, editor, *Baylor College of Medicine Cardiology Series*, Vol. I, Part III. Northfield, Ill.: Medical Communications, Inc., 1976b.

Stamler, J.: Research related to risk factors. *Circulation* 60:1575, 1979a.

Stamler, J.: Population studies, in R.I. Levy, B. Rifkind, B. Dennis, and N. Ernst, editors, *Nutrition, Lipids, and Coronary Heart Disease.* New York: Raven Press, 1979b, pp. 25–28.

Stamler, J.: Primary prevention and lifestyles, in R.M. Lauer and R.B. Shekelle, editors, *Childhood Prevention of Atherosclerosis and Hypertension.* New York: Raven Press, 1980a, p. 3.

Stamler, J.: The fat-modifid diet: its nature, effectiveness, and safety, in R.M. Lauer and R.B. Shekelle, editors, *Childhood Prevention of Atherosclerosis and Hypertension.* New York: Raven Press, 1980b, p. 387.

Stamler, R., and Stamler, J., editors: Asymptomatic hyperglycemia and coronary heart disease. *J. Chron. Dis.* 32:683–837, 1979.

Steinberg, D.: Research related to underlying mechanisms in atherosclerosis. *Circulation* 60:1559, 1979.

Stern, M.P.: The recent decline in ischemic heart disease mortality. *Ann. Intern Med.* 91:630–640, 1979.

Strong, J.P.: *Atherosclerosis in Primates.* Basel: Karger, 1976.

Symposium on Alcohol and Cardiovascular Diseases, March 5–6, 1980, San Diego, Calif.

Task Force on Arteriosclerosis of the National Heart and Lung Institute, in *Arteriosclerosis,* Vol. I. Washington, D.C.: DHEW, Public Health Service, DHEW Publication No. (NIH) 72-137, 1971.

Thompson, G., Kilpatrick, D., Oakley, C., Steiner, R., and Myant, R.: Reversal of cholesterol accumulation in familial hypercholesterolemia by long-term plasma exchange (Abstr.). *Circulation* 58(II):181, 1978.

Truswell, A.S.: Diet and plasma lipids—a reappraisal. *Am. J. Clin. Nutri.* 31:977–989, 1978.

Turpeinen, O.: Effect of cholesterol-lowering diet on mortality from coronary heart disease and other causes. *Circulation* 59:1, 1979.

U.S. Department of Health, Education, and Welfare USDHEW (PHS): Surgeon General's Report on Health Promotion and Disease Prevention, Pub. No. 79–55071. Washington, D.C.: U.S. GPO, 1979.

U.S. Senate Select Committee on Nutrition and Human Needs: Dietary goals for the United States. Washington, D.C.: U.S. GPO, 1977.

Vesselinovitch, G., Wissler, R.W., Hughes, R., and Borensztajn, J.: Reversal of advanced atherosclerosis in rhesus monkeys. I. Light-microscopic studies. *Atherosclerosis* 23:155–176, 1976.

Wagner, W.D., and Clarkson, T.B.: Comparative primate atherosclerosis. II. A biochemical study of lipids, calcium, and collagen in atherosclerotic arteries. *Exp. Mol. Pathol.* 23:96–121, 1975.

Wilbur, C.S., Zifferblatt, S.M., Tillotson, J.L., and Raab, C.: Putting good nutrition counseling into practice. National Heart, Lung and Blood Institute Publication (in press), 1980.

Wilson, D.E., and Lees, R.S.: Metabolic relationships among the plasma lipoproteins. Reciprocal changes in the concentrations of very low density lipoproteins in man. *J. Clin. Invest.* 51:1051, 1972.

Wissler, R.W., and Vesselinovitch, D.: The effects of feeding various dietary fats on the development and regression of hypercholesterolemia and atherosclerosis, in C. Sirtori, G. Ricci, and S. Gorin, editors, *Diet and Atherosclerosis*. New York: Plenum Press, 1975, p. 65.

Wissler, R.W., Chairman: Laboratory-Experimental Section, Conference on the Health Effects of Blood Lipids. *Prev. Med.* 8:715–732, 1979.

Wood, P.D., and Haskell, W.L.: The effect of exercise on plasma high density lipoproteins. *Lipids* 14:417–427, 1979.

World Health Organization European Collaborative Group: An international controlled trial in the multifactorial prevention of coronary heart disease. *Int. J. Epidemiol.* 3:219, 1974.

World Health Organization: *World Health Statistics Annual 1973. Volume I: Vital Statistics and Causes of Death.* Geneva: WHO, 1976.

Wynder, E.L., Chairman: Conference on the Health Effects of Blood Lipids: Optimal distribution for populations. *Prev. Med.* 8:609–759, 1979.

Yano, K., Rhoads, G.G., and Kagan, A.: Coffee, alcohol, and risk of coronary heart disease among Japanese men living in Hawaii. *N. Engl. J. Med.* 297:405, 1977.

Yudkin, J.: Diet and coronary thrombosis—hypothesis and fact. *Lancet* 2:155–162, 1957.

Zifferblatt, S.M., and Wilbur, C.S.: Dietary counseling: Some realistic expectations and guidelines. *J. Am. Diet. Assoc.* 70:591–595, 1977a.

Zifferblatt, S. M., and Wilbur, C.S.: Maintaining a healthy heart: Guidelines for a feasible goal. *Prev. Med.* 6:514–525, 1977b.

CHAPTER 6

Cigarette Smoking among Children and Adolescents: Causes and Prevention

GILBERT BOTVIN, PH.D.   ALFRED MCALISTER, PH.D.

Health Consequences

A vast and ever-growing literature of clinical, experimental, pathological, and epidemiological studies has provided compelling evidence of the negative health consequences of cigarette smoking. Much of this evidence is summarized in the recent Surgeon General's Report (USPHS, 1979). Cigarette smoking has been associated with a number of chronic diseases including cardiovascular disease, various cancers, chronic obstructive lung disease, and peptic ulcers. On the average, smokers have a 70 percent greater risk of mortality than nonsmokers and there is a direct relationship between the number of years they have been smoking and the extent of their risk.

Although the morbid or fatal consequences of smoking may not emerge until later in life, there is growing evidence that the health effects of smoking evolve over a lifetime. Autopsy studies have indicated, for example, that smoking is associated with more severe and extensive atherosclerosis of the aorta and coronary arteries. Moreover, a number of scientific questions have been raised concerning the effects of smoking on the severity of atherosclerosis in childhood and adolescence and the premature development of adult forms of these lesions. Clinical, experimental, pathological, and epidemiological studies in humans and animals demonstrate that smoking produces measurable lung damage in the very young. Young cigarette smokers, even those without respiratory symptoms, have evidence of small airway dysfunction more frequently than nonsmokers. Young smokers also have a higher prevalence of regular coughing, phlegm production, wheezing, and other respiratory symptoms than their nonsmoking peers.

Prevalence and Current Trends

In recent years cigarette smoking has declined among the adult population to a current level of about 33 percent. Yet cigarette smoking continues to be a significant problem among children and adolescents. According to a recent national survey, about 12 percent of teenagers between the ages of 12 and 18 are regular cigarette smokers (DHEW, 1979). This represents about a 3 percent reduction from the 1974 level of 15 percent. Smoking has decreased since 1974 in all age groups except for women in the 17- to 18-year-old category, for whom smoking remains about the same (26 percent). Furthermore, smoking has increased among women in the 17- to 24-year-old category, and now exceeds that of males.

Need for Prevention

Based on the existing evidence, few people would dispute the fact that cigarette smoking seriously jeopardizes the health and well-being of the smoker. However, while estimates indicate that the majority of current smokers would like to quit, few of these efforts have been successful (Gallup, 1974). Recent reviews of the smoking cessation literature have indicated that once the smoking habit is firmly established, it is extremely difficult to break (Bernstein, 1969; Bernstein and McAlister, 1976; Lichtenstein and Danaher, 1976; Schwartz, 1969). A logical alternative to smoking cessation, naturally, would involve preventing individuals from becoming cigarette smokers. However, it is only through an understanding of the factors involved in promoting the onset of cigarette smoking that successful approaches to prevention can be formulated. Therefore, before going on to review some of the strategies used to attempt to prevent the onset of cigarette smoking, we shall breifly outline some of the major factors which appear to play a role in smoking onset and describe the process of becoming an habitual cigarette smoker.

DEVELOPMENT OF THE SMOKING HABIT

The initiation and development of tobacco use is predominantly an adolescent phenomenon which begins in the early teens, increases in the middle teens, and levels off by the late teens (McKennell, 1968).

Although smoking begins innocuously enough as part of the adolescent's social rites of passage, for all too many teenagers early experimentation is just the first step in a gradual but inexorable process that ultimately leads to regular habitual cigarette smoking. For the most part, regular smoking does not begin until midadolescence (Matarazzo and Matarazzo, 1968). Experimentation, on the other hand, may begin much earlier. In a recent study approximately 20 percent of the individuals surveyed had their first cigarette before the age of 12 and 6 percent had their first cigarette before the age of 10 (Botvin, Eng, and Williams, 1978). Generally, if one has not become a cigarette smoker by age 20, he or she is likely to remain a nonsmoker for life (McKennell, 1968).

Whatever the reasons for becoming a cigarette smoker, there appear to be three discrete states in the acquisition of the smoking habit. For most smokers, the first stage habit involves experimentation within social groups. at this stage of smoking adolescents smoke almost exclusively with their friends and, in general, solitary smoking is relatively infrequent (Palmer, 1970). During the next stage, the neophyte smoker continues smoking within a social setting but also begins to smoke alone. At this stage the smoker appears to begin deriving some physiological gratification from tobacco so that it is no longer merely the act of smoking that is reinforcing but also the nicotine and other properties of the tobacco. This appears to be the transition from being an experimenter to being an habitual smoker. The adolescent at this point seems to be well on the way to becoming a regular smoker, although the pattern of smoking may still be somewhat sporadic.

After about three or four years of occasional smoking, regular adult-type smoking occurs (Russell, 1974). The smoking pattern may vary from light (fewer than ten cigarettes per day) to heavy (over 40 cigarettes per day). At this point the smoker has acquired the smoking habit and, in the view of some researchers, may be both psychologically and physiologically dependent on tobacco (Russell, 1974). Overall, the development of the smoking habit and the general pattern of tobacco use is strikingly similar to that associated with other forms of tolerance leading to increased dosages and a desire for repeated administrations and ultimately psychological dependence (Bradshaw, 1973).

FACTORS ASSOCIATED WITH TOBACCO USE

What are the factors promoting the acquisition of the smoking habit?

Are some people more likely to become cigarette smokers than others? Is there a single etiologic pathway to chronic cigarette smoking? Numerous researchers have attempted to answer these and other questions regarding the causes underlying the development of the smoking habit. With few exceptions, these researchers have employed a single methodology which has involved the comparison of smokers and nonsmokers in terms of one or more variables. The basic premise of studies cast in this mold is that if it were possible to discriminate accurately between smokers and nonsmokers on the basis of a given variable or cluster of variables then it could be inferred that this variable or variables played a major role in the etiology of the smoking habit. Below we shall briefly summarize some of the variables that have been found to be associated with cigarette smoking. In general, these variables fall into four categories: sociodemographic variables, personality variables, behavioral variables, and cognitive/attitudinal variables.

Sociodemographic Variables

A number of researchers have noted an association between a variety of sociodemographic variables and smoking behavior. Of these, the most frequently observed variables include the smoking status of family and friends, parental attitudes toward smoking, and socioeconomic status.

Smoking Status of Family Members. One of the earliest influences on the young smoker comes from his parents. This influence generally takes the form of parent modeling, although parental attitudes toward smoking may also affect an individual's decision to smoke (Thomas and Wake, 1969). One of the most consistently observed differences between smokers and nonsmokers is that smokers generally have at least one parent who smokes (Borland and Rudolph, 1975; Levitt and Edwards, 1969; Newman, 1971; Williams, 1973; Wohlford, 1970). Not surprisingly, if both parents smoke the child is more likely to smoke than if only one parent smokes (DHEW, 1976). While either parent may exert an influence on a child's smoking (or nonsmoking) behavior, the same-sex parent appears to be somewhat more influential (Bewley, Bland, and Harris, 1974; Wohlford, 1970). That is, a girl is more likely to smoke if her mother smokes, and a boy is more likely to smoke if his father smokes.

Other family variables have been found to be associated with smoking behavior in a child or adolescent. For example, children living in single parent homes are much more likely to smoke than those living in homes with both parents (DHEW, 1976). Also, individuals having older siblings who smoke are more likely to smoke, and individuals from families in which both a parent and an older sibling smoke are four times as likely to smoke as those from families where no one smokes (DHEW, 1976).

Furthermore, parental approval may also be an important determinant of an adolescent's smoking status. One study indicated that 11 percent of the smokers surveyed had been given their first cigarette by a parent (Botvin et al., 1978). Conversely, in cases where parents clearly disapprove of their children smoking, the children smoked much less frequently than children whose parents had more tolerant attitudes toward smoking (McRae and Nelson, 1971). Similarly, children whose parents were ex-smokers (and presumably had strong anti-smoking attitudes) have been found to be even less likely to smoke than children whose parents never smoked (Thomas and Wake, 1969).

In summary, a variety of family variables appear to influence the decision to smoke. The greater the number of these variables, the more likely a child is to become a smoker. Overall, these findings are consistent with those regarding the use of a variety of other substances. For example, in the case of alcohol, drinkers also tend to have parents who drink (Braucht et al., 1973). Furthermore, other studies have shown that there is tendency for members of the same family to use the same drug (Annis, 1974).

Smoking Status of Friends. Perhaps the strongest relationship between a sociocultural variable and smoking status concerns the smoker's peer or reference group. Countless studies have noted that most smokers have friends who smoke (Bewley and Bland, 1977; Bewley et al., 1974; Eisinger, 1971; Foss, 1973; Horn and Waingrow, 1966; Jessor, Carman, and Grossman, 1968; McKennell, 1968). In a 1974 survey, 87 percent of the teenage smokers indicated that at least one of their best friends was a regular smoker (DHEW, 1976). There also appears to be a direct relationship between the number of friends individuals have who smoke and the likelihood that they too will smoke. In other words, the more friends individuals have who smoke, the more likely they are also to smoke (McKennell, 1969; McRae and Nelson, 1971). On the other hand, nonsmokers and exsmokers tend to have fewer friends who smoke than smokers (McKennell, 1969).

Although the precise reason for the relationship between individuals' smoking status and that of their friends is not known, it has been suggested that an individual's peer or reference group maintains and enforces conformity to group norms and standards regarding a variety of behaviors which may or may not include smoking (DHEW, 1976). An alternative explanation suggests that individuals may simply choose friends who are similar to themselves along a variety of dimensions (Reeder, 1977). Thus, it may *not* be that peers influence teenagers to smoke; rather, smokers may merely tend to associate with other smokers because of perceived commonalities and mutually accepted values.

One argument for the former explanation comes from the observation that changes in the smoking habits of the members of individuals' reference group are frequently accompanied by a corresponding change in their smoking behavior. For example, in one study ex-smokers reported that 78 percent of their friends smoked when they started but that at the time of the survey only 20 percent of their friends were smokers (Eisinger, 1971).

Socioeconomic Status. Another sociodemographic variable found to differentiate between smokers and nonsmokers concerns socioeconomic status (SES). In general, researchers have reported an inverse relationship between SES and smoking behavior among teenagers (Borland and Rudolph, 1975). However, this relationship among adults is somewhat more complex and needs to be qualified. In terms of educational level, there is an inverse relationship between SES and smoking behavior, although this relationship is much less pronounced among families. Yet in terms of both occupational status and income level, there is a divergence between males and females with an inverse relationship among males and a direct relationship among females (DHEW, 1976).

Several variables related to SES have been found to be associated with smoking among teenagers. two of these concern parental education and students' educational aspirations. There is an inverse relationship between both parental education and educational aspirations and smoking status. More specifically, children from homes where one or both parents went to college are less likely to smoke; and children who plan to go to college and are enrolled in college preparatory courses also tend not to smoke (DHEW, 1976). Closely related to educational aspiration is social mobility. For the most part, individuals who are upwardly mobile (i.e., attempting to improve their SES) are less likely to smoke, while downwardly mobile individuals tend to smoke heavily (Clausen, 1968; Srole and Fischer, 1973).

Personality Variables

Relationships between a number of personality variables and smoking have been noted by a great number of investigators. In fact, this appears to be one of the most widely researched areas related to smoking. For convenience, these personality variables have been grouped into two general categories: (1) variables relating to general personality characteristics and (2) variables relating to psychological adjustment.

General Personality Characteristics. Among variables relating to personality, smoking has been correlated with an external locus of control (Williams, 1973), high impulsivity (Fracchia, Sheppard, and Merlis, 1974; Williams, 1973), and an impatience to grow up (Fracchia et al., 1974). However, of these variables, locus of control appears to be the most significant both concerning initial smoking and quitting. Although in general smokers are more externally oriented than nonsmokers, those who eventually quit tend to be somewhat more internally oriented than those who continue to smoke (Foss, 1973; Mlott and Mlott, 1975). Furthermore, adult smokers tend to be more extroverted (Matarazzo and Saslow, 1960; Matarazzo and Matarazzo, 1968; Smith, 1970) and teenage smokers have a stronger peer orientation (Fracchia et al., 1974) than nonsmokers.

Another consistent finding regarding the smoker's personality concerns self-image. Mausner and Platt (1971) have observed the role smoking plays in establishing a sense of identity, and other investigators have suggested that smoking may be an attempt to compensate for a poor self-image (Borland and Rudolph, 1975; Fracchia et al., 1974). Indeed, smoking has been associated with low self-esteem (Newman, 1971) and smokers reportedly view themselves as being inferior to nonsmokers (McKennell, 1968). Similarly, smokers have been found to have a higher degree of self-dissatisfaction (Coan, 1973), and many smokers also have been found to lack social confidence (McKennell, 1969).

Psychological Adjustment. Some studies have attempted to differentiate between smokers and nonsmokers on a variety of measures relating to psychological functioning. For the most part, psychological adjustment has been found to be inversely related to smoking, with individuals who quit somewhere between habitual smokers and nonsmokers (Coan, 1973; Reynolds and Nichols, 1976). Among smokers, those with low smoking frequencies generally cluster closer to the "well" end of the mental health continuum, whereas smokers with higher smoking frequencies fall closer to the "impaired" end (Srole and Fischer, 1973). Smokers have also been reported to be highly anxious (Coan, 1973; Matarazzo and Matarazzo, 1968) and neurotic (Matarazzo and Saslow, 1960; Matarazzo and Matarazzo, 1968; Smith, 1970). And in a study of college students, Cattell and Krug (1967) found that smokers could be differentiated from nonsmokers based on the results of a psychological assessment.

Behavioral Correlates

Smokers and nonsmokers also appear to differ along several behavioral dimensions with specific behaviors being associated with individuals who smoke. These behavioral differences fall into four basic categories: academic performance, leisure activities, antisocial tendencies, and employment.

Academic Performance. Several studies have shown that smokers are less academically successful than their peers (Bewley and Bland, 1977; Borland and Rudolph, 1975; Lieberman Research Inc., 1969; Matarazzo and Saslow, 1960; Newman, 1971). However, since there are no apparent differences between smokers and nonsmokers in terms of intelligence, the differences in academic performance are assumed to reflect a difference in orientation and aspirations.

Leisure Activities. In addition to the smoker's lower involvement scholastically, there is a commensurate lack of participation in extracurricular activities such as sports or clubs (Matarazzo and Matarazzo, 1968; Newman, 1971). In fact, in general, smokers tend to spend their leisure time quite differently than nonsmokers. Smokers are rarely involved in organized activities but, instead, prefer to "hang out" with their friends (DHEW, 1976).

Antisocial Tendencies. Moreover, smokers are frequently characterized as being hostile and having antisocial tendencies. In a study conducted by Reynolds and Nichols (1976), they found that smokers were more likely than nonsmokers to engage in a variety of activities that broadly fall in the category of antisocial activities. Specifically, smokers were more likely to have engaged in fighting, quarrelling, swearing, lying, cutting class, ditching dates, gambling, and drinking. Conversely, they were less likely to have been involved in altruistic or religious activities. Other studies have reported that smokers are frequently disciplinary problems (Newman, 1971). Additionally, smokers are more likely to indulge in risk-taking behaviors (DHEW, 1976).

Work Experience. Another aspect of teenage lifestyle that has been correlated with smoking behavior concerns employment. According to a recent government study, teenagers who work either full- or part-time are twice as likely to be smokers as those who do not work (DHEW, 1976). It has been suggested that because of their proximity to adults in the work environment, teenagers are more likely to experiment with smoking and other adult behaviors.

Attitudes and Beliefs about Smoking

The major premise of traditional smoking education programs has been that there is a relationship between attitudes and beliefs about smoking and smoking status. Thus, if students believed that smoking was dangerous to their health and generally held negative attitudes toward smoking, it was assumed that they would choose not to smoke. To date, the data have not supported this position with respect to knowledge and use. In fact, some research has suggested that the more students know about a particular substance, the more likely they are to use it (Halpern and Whiddon, 1977).

Whether or not this is so, there is a preponderance of evidence demonstrating that the awareness that smoking is a health hazard does not prevent individuals from smoking (Albino and Davis, 1975; James, 1972; Rabinowitz and Zimmerli, 1974). The vast majority of students (estimates range from 94 percent to 99 percent) are aware of the dangers of cigarette smoking; however, many still choose to smoke. Although one recent survey did find that a greater proportion of nonsmokers believed that smoking was dangerous, still 90 percent of the smokers reportedly recognize the health hazard of smoking (DHEW, 1976) and have apparently chosen to ignore this fact.

It has also been suggested that attitudes and beliefs about smoking can (1) differentiate between smokers and nonsmokers and (2) predict future smoking status. To some extent, the results of one two-year longitudinal study support this hypothesis since nonsmokers who remained nonsmokers had stronger anti-smoking attitudes than smokers or nonsmokers who subsequently became smokers (Downey and O'Rourke, 1976). Related research has shown that a shift from a positive attitude concerning the social acceptability of smoking toward a more negative attitude accompanied changes from smoking to nonsmoking behavior (Erickson and Cramer, 1976).

However, while it seems apparent that for the most part there is some sort of relationship between smoking status and attitudes about smoking, it is unclear whether attitudes determine smoking status or smoking status affects attitudes. Unfortunately, the evidence appears to suggest the latter. As a national survey conducted by HEW indicates, most teenagers have no intention of becoming cigarette smokers (DHEW, 1976), yet many of them do. One reason for this may be the fact that students' attitudes toward smoking tend gradually to become less negative as they approach adolescence; and while they are cognizant of the fact that cigarette smoking is a serious health threat, as they get older they begin to take the threat less seriously (Schneider and Vanmastrigt, 1974). Thus, although nearly all elementary school students possess anti-smoking attitudes and beliefs, as they approach adolescence a variety of factors appear to promote a more tolerant disposition toward smoking.

Developmental Variables

In addition to the variables discussed above, a number of factors resulting from the normal course of psychological development appear to play a role in the promotion of cigarette smoking. For the most part, these developmental factors concern changes in children's "moral" orientation, the declining influence of parents and authority figures, and increasing reliance on and conformity to the peer group.

Moral Development. According to Piaget (1932), sometime between the ages of five and twelve (usually around seven or eight) children's moral orientation shifts from a rigid and inflexible notion of right and wrong to one that takes into account a myriad of situational factors. Simply put, children's moral standards gradually become less absolutistic and more flexible and relativistic. With this new orientation children can accept deviations from the established rules and norms and come to recognize that, for example, lying may be justified in certain situations. Furthermore, as children mature they become more autonomous and their moral judgments and conduct become less influenced by parental authority and more the result of their own experience (Kohlberg, 1969). In fact, there is a general decline in the acceptance of authority and in the subordination to adult norms and dictates (Mussen, Conger, and Kagan, 1974).

Sources of Influence. Although during early childhood parents exert the most powerful influence on their children, upon entry into the school environment this influence decreases somewhat and peers and other socializing agents (e.g., teachers) become increasingly important (Mussen et al., 1974). Generally speaking, in the event of a conflict between the advice provided by parents or peers, there is a progressive decline with age concerning compliance with parental advice (Russell, 1974). However, this is not to say that parents are unable to influence their children; quite simply it depends on the area of concern. While peers may be more influential with regard to matters of clothing, music, etc., parents are generally more influential than peers or even best friends concerning areas like career and educational choices. Moreover, there is considerable overlap between the values of parents and peers because of commonalities in their background (Mussen et al., 1974).

Conformity. Increased dependence on the peer group is typically accompanied by a corresponding rise in conformity behavior. Pre-school children are almost totally impervious to pressure to conform (Hartup, 1970), but the tendency to conform to group norms increases during middle childhood (Costanzo and Shaw, 1966; Piaget, 1932). Conformity needs and behavior increase rapidly during pre-adolescence and early adolescence and decline steadily from middle to late adolescence (Mussen et al., 1974). However, despite this general developmental trend toward increased conformity, individual susceptibility may vary greatly. Thus, if the values of the peer group should be in conflict with those held by the child, the child's susceptibility to change will to a large extent depend on the relative importance of peer acceptance. Furthermore, differential susceptibility to conformity pressure has been shown to be a function of sex and personality characteristics. Girls tend to be more conforming to peer group pressure than boys (Maccoby and Masters, 1970); and individuals who are more dependent and anxious (Walters, Marshall, and Shooter, 1960) and who have low self-esteem and high social sensitivity (Hartup, 1970) tend to be more conforming.

SMOKING PREVENTION STRATEGIES

As with adults, it is extremely difficult for most teenagers who smoke regularly to quit. In fact, it may actually be more difficult for teenagers to quit smoking since they are still living in the same environment that led them to smoke in the first place. It is interesting to note in this connection that most young cigarette smokers do not realize the extent to which they are dependent on cigarettes. Unless they have attempted to quit themselves, teenage smokers tend to believe that they can stop whenever they want.

Given the attendant dangers of cigarette smoking and the difficulty of quitting once the habit is acquired, the most propitious approach to the problem of cigarette smoking is prevention. A variety of strategies have been utilized to reduce the number of youth joining the ranks of smokers. The major approaches will be discussed briefly below. This review is not meant to be comprehensive but rather representative of the kind of smoking prevention programs that have been conducted to date.

Smoking Education Programs

By and large, elementary and junior high school anti-smoking programs have been informational in nature. That is, schools or voluntary organizations have developed programs that provide students with factual information concerning the long-term physiological effects of cigarette smoking. The main purpose of these programs has generally been to decrease the incidence of smoking among students by effectuating changes in their knowledge, attitudes, and beliefs about cigarette smoking. The fundamental premise of such programs is that students will choose *not* to smoke if they are well-informed about the harmful effects of cigarette smoking.

Some of these programs have been targeted at elementary school students. One such program contained a series of modules designed to teach students information about good health (Albino and Davis, 1975). Other programs have been developed primarily for junior high school students. These programs generally include a strong anti-smoking component within the context of a more general health education curriculum (Rabinowitz and Zimmerli, 1974). Furthermore, voluntary organizations such as the American Cancer Society have supported the anti-smoking efforts of teachers by providing a variety of pamphlets, posters, and films.

In contrast to the relatively passive role of students participating in the majority of programs, some anti-smoking programs have attempted to involve students more actively in both the organization and administration of these programs. In some programs student involvement has taken the form of organizing movies, poster contests, and other anti-smoking activities (Grigson, 1970), while other programs have recruited older peers to talk with younger students in an attempt to dissuade them from becoming smokers (Harnett, 1973; Rosner, 1974). The assumption of the latter approach has been that students would be more receptive to anti-smoking messages from peers than they would be to similar messages from teachers or other authority figures. Unfortunately, the majority of the peer leadership programs have failed to include an evaluation component, making it impossible to determine the effectiveness of student-led programs for preventing the onset of cigarette smoking.

Given the power and complexity of the factors promoting tobacco use, it is not surprising that programs which focus on education regarding the health effects of smoking and aimed at primary grade students not yet exposed to smoking pressure do not appear to have much effect on eventual smoking behavior. Data on the few intervention programs which have been evaluated are well-reviewed by Evans and co-workers (1979) and Thompson (1978). Strictly health-related education is clearly necessary to prepare the young person with reasons for not smoking but, as one of the originators of the "Berkeley Project" has agreed (Foster, 1976), it requires carefully designed supplementary intervention to provide a sophisticated counter to the strong social influences encountered during early adolescence. Almost all elementary school students will state that they do not want to start smoking, but they may not be equipped to resist social pressure toward smoking, and thus may not be able to fulfill that intention as they enter the teen years.

Psychosocial Prevention Strategies

More recently, several different groups have developed and tested prevention strategies that focus primary attention on the psychosocial factors promoting cigarette smoking. A feature shared by all these strategies involves making students aware of the various social pressures to smoke and teaching them how to cope with these effectively. In all of these programs there is an attempt to teach students techniques for resisting peer pressure to smoke. However, these programs differ in terms of the way in which this is accomplished and the extent to which coping with peer pressure is emphasized.

Psychological Inoculation. Pioneering work in the development and testing of a strategy for countering social influences to smoke has been conducted by Evans and his students and colleagues at the University of Houston and the Baylor School of Medicine (Evans, 1976; Evans et al., 1978). Part of Evans' work is based on the theory of psychological "inoculation" as originated by McGuire (1964, 1972). The concept of psychological inoculation is analogous to the concept of inoculation in traditional preventive medicine. The idea is that if an individual is expected to encounter the cultural analogue of "germs" (i.e., social pressures toward adoption of a behavior detrimental to health), then "infection" can be prevented by exposing the person to a weak dose of those "germs" in a way that facilitates the development of "antibodies" (i.e., skills for resisting pressures toward adoption of unhealthy behaviors).

The applicability of the concept of inoculation as a way of intervening in the smoking adoption process is fairly straightforward. If youngsters are likely to be called "chicken" for refusing to try cigarettes, they can be forewarned of pressures of that sort and provided with the necessary skills to counter those pressures. For example, they can be trained to reply: "If I smoke to prove to you that I'm not a chicken, all I'll really be showing is that I'm afraid not to do what you want me to do. I don't want to smoke." If young people are likely to see older youth posturing and acting "tough" by smoking, they can be taught to think to themselves: "If they were really 'tough,' they wouldn't have to smoke to prove it."

Evans' research has also involved intervention components which provide students with feedback concerning the rate of smoking among their peers and communicate immediate physiological effects of smoking (Evans et al., 1978; Evans, Hansen, and Mittelmark, 1977). Every two weeks, students are required to submit saliva samples along with self-reports (questionnaires) of smoking. Before the first administration of the questionnaires, students are shown a film illustrating how their smoking can be detected from the saliva sample. Since the saliva assay is too expensive to analyze more than a few samples, the students are shown the film prior to completing the questionnaire in order to improve the validity of their self-reports. The students' samples and self-reports are identified by code numbers. Although no individual feedback is actually given to parents or school authorities, the proportion of self-reported smokers in each classroom is publicly announced as objective data at frequent intervals.

Evans' group has conducted a well-designed pilot test of these interventions, comparing monitoring/feedback and monitoring/feedback plus inoculation to a control group (Evans et al., 1978). The results show that monitoring reduces onset rates of experimental smoking to roughly half of that observed in the control group during the first two-and-a-half months of the school year in a seventh grade study population. Disappointingly, however, the inoculation treatment produced no additional reduction in the onset of experimentation with tobacco.

There are several reasons why the way that the inoculation procedure was conducted would make it less than optimally effective. First, films may be only inattentively viewed by adolescents in a classroom setting. Second, the fact that the films are presented by adults working

in concert with school authorities and are followed by teacher-led discussion may reduce their influence among the young people who are
most likely to start smoking, i.e., those who are seeking ways to assert
their independence from adult authorities. These young people may
tend to express hostility toward even the most well-intentioned teachers and may reject the inoculation films simply because of their source.
Finally, films followed by discussions do not provide opportunities for
the kind of guided practice and role-playing which is most effective in
promoting skill acquisition (Bandura, 1977). Without actual practice,
young people may be somewhat uncertain and hesitant about applying
the pressure-resistance tactics displayed in the films.

Psychological Inoculation and Training. Studies begun at the Stanford University School of Medicine and continuing there and at the
Harvard University School of Public Health are exploring a somewhat
more intensive approach to applying the concept of inoculation to the
prevention of smoking and other behaviors detrimental to health (Mc-
Alister, Perry, and Maccoby, 1979). The distinctive features of this
work are (1) the employment of older young people (*peer leaders*) as
the primary agents delivering the intervention and (2) the use of role-
playing and other techniques to enhance the learning of pressure-
resistance skills. These ideas have been suggested in recent publications by Hartup and Louge (1975) and Bandura (1977).

It is well known that during early adolescence, peers tend to over-
take adults as sources of influence. Peer teaching has become recognized as a highly effective way for stimulating poorly motivated
learners (Vriend, 1969), and peer teaching teams have been formed as
a way of efficiently providing more traditional health education to
large numbers of elementary school children (McRae and Nelson,
1971). Peer counseling, in which young people are trained to help
peers seeking advice on how to handle personal problems, has also
been successfully applied in several settings (Hamburg and Varenhorst, 1972; Alwine, 1974). The "teen-challenge" or "mod squad"
approach to drug abuse prevention was in vogue in recent years, but
beyond the Stanford and Harvard studies referred to here, no serious
research has been conducted to determine how this approach can be
employed to apply the concept of inoculation to the prevention of
smoking and other behaviors detrimental to health.

Other techniques and theories that are being systematically employed in this work include elicitation of a public commitment not to
smoke (Kiesler, Collins, and Miller, 1969) and induction of reactance
(Brehm, 1966) against predictions that many young people will start
smoking whether they want to or not. Behavioral training to resist

specific pressures to smoke utilized procedures systematized by Bandura (1977).

Over the course of a year of intensive development and pretesting, a seven-session peer leadership curriculum designed for implementation in sixth or seventh grade classrooms has been developed. The first session is aimed at strengthening the students' commitment not to become dependent on tobacco and demonstrating the overt and subtle social influences which favor smoking. During the second session, verbal or cognitive responses appropriate to various pressures (e.g., advertising, dares from friends) are demonstrated and students are encouraged to develop and present their own ideas on how to handle those situations. For example, students learn to respond to advertisements depicting women smokers as "liberated" by thinking: "She's not really independent if she's hooked on tobacco." During the third session students create skits in which they role-play verbal responses to various inducements to smoke. For example, when called "chicken" for not accepting a cigarette, they learn to respond by saying: "I would be a chicken if I smoked just to impress you." Subsequent sessions are essentially "boosters" in which activities from previous sessions are repeated in variations. The first three sessions occur on subsequent days during the first month of school, with the remaining four spread out during the year.

Peer leaders implementing the program are recruited from a nearby high school by a popular teacher on the basis of their communication skills and judged attractiveness to the kind of young people who are likely to start smoking—"Fonzie" or "Modsquad" types who are adventurous and unconventional but not unhealthy in their behavior. They are trained in a series of three two-hour sessions of demonstration and guided practice. Selection of the popular teacher to coordinate the program is according to a recommendation from the school's principal. Selection of the peer leaders is purely by subjective judgment on the basis of the quality and appropriateness of their written answer to a question about their reasons for volunteering for the program and feelings about how they can contribute to it.

The peer leadership curriculum is intended to be a part of regular school-sponsored, educational activities, rather than an externally administered intervention. Since it is designed to provide a positive but noncoercive counter to social pressures toward smoking and uses methods created to help young people become more independent and assertive, school officials are more than willing to sponsor the program. With the school itself accepting responsibility for the voluntary experimental activities, the issue of informed consent is not critical. However, parents are notified of the program and given the opportunity to withdraw their children.

The effectiveness of this type of intervention was assessed in a pilot experiment near San Jose, California, conducted during the 1977–1978 school year. One school served as a control, while another received the experimental program. The two schools served middle- and upper-middle-class populations and their baseline rates of smoking were nearly identical. The percent of students who reported that one or more of their parents smoked was approximately 42 percent in both schools. Students in the control school seemed initially less likely to start smoking, as they had been exposed to intensive primary grade health education (School Health Curriculum Project) (Edson, 1973). The principal of the control school expressed the view that few students smoked in this school, whereas the principal of the treatment school considered smoking to be a problem. Both schools had identical rules and disciplinary procedures regarding smoking and their enforcement was equally stringent in both. More infractions had been observed in the treatment school in the year preceding our pilot study.

A baseline and two follow-up surveys were supplemented with random samplings of exhaled breath conducted in a method that was similar to Evans' procedure for increasing self-report accuracy (1977) except that anonymity was insured in order to reduce perceived threat of individual monitoring and to help respondents feel safe in providing truthful answers. Over two years of study, students in the school which received the experimental program began smoking at less than half the rate of those in the comparison school. Moreover, fewer frequent alcohol and marijuana users were found at follow-up in the program school.

These encouraging data suggest that a useful way of applying the inoculation strategy may indeed have been formulated. In fact, intensive interviews with a few of the 11- and 12-year-olds who participated in the study indicate that the intervention may have influenced the entire "social atmosphere" regarding smoking. The students report that "hardly anybody smokes now" and this "it's not 'cool' to smoke any more." Evidently cigarette use is no longer viewed as an effective way of appearing "tough" or "cool" among the young people who were exposed to the intensive peer leadership program. The school principal also thinks that the program worked and reports that not a single seventh grader has been caught smoking, although many older students (not exposed to the program) have been, and many seventh graders were found smoking during the previous year.

Broad-Spectrum Intervention. A third smoking prevention strategy called Life Skills Training (LST) was developed and tested in New

York at the American Health Foundation. Although in some respects similar to the above strategies, the notion of inoculation is not the only aspect of this approach. Instead, this prevention strategy is based on a model of smoking onset that emphasizes the interaction of environmental (social) and personal factors. According to this model, cigarette smoking is promoted by pro-smoking social influences, with specific individual characteristics determining the extent to which one is susceptible to these influences. Social pressures to smoke may come from family members, peers, and the media. However, *not all individuals are equally susceptible to these social influences*. Researchers have noted that certain psychological characteristics of individuals determine the extent to which they are susceptible to social influence (Bandura, 1969; Rotter, 1972; Tedeschi and Bonoma, 1972). Interestingly enough, some of these same characteristics have been associated with cigarette smoking (e.g., an external locus of control, a low self-esteem, a lack of self-confidence, and anxiety).

The main thrust of the LST program is to increase students' resistance to the various pro-smoking social influences. In more specific terms, the LST program is designed: (1) to provide students with the requisite knowledge, skills, and awareness to deal with direct pressures to smoke (e.g., peer pressure); (2) to decrease their general susceptibility to indirect social influences (e.g., the desire to emulate attractive models) by increasing their sense of self-mastery, self-esteem, self-confidence, independence, and autonomy; (3) to enable them to cope effectively with anxiety, particularly that induced by social situations; and, to a lesser extent, (4) to increase students' knowledge of the immediate consequences of smoking.

Thus, the LST approach is designed to focus in a comprehensive fashion on the key determinants of smoking onset, with primary attention given to the social and psychological factors believed to influence teenagers to smoke. Students participating in the program meet weekly for approximately three months. The main emphasis of the program is on the acquisition of basic life skills relevant to the problems and concerns of teenagers. The program utilizes a combination of lecture, discussion, demonstration, and role-playing and includes sessions on self-image and self-improvement, decision-making and independent thinking, advertising techniques, coping with anxiety, communication skills, social skills, assertiveness training as well as myths and realities about cigarette smoking. Table 6-1 provides a brief description of each session. A more complete description of each session is provided elsewhere (Botvin and Eng, 1979).

An integral part of the program involves participation in a self-

Table 6-1
Description of Life Skills Training Program

Session	Material Covered
Orientation	General introduction to the program; administration of pretest questionnaire; overview of forthcoming sessions.
Smoking: Myths and Realities	Common attitudes and beliefs about smoking; prevalence of smoking, reasons for and against smoking, the process of becoming an addicted smoker, and the decreasing social acceptability of smoking.
Self-Image and Self-Improvement	Self-image and how it is formed, the relationship between self-image and behavior, the importance of positive self-image, and ways of improving self-image.
Decision Making and Independent Thinking	A general decision making strategy; decision making and sources of influence affecting decisions, resisting persuasive tactics, and the importance of independent thinking.
Advertising Techniques	Use and function of advertising, ad techniques, identifying ad techniques used in cigarette advertising and how they are designed to affect consumer behavior, alternative ways of responding to these ads.
Coping with Anxiety	Situations causing anxiety, demonstration and practice of techniques for coping with anxiety.
Communication Skills	Verbal and nonverbal communication, techniques for avoiding misunderstandings, basic conversational skills, giving and receiving compliments, making introductions, etc.
Dating Skills	Boy-girl relationships, conversing with the opposite sex, the nature of attraction, asking or being asked out for a date.
Assertiveness	Difference between assertion and aggression, standing up for one's rights, common situations calling for an assertive response, reasons for not being assertive, responding to peer pressures to smoke.
Conclusion	Brief review, conclusions, posttest.

improvement project which is designed to be completed by the end of the program. Students are asked to select a personal skill or behavior that they would like to change, decide on a realistic long-term goal, and work in a systematic fashion toward achieving that goal. Progress is evaluated weekly to enable students to gradually shape their own behavior and chart their progress. Furthermore, students are expected to complete "homework" assignments (written or behavioral) in order to prepare them for the next session or to reinforce material already covered.

Two studies employing the LST strategy have been conducted over the past two years. Both studies randomly assigned schools to treatment conditions, and in both studies experimental and control schools were comparable with respect to SES and smoking prevalence. The initial pilot study (Botvin, Eng, and Williams, 1980) involved testing a ten-session version of the LST program. The program was implemented by two outside specialists (a psychologist and health educator) with eighth, ninth, and tenth graders (N = 281). There were significantly fewer students beginning to smoke in the group which had participated in the program than in the control group both at the end of the program (4 percent vs. 16 percent) and at the three month follow-up (6 percent vs. 18 percent).

The second study (Botvin and Eng, 1980) involved testing a 12-session version of the LST program. In addition to the original ten sessions, a session dramatizing the immediate physiological effects of smoking based on the work of the New Hampshire Lung Association (Eckdahl, 1979) was included as well as an additional session on social skills. In this study, 11th and 12th grade peer leaders were trained to conduct the LST program with seventh graders (N = 426). Furthermore, saliva samples were collected prior to administration of the self-report questionnaire in a variant of the "bogus pipeline" procedure used by Evans and his co-workers (1977). As with the first study, there were significantly fewer new smokers among the students who had participated in the program compared to those in the control group (8 percent vs. 19 percent).

Overall, both studies demonstrated the efficacy of the LST strategy for reducing the number of new experimental smokers as well as promoting the kind of cognitive and personality changes hypothesized to be related to decreased susceptibility to pro-smoking influences. The program appears to be effective when implemented either by outside specialists or older students. Since the program is oriented around the notion of self-improvement and deals with areas of general concern to teenagers, the students have responded positively and enthusiastically to the LST program, frequently suggesting that it be extended to an entire year. Presumably the fact that students found the program interesting and relevant contributed to its success. An additional benefit of the LST program is that its emphasis on self-improvement and the acquisition of basic coping skills makes it applicable to other health-related concerns such as substance abuse and mental health.

SUMMARY AND CONCLUSION

Based on the rather extensive evidence that has been amassed since the time of the initial Surgeon General's Report (USPHS, 1964), there can be no doubt of the health hazards posed by cigarette smoking. The growing awareness of the adverse health consequences of cigarette smoking has led many adults to quit smoking. As the prevalence of smoking has decreased, the social acceptability of smoking has also decreased. Nonsmokers have become increasingly outspoken concerning their rights as nonsmokers, and some states have passed "clean indoor air" acts prohibiting cigarette smoking in certain public places.

However, notwithstanding the tremendous strides that have been made in recent years among adults, cigarette smoking among teenagers continues to be a major concern. Programs developed to prevent students from acquiring the smoking habit have generally not been rigorously evaluated and those few which have been evaluated have produced rather disappointing results. Most of these programs have attempted to dissuade students from smoking by making them aware of the deleterious effects of smoking. However, the vast majority of teenagers are fully cognizant of the dangers of smoking and still begin to smoke. Fear arousal or knowledge-based approaches do not appear to be effective means of deterring smoking onset. The more immediate social consequences of smoking appear to be more powerful for most teenagers than the kind of delayed consequences associated with health.

The reasons why some individuals become smokers while others do not are not well understood. Indeed, the process of becoming a cigarette smoker is complex and, like other forms of human behavior, undoubtedly involves the interaction of a variety of factors. Our brief review of the factors which appear to be involved in the onset of smoking indicates that sociodemographic factors, personality, knowledge, attitudes and beliefs all, to some extent, play a role. In addition, smoking has been found to be associated with several other forms of behavior. The relative importance of these various factors may vary from individual to individual. Moreover, factors relating to normal psychosocial development may potentiate pro-smoking factors, making most teenagers particularly susceptible to social (environmental) pressures to smoke.

Existing knowledge of the smoking onset process combined with an understanding of adolescence suggest that the most efficacious prevention strategies would be those that focus on the psychosocial factors promoting smoking. This may be accomplished by making teenagers aware of the social influences to smoke and decreasing their susceptibility to these influences. The three strategies discussed in this chapter are examples of the kinds of smoking prevention approaches that show the greatest potential for success. Two of the strategies discussed are based on the notion of inoculation and teach students ways of effectively coping with peer pressures to smoke. The third strategy also includes aspects of the other two approaches, but focuses primarily on teaching more general coping skills. Despite the differences among these approaches, they share a common focus in providing teenagers with the requisite skills to deal more effectively with the pressures to smoke originating from their social environment. Results of pilot studies of these techniques demonstrate at least short-term success.

Although knowledge of the long-term consequences may not play a major role in determining smoking status, it is nevertheless important that students have enough information to make an informed decision. Furthermore, knowledge of the immediate consequences of smoking along with an awareness of the actual prevalence of smoking among both adults and teenagers may help to deter smoking onset. Yet smoking prevention programs must be developed with the recognition that the various social and psychological pressures affecting teenagers may be powerful enough to override an awareness of the negative consequences of smoking as well as conventional anti-smoking attitudes and beliefs.

As our understanding of the processes through which individuals become cigarette smokers grows, it becomes increasingly clear that the complex nature of the problem requires broad and complex approaches to its solution. Beyond merely informing students of the harmful immediate and long-range consequences of smoking, they must also be taught techniques for resisting social pressures to smoke. Furthermore, students' general susceptibility to pro-smoking influences must be decreased by helping them to develop a sense of self-mastery, self-confidence, self-esteem, and independence. However, to be completely successful in promoting healthy lifestyles, it may be necessary to go beyond solutions aimed at the individual toward those which deal with the social environmental factors promoting unhealthy behaviors. Thus, the ultimate solution of the problem of cigarette smoking may require the creation of a more hopeful and healthy environment.

RECOMMENDATIONS

School Programs

Based on what we know at this time, we can confidently recommend that smoking prevention strategies similar to the ones described in this chapter should be integrated into existing school health programs. Ideally, such programs should follow a strong elementary school health education program which can provide students with reasons for not smoking as well as a sense of responsibility for their own health. Psychosocial smoking prevention programs should begin during sixth or seventh grade and continue throughout the junior high school period. Thus, beyond merely educating students about the dangers of smoking, educators should feel responsible to train students to resist social pressures and overcome personal susceptibilities toward smoking.

Community Role

In addition, parents and health professionals along with other members of the community can contribute to the prevention of cigarette smoking. Although this can be done by supporting the kind of intervention programs described above, perhaps the most important contribution would involve providing children with good nonsmoking role models by not smoking themselves. Similarly, it is important that they convey to children anti-smoking attitudes and beliefs by making their views on cigarette smoking known to them.

Finally, the likelihood that children will become cigarette smokers can be decreased by providing them with opportunities to develop a sense of self-mastery, self-confidence, and self-reliance (e.g., by participation in extracurricular activities such as sports, hobbies).

Future Research

Certainly much more research is needed in this important public health area. We need to learn more about the reasons for becoming an habitual smoker as well as the process that leads from nonsmoking to smoking. Although the psychosocial prevention strategies discussed in this chapter are among the most promising available approaches, further testing of these methods and their various components is necessary.

The length of such programs, the most effective modes of intervention, the optimal age of intervention, and the differential effect of these programs on males and females, high-risk versus low-risk students, and so on, are issues that need to be subjected to careful research. However, while it would be desirable to understand these and other issues fully, it is important to recognize that strategies do currently exist which can deter the onset of cigarette smoking in a substantial proportion of junior high school students.

REFERENCES

Albino, J., and Davis, R.: A health education program that works. *Phi Delta Kappa* 57:256–259, 1975.

Alwine, G.: If you need love, come to US—an overview of a peer counseling program in a senior high school. *J. School Health* 44:463–464, 1974.

Annis, H.M.: Patterns of intra-familial drug use. *Br. J. Addiction* 69:361–369, 1974.

Bandura, A.: *Principals of Behavior Modification.* New York: Holt, Rinehart and Winston, 1969.

Bandura, A.: *Social Learning Theory.* Englewood Cliffs, N.J.: Prentice-Hall, 1977.

Bernstein, D.A.: Modification of smoking behavior: an evaluative review. *Psychol. Bull.* 71:418–440, 1969.

Bernstein, D.A. and McAlister, A.: The modification of smoking behavior: process and problems. *Addictive Behaviors* 1:89–102, 1976.

Bewley, B., and Bland, J.: Academic performance and social factors related to cigarette smoking by school children. *Br. J. Prev. Soc. Med.* 31:18–24, 1977.

Bewley, B., Bland, J., and Harris, R.: Factors associated with the starting of cigarette smoking by primary school children. *Br. J. Prev. Soc. Med.* 28:37–44, 1974.

Borland, B.L., and Rudolph, J.P.: Relative effects of low socioeconomic status, parental smoking and poor scholastic performance on smoking among high school students. *Soc. Sci. Med.* 9:27–30, 1975.

Botvin, G., and Eng, A.: *Life Skills Training: Teacher's Manual.* American Health Foundation, 1979.

Botvin, G., and Eng, A.: The efficacy of a multi-component smoking prevention program implemented by older peer leaders. Paper presented at the annual meeting of the Eastern Psychological Association, Hartford, April, 1980.

Botvin, G., Eng, A., and Williams, C.: The ethnography of teenage cigarette smoking. Paper presented at the annual meeting of the American Public Health Association. Los Angeles, October, 1978.

Botvin, G., Eng, A., and Williams, C.: Preventing the onset of cigarette smoking through life skills training. *Prev. Med.* 9:135–143, 1980.

Bradshaw, P.W.: The problem of cigarette smoking and its control. *Informational J. Addiction* 8:353–371, 1973.

Braucht, G.N., Brakarsh, D., Follingstad, D., and Berry, K.L.: Deviant drug use in adolescence: A review of psychosocial correlates. *Psychol. Bull.* 79:92–106, 1973.

Brehm, J.: *A Theory of Psychological Reactance.* New York: Academic Press, 1966.

Cattell, R.B., and Krug, S.: Personality factor profile peculiar to the student smoker. 14:116–121, 1967.

Clausen, J.A.: Adolescent antecedents of cigarette smoking: Data from the Oakland Growth Study. *Soc. Sci. Med.* 1:357–382, 1968.

Coan, R.W.: Personality variables associated with cigarette smoking. *J. Personality Soc. Psychol.* 26:86–104, 1973.

Costanzo, P., and Shaw, M.: Conformity as a function of age level. *Child Dev.* 37:967–975, 1966.

Department of Health, Education and Welfare: Teenage Smoking: National Patterns of Cigarette Smoking, Age 12 through 18, in 1972 and 1974. DHEW Publication No. (NIH) 76-931, 1976.

Department of Health, Education and Welfare. Teenage Smoking: Immediate and Long-term Patterns, National Institute of Education, November, 1979.

Downey, A., and O'Rourke, T.: The utilization of attitudes and beliefs as indicators of future smoking behavior. *J. Drug Educ.* 6:283–295, 1976.

Eckdahl, V.: School health education project: The use of biofeedback machines in the prevention of smoking. Paper presented at the National Interagency Counsel on Smoking and Health, San Francisco, April, 1979.

Edson, L.: Schools attacking the smoking problem. *Am. Educ.* 9:10–14, 1973.

Eisinger, R.: Psychosocial predictors of smoking recidivism. *J. Health Soc. Behav.* 12:355–362, 1971.

Erickson, L., and Cramer, J.: Smoking behavior development and modification: an empirical application of three social psychological theories. *J. Appl. Soc. Psychol.* 6:369–386, 1976.

Evans, R.I.: Smoking in children: Developing a social psychological strategy of deterrence. *J. Prev. Med.* 5:122–127, 1976.

Evans, R.I., Hansen, W.B., and Mittlemark, M.B.: Increasing the validity of self-reports of smoking behavior in children. *J. Appl. Psychol.* 62:521–523, 1977.

Evans, R.I., Rozelle, R.M., Mittelmark, M.B., Hansen, W.B., Bane, A.L., and Havis, J.: Deterring the onset of smoking in children; knowledge of immediate physiological effects and coping with peer pressure, media pressure and parent modeling. *J. Appl. Soc. Psychol.* 8:126–135, 1978.

Evans, R.I., Henderson, A.H., Hill, P.C., and Raines, B.E.: Current psychological, social and educational programs in control and prevention of smoking: A critical methodological review, in Gotto and Paolelli, editors, *Atherosclerosis Rev.* 6:203–243, 1979.

Foss, R.: Personality, social influence and cigarette smoking. *J. Health and Soc. Behav.* 14:279–286, 1973.

Foster, R.: Personal communication. September, 1976.

Fracchia, J., Sheppard, C., and Merlis, S.: Early cigarette smoking and drug use: Some comments, data and thoughts. *Psychol. Rep.* 34:371–374, 1974.

Gallup Opinion Index Report #108, June, 1974, pp. 20–21.

Grigson, W.H.: Smoking: The problem and a solution. *Physical Educators* 27:11–13, 1970.

Halpern, G., and Whiddon, T.: Drug education: Solution or problem? *Psychol. Rep.* 40:372–374, 1977.

Hamburg, B.A., and Varenhorst, B.B.: Peer counseling in the secondary schools: A community mental health project for youth. *Am. J. Orthopsychiatry* 42:566–581, 1972.

Harnett, A.L.: Suggested guidelines for a high school smoking intervention clinic. *J. School Health* 43:221–224, 1973.

Hartup, W.: Peer interaction and social organization, in P. Mussen, editor, *Carmichael's Manual of Child Psychology*, 3rd ed., Vol. 2. New York: Wiley, 1970.

Hartup, W., and Louge, R.: Peers as models. *School Psychol. Dig.* 4:11–21, 1975.

Horn, D., and Waingrow, S.: Some dimensions of a model for smoking behavior change. *Am. J. Public Health* 56:20–26, 1966.

James, W.: Where did we go wrong? *J. Health, Physical Education Recreation* 43:21–22, 1972.

Jessor, R., Carman, R., and Grossman, P.: Expectations of need satisfaction and drinking patterns of college students. *Q. J. Stud. Alcohol* 29:101–116, 1968.

Kiesler, C.A., Collins, B.E., and Miller, N.: *Attitude Change: A Critical Analysis of Theoretical Approaches*. New York: John Wiley, 1969.

Kohlberg, L.: A cognitive development approach to socialization, in D. Gosline, editor, *Handbook of Socialization Theory and Research*. Chicago: Rand McNally, 1969.

Levitt, E., and Edwards, J.A.: A multivariate study of correlative factors in youthful cigarette smoking. *Dev. Psychol.* 2:5–11, 1969.

Lichenstein, E., and Danaher, B.G.: Modification of smoking behavior: a critical analysis of theory, research, and practice, in Hersen, Eisler, and Miller, editors, *Progress in Behavior Modification* Vol. 3. New York: Academic Press, 1976.

Lieberman Research, Inc.: The teenager looks at smoking. Lieberman Research, Inc., conducted for the American Cancer Society, 1969.

Maccoby, E., and Masters, J.: Attachment and dependency, in P.H. Mussen, editor, *Carmichael's Manual of Child Psychology*, 3rd ed., Vol. 2. New York: Wiley, 1970.

Matarazzo, J., and Matarazzo, R.: Smoking, in D. Sills, editor, *International Encyclopedia of the Social Sciences*, Vol. 14. New York: MacMillan and Free Press, 1968, pp. 335–340.

Matarazzo, J., and Saslow, G.: Psychological and related characteristics of smokers and nonsmokers. *Psychol. Bull.* 57:493–513, 1960.

Mausner, B., and Platt, E.S.: *Smoking: A Behavioral Analysis*. New York: Pergamon Press, 1971.

McAlister, A., Perry, C., and Maccoby, N.: Adolescent smoking: Onset and prevention. *Pediatrics* 63:650–658, 1979.

McGuire, W.J.: Inducing resistance to persuasion: Some contemporary approaches, in L. Berkowitz, editor, *Advances in Experimental Social Psychology, Vol. I. New York: Academic Press, 1964.*

McGuire, R.: Psychological components of social influence, in J.T. Tedeschi, editor, *The Social Influence Processes*. New York: Aldine-Atherton, 1972.

McKennell, A.: British research into smoking behavior, in E. Borgatta and R. Evans, editors, *Smoking, Health, and Behavior,* Chicago: Aldine Publishing Co., 1968.

McRae, C.F., and Nelson, D.M.: Youth to youth communication on smoking and health. *J. School Health* 41:445–447, 1971.

Mlott, S.R., and Mlott, Y.D.: Dogmatism and locus of control in individuals who smoke, stopped smoking and never smoked. *J. Community Psychol.* 3:53–57, 1975.

Mussen, P., Conger, J., and Kagan, J.: *Child Development and Personality,* 4th ed. New York: Harper and Row, 1974.

Newman, I.: Ninth grade smokers—two years later; University of Illinois antismoking educational study. *J. School Health* 41:497–501, 1971.

Palmer, A.B.: Some variables contributing to the onset of cigarette smoking among junior high school students. *Soc. Sci. Med.* 4:359–366, 1970.

Piaget, J.: *The Moral Judgment of the Child.* London: Routledge and Kegan Paul, 1932.

Rabinowitz, H.S., and Zimmerli, W.H.: Effects of health education program on junior high school students' knowledge, attitudes and behavior concerning tobacco use. *J. School Health* 44:324–330, 1974.

Reeder, L.G.: Sociocultural factors in the etiology of smoking behavior: An assessment, in *Research in Smoking.* NIDA Research Monograph Series, 1977.

Reynolds, C., and Nichols, R.: Personality and behavioral correlates of cigarette smoking: One year follow-up. *Psychol. Rep.* 38:251–258, 1976.

Rosner, A.: Modifying attitudes of upper elementary students toward smoking. *J. School Health* 44:97–98, 1974.

Rotter, J.B.: Generalized expectancies for internal versus external control of reinforcement, in J.B. Rotter, J.E. Chance, and E.J. Phares, editors, *Applications of a Social Learning Theory of Personality.* New York: Holt, Rinehart and Winston, 1972, pp. 260–295.

Russell, M.A.H.: Realistic goals for smoking and health: a case for safer smoking. *Lancet* 1:254–258, 1974.

Schneider, F.W., and Vanmastright, L.A.: Adolescent–pre-adolescent differences in beliefs and attitudes about cigarette smoking. *J. Psychol.* 87:71–78, 1974.

Schwartz, J.L.: A critical review and evaluation of smoking control methods. *Public Health Rep.* 84:489–506, 1969.

Smith, G.: Personality and smoking: A review of the empirical literature, in W. Hunt, editor, *Learning Mechanisms in Smoking.* Chicago: Aldine, 1970, p. 42.

Srole, L., and Fischer, A.K.: The social epidemiology of smoking behavior, 1953–1970: The midtown Manhattan study. *Soc. Sci. Med.* 7:341–358, 1973.

Tedeschi, J.T., and Bonoma, T.V.: Power and influence: An introduction, in J.T. Tedeschi, editor, *The Social Influence Processes.* New York: Aldine-Atherton, 1972, pp. 1–49.

Thomas, E.M., and Wake, F.R.: Effects of health education on smoking habits in school students: A longitudinal study, Part I—Smoking behavior and attitudes of grade 7 Ottawa students, A report to the Department of National Health and Welfare, 1969.

Thompson, E.L.: Smoking education programs. *Am. J. Public Health* 68:250–257, 1978.

U.S. Public Health Service: Smoking and Health. Report of the Advisory Committee to the Surgeon General of the Public Health Service, Center for Disease Control, PHS Publication No. 1103, 1964.

U.S. Public Health Service: Smoking and Health: A Report of the Surgeon General. U.S. Department of Health, Education and Welfare. PHS Publication No. 79-50066, 1979.

Utech, D., and Hoving, K.L.: Parents and peers as competing influences in the decisions on children of differing ages. *J. Soc. Psych.* 78:267–274, 1969.

Vriend, T.: High-performing inner-city adolescents assist low-performing peers in counseling groups. *Personnel Guidance J.* 48:897–904, 1969.

Walters, R., Marshall, W., and Shooter, J.: Anxiety, isolation, and susceptibility to social influence. *J. Personality* 28:518–529, 1960.

Williams, A.F.: Personality and other characteristics associated with cigarette smoking among young teenagers. *J. Health Soc. Behav.* 14:374–380, 1973.

Wohlford, P.: Initiation of cigarette smoking: Is it related to parent smoking behavior? *J. Consult. Clin. Psychol.* 2:148–151, 1970.

CHAPTER 7

Mechanisms in Juvenile-Onset Diabetes Mellitus: Current Concepts

HOWARD A. FISHBEIN, DR.PH   ALLAN L. DRASH, M.D.
LEWIS H. KULLER, M.D., PH.D.

Diabetus mellitus is a systemic disorder of energy metabolism with a multiplicity of probable etiological factors and with extremely variable clinical expression and course. The weight of accumulating evidence strongly supports the thesis that the term *diabetes mellitus* covers several diseases that should be considered separate and distinct entities. These would include maturity-onset diabetes, usually associated with obesity; carbohydrate intolerance associated with the aging process; carbohydrate intolerance secondary to endocrine excess, such as occurs in acromegaly and Cushing's syndrome; and insulin-deficiency diabetes, seen most typically in otherwise healthy children, but also occurring in the young adult and in patients with primary pancreatic diseases such as cystic fibrosis.

Diabetes mellitus is seen in its purest form in the child. The disease is almost invariably one of primary insulin deficiency, and the metabolic derangements are a consequence of this insulin lack. Major disturbances in carbohydrate, lipid, and protein metabolism result, which lead to predictable clinical features. Far less commonly, maturity-onset type diabetes with normal or excessive insulin levels, often associated with obesity, is also seen childhood.

THE FACES OF DIABETES IN CHILDHOOD

Transitory Neonatal Diabetes

The expression of permanent diabetes mellitus in the neonatal period is extraordinarily rare. When hyperglycemia within the first two weeks of life occurs, the syndrome of transitory neonatal diabetes (Cornblath and Schwartz, 1976) must be considered as the likely diagnosis. These infants are usually the products of difficult pregnancies with an increased incidence of maternal hypertension, proteinuria, and premature delivery. The infants are usually very small, due to both prematurity and placental insufficiency. Hyperglycemia, glucosuria, and dehydration may develop within the first few days of life. Ketonemia and ketonuria are uncommon but do occur. These infants appear to have defective insulin synthesis and/or release secondary to intrauterine malnutrition. They are exceptionally insulin-sensitive, but must be treated with insulin like any other diabetic, until such time as the islet tissue responsiveness returns to normal. This may take several weeks or two or three months. The diagnosis of the transitory syndrome can be made only in retrospect after the infants have gone into a complete remission and no longer require insulin therapy. These infants are not known to have an increased risk for later development of permanent diabetes.

Chemical Diabetes Mellitus in Childhood

It is accepted that maturity-onset diabetes represents a progression of carbohydrate intolerance from a so-called stage of prediabetes to asymptomatic chemical diabetes and eventually to overt symptomatic diabetes. Until recently, there has been little appreciation that the same or a similar course of events may be seen in the child (Rosenbloom, 1973). Based on studies by a number of investigators, 10–15 percent of the normal-weight, asymptomatic, healthy siblings of children with insulin-requiring diabetes mellitus have chemical diabetes mellitus when tested with a standard oral glucose tolerance test (Drash, 1973a). Most of these children have insulin responses to glucose and tolbutamide that are excessive when compared with those of normal children without a family history of diabetes, although decreased insulin secretion has also been reported (Drash, 1973a; Murthy, Guthrie, and Womack, 1969; Rosenbloom, 1970; Rosenbloom, Drash, and Guthrie, 1973). The mechanism for this interval of "insulin resistance" is unclear. The general opinion has been that detection of carbohydrate intolerance in the child will be followed rapidly and almost inevitably by the development of overt diabetes. This is now known not to be true. The progression from asymptomatic chemical diabetes in the child to overt diabetes is highly unpredictable. A follow-up study of more than 200 such children showed conversion to symptomatic, insulin-requiring diabetes in less than 10 percent of the group in an observation period greater than six years (Rosenbloom et al., 1973). The only apparent predictors for an accelerated course are low insulin responses to glucose challenge and a declining growth rate. Therapy during the interval of asymptomatic chemical diabetes, whether with small doses of insulin, oral sulfonylurea agents, or diet, has not been shown to be effective in altering the course of the disorder (Rosenbloom et al., 1973). HLA typing and detailed study of the immune system may prove to be of value in more definitive classification of such patients.

Obesity-Related Diabetes in Childhood

A maturity-onset type of diabetes is occasionally seen in the child (Pildes, 1973). These individuals are not invariably overweight, have high basal and stimulated insulin responses to glucose, glucagon, and arginine, and have generally mild symptoms (Drash, 1973b). Such patients make up probably less than 2 percent of the patients who developed diabetes under 16 years of age. In our experience they are most commonly black adolescent females. Their response to therapy is as frustrating and difficult as that of the classical adult maturity-onset obese patients. A very special form of obesity-related diabetes in childhood is the Prader-Willi syndrome. These are mentally retarded children with short stature, gross obesity, characteristic facial features, and an uncontrollable appetite. They have an unusual timing of adolescence, including premature but incomplete sexual development or very delayed sexual maturation, and eventually develop diabetes, usually during the adolescent years.

Gross obesity is frequently associated with asymptomatic carbohydrate intolerance. In our studies of teenagers evaluated for obesity, we find that approximately 40 percent of those who are 100 percent over ideal body weight for age and height have carbohydrate intolerance (Drash, 1973b). This is completely reversible by significant reduction in body weight (A.L. Drash et al., unpublished observations). Persistence of obesity in such patients will probably be associated with the eventual development of symptomatic diabetes. However, we have not seen such patients go on to insulin requirement during a period of observation of approximately ten years.

Cystic Fibrosis and Diabetes Mellitus

With improvement in medical care, many children with cystic fibrosis are not living into the late teens and early adult years. With this increased longevity, more and more investigators are documenting the presence of carbohydrate intolerance in children with cystic fibrosis and the development of overt diabetes in a small percentage of such patients (Lippe, Sperling, and Dooley, 1977; Handwerger and Roth, 1975). Children with cystic fibrosis who develop symptomatic diabetes usually do so in the adolescent years. They generally have mild diabetes that can be easily controlled by small doses of insulin, and ketoacidosis is uncommon. Diabetes in these individuals is considered to be secondary to the inflammatory process in the pancreas, resulting from the fibrocystic changes. In our experience, diabetes of the more usual type—that is, ketoacidosis-prone with a requirement for more standard insulin dosage—is seen more often in children with cystic fibrosis than in the population at large.

Miscellaneous Causes of Carbohydrate Intolerance in the Child

As in the adult, carbohydrate intolerance and occasionally symptomatic diabetes mellitus may be seen in the child secondary to excessive production of "anti-insulin" hormones such as growth hormone, ACTH, cortisone, epinephrine, or glucagon. The stress of an infectious disease with a temperature elevation may lead to transitory hyperglycemia and glucosuria. This is particularly true in small children following a generalized seizure and dehydration with acidosis. It is not known whether such patients have an increased likelihood of eventually developing diabetes. Follow-up studies should be carried out after the child has returned to a normal state of health. Chronic malnutrition is frequently accompanied by carbohydrate intolerance (Pimstone et al., 1975), and even in the well-nourished child inadequate carbohydrate for a few days prior to glucose tolerance testing may result in a falsely abnormal test result (Seltzer, 1970).

Classical Diabetes Mellitus in the Child

Well over 95 percent of children with diabetes mellitus have the condition that is generally referred to as juvenile diabetes mellitus. These patients have an absolute deficiency in the production of insulin, resulting in hyperglycemia and glucosuria. In addition, hypercholesterolemia and hypertriglyceridemia may be present, and in some patients there may be evidence of impaired protein synthesis. The usual clinical story includes a history of a recent respiratory illness followed by progressive polyuria, polydipsia, and polyphagia. Weight loss is common, and ketoacidosis will develop if therapy is not instituted. The duration of the clinical symptoms may vary from as little as two or three days prior to diagnosis to as long as several months. The great majority of children have a clinical history less than three weeks in duration. In our experience, ketoacidosis as a presenting complication is becoming less common. Less than 20 percent of our newly diagnosed patients require acute treatment for ketoacidosis at the time of admission. The remaining 80 percent are in varying degrees of metabolic derangement short of significant acidosis. These patients are readily managed by administration of short- or intermediate-acting insulins and dietary alteration.

EPIDEMIOLOGICAL ASPECTS

Information on both the nature and the frequency of juvenile-onset diabetes (JOD) or any other disease in the population is important. The identification of groups of people at high risk to particular diseases, coupled with observations of secular trends are helpful in developing hypotheses regarding the etiology and treatment of disease and may have implications for social policy, medical education, secondary prevention, and research strategy.

An epidemiolgic description of JOD must start with a definition of the entity. Working definitions based on current knowledge support classifying diabetes into two major types. JOD is generally an insulin dependent, relatively severe disease in which the affected individual is ketosis prone; it usually has its onset in young individuals. Maturity-onset diabetes (MOD) is generally non-insulin dependent, relatively mild (as determined by the degree of glycemia and ketosis), and shows increasing prevalence and incidence with increasing age. It should be emphasized that these are broad definitions and that within these two divisions other special types of diabetes exist. For example, it is now recognized that mild non-insulin dependent diabetes with onset in the young does occur. The term MODY (maturity onset diabetes of youth) has been given to this group of patients of mild hyperglycemia with onset during youth (West, 1978). Individuals with MODY are variable in that some are obese and some have a familial diabetes history, while others are lean with no family history of diabetes. The prevalence of MODY in any population has not been elucidated. It is likely that such ascertainment would rely greatly on criteria for defining the disorder. While recognizing the variability of diabetes, the present chapter will concentrate principally on JOD as defined above.

Descriptive Epidemiology

Prevalence studies have been conducted around the world; Table 7-1 presents some of the available data. It is apparent that international comparisons are difficult, because methods of ascertainment and age grouping differ from study to study. Very few U.S. studies exist on the prevalence and incidence of diabetes. The 1973 U.S. National Health Interview Survey (U.S. HEW, 1975) reported prevalence and incidence rates for juvenile diabetics under 17 years of age. These data were used in the National Diabetes Commission Report of 1976 (U.S. HEW, 1975). For the U.S. population under 17 years of age, roughly 20,000 new cases per year or 3 per 10,000 population was the estimated incidence rate. The prevalence rate was estimated at 13 per 10,000. These data have major problems. Participant responses in the survey was not verified through any follow-up of medical record review. Second, the survey did not attempt to distinguish between insulin dependent and insulin independent diabetics. Third, large age groupings were used in compiling the data, providing no opportunity for generation of age-specific rates.

Hospital medical records were reviewed from the 16-year period 1946 to 1961 to analyze disease patterns of children in Erie County, New York (Sultz, 1968). JOD was the most frequent disorder identified. Incident rates for children under 16 years of age varied from 0.7 to 1.1 per 10,000 population, depending on age and year. The method of study employed precluded the identification of nonhospitalized cases. Only JOD cases 16 years of age or younger were included. In another attempt at determining the frequency of JOD, Michigan's school district superintendents completed a questionnaire identifying diabetic school children (Gorwitz, 1976). A prevalence rate of 16 and an incidence rate of 1.6 per 10,000 population was reported. Major problems in ascertaining cases should also be recognized as existing in this study. Not all of the Detroit school area responded to the questionnaire; a response rate of only 75 percent was attained. In addition, the reliability of whether or not schools were aware of all diabetic children enrolled was not raised. Gorwitz did collect age-specific data and year of onset of identified cases. This had not been done in previous studies, but should be standard procedure when obtaining incidence and prevalence data. A re-

Table 7-1
Prevalence of Youth-Onset Diabetes

U.S. STUDIES

INVESTIGATORS AND YEAR OF REPORT	POPULATION	AGES	RATE PER 1,000	METHOD OF ASCERTAINMENT
National Center for Health Statistics (1973)	U.S.(representative sample)	0-16	1.3	Household interview method, 1973
Sultz, et. al. (1968)	Erie County, N.Y.	0-16	0.6	Count of known cases including records
Corwitz, et. al. (1976)	Michigan school children	5-18	1.6	Questionnaire survey of school personnel
Kyllo (1978)	Minnesota	6-18	1.89	Known cases
Palumbo, et. al. (1976)	Rochester, Minn. children	5-18	1.0	Survey of clinical records

EUROPEAN STUDIES

INVESTIGATORS AND YEAR OF REPORT	POPULATION	AGES	RATE PER 1,000	METHOD OF ASCERTAINMENT
Teuscher (1975)	Canton of Berne, Switzerland	0-19	0.59	Known cases plus urine screening
Breadmore and Reid (1966)	North Hamptonshire, England	5-16	0.8	Diagnosed cases
Wadsworth and Jarrett (1974)	Britain	11	0.1	Diagnosed cases in a cohort
Schliack (1973) cited by Wadsworth (1974)	East Germany	0-9	0.2	Diagnosed cases
		10-19	0.8	
		20-29	1.6	Registry (insulin
Lestradet	France	0-19	0.3	treated only)
Rostlapil, et. al. (1976)	Czechoslovakia	0-15	0.39	Registry
Holmgran, et. al. (1974)	Vasterbotten County, Sweden	0-15	2.2	Known cases
Christau, et. al. (1976)	Denmark	0-29	0.7	Registry

Adapted with permission from K. West, *The Epidemiology of Diabetes and Its Vascular Lesions,* Elsevier North Holland, Inc., New York, 1978.

256

analysis of the data of Gorwitz and Sultz suggested that the studies showed an increase in the incidence and prevalence of JOD over time (North, 1977). The possibility of an actual increase in frequency of diabetes deserves great attention; yet accurate longitudinal-epidemiologic studies of JOD to assess change over time are lacking.

Currently, we are aware of only two places in the U.S. where a comprehensive registry for those with JOD is being established. These programs are located in Pittsburgh, Pennsylvania, at Children's Hospital (Drash, 1979) and at the Department of Health, Diabetes Control Project, of the state of Rhode Island (Fishbein, Faich, and Belloni, 1979). Data from both of these programs will be available within the coming year. Such data bases should generate reliable frequency information. Information generated from these registries will be of considerable interest for those examining JOD etiologies. An identified group of patients with JOD will also facilitate future etiologic investigations by providing a defined population.

Genetic Considerations

The familial nature of diabetes has been noticed for centuries. There is little doubt that genetic factors are strong determinants for the development of the disease. While there is a paucity of literature available on the incidence of diabetes, the converse is true for the genetics of the disease. Although the precise mode of diabetes inheritance has remained controversial, it is clear that a single genetic mechanism is not sufficient to describe diabetes occurrence. One of the major confounding factors in studies of diabetes inheritance is the varied presentations of the disease. There is a wide spectrum of subclinical disease profiles: variance in age of onset; diverse incidence rates in different ethnic and geographic groups with no definite relationship to diet, phenotype, or residence; and perhaps most important, there is no consistent available genetic maker for the disease.

Several reports on the genetics of diabetes are based on series of hospital or clinic patients without reference to a defined population at risk (Rosenbaum, 1967; White, 1956; Rippy, 1964). Without defining the population at risk, the data and corresponding inferences gathered from one group of diabetics is specific to that group and cannot be generalized. Implications from such data may or may not be applicable to other diabetics not of the defined group. Perhaps this has been part of the explanation for the existence of many genetic hypotheses about diabetes.

Genetic heterogeneity in diabetes mellitus has been offered as the explanation for the marked familial and clinical variations of the disease. Heterogeneity implies that different genetic and/or environmental factors can produce similar phenotypes. In diabetes, multiple distinct genetic factors may result in glucose intolerance among those affected. Clinical, biochemical, pathological, and immunological findings have led researchers toward a heterogeneity viewpoint.

Historically, classic studies concluded that the diabetic genotype consisted of a double dose of one mutant gene at a single locus (Pincus and White, 1933; Allan, 1933). This simple autosomal recessive theory has recent ardent supports (Post, 1962; Steinberg, 1961; Barrai, 1965).

One alternative hypothesis to this recessive theory has been suggested (Simpson, 1962). Families which contained a juvenile onset diabetic were examined. Findings showed an increase in familial incidence of diabetes among young parents, sibs, and offspring of JOD cases. In different generations, an excess of young diabetics was found, suggesting a possible hereditary influence that predisposes to diabetes at an early age. This is an intriguing finding; for even if parents, grandparents, or great grandparents did not have diabetes, this still does not eliminate the possibility of a hereditary predisposition to diabetes. Many who were latent diabetics may have died from other causes before the disease developed. Children of these individuals may have been predisposed to diabetes even though their parents would seem to have been normal. Simpson's data do not support a single-recessive-gene hypothesis. She concluded that there is either multiple gene control or genetic heterogeneity operative in the disease inheritance.

It has been suggested (Rimoin, 1971) that if diabetes is genetically heterogeneous, many of the inconsistencies and disagreements in genetic studies could be explained. Monozygotic twins provide a natural human model for the segregation of genetic versus nongenetic factors in the etiology of diabetes. A 100 percent concordance rate for the disease would be hypothesized if the development of diabetes was determined solely by genetic factors. Various studies on twins have shown that the concordance rate falls far short of 100 percent. For example, a higher concordance for MOD diabetes in monozygotic twins then in dizygotic twins was found; however, the figures were only 70 percent versus 35 percent (Gottlieb and Root, 1968). This supports some genetic role, but suggests environment may also be acting. For JOD the concordance was even lower; 10 percent versus 3 percent in JOD monozygotic versus dizygotic twins.

When diabetes developed in the index twin before the age of 40, one-half the pairs were found to be discordant. In twins developing the disease after 40 years of age, nearly all pairs were found to be concordant (Tattersall, 1972). The high rate of concordance found in identical twins when onset in the index twin develops after age 40 attests to the strong effect of heredity on maturity onset diabetes. However, it should be noted that environmental factors often tend to be very similar in twins. In addition, obesity is recognized as being strongly genetic (Seltzer, 1968). Furthermore, the sample size used by Pyke and Tattersall was small. With sparse data available on obesity in twin studies, the degree to which concordance of maturity-onset diabetes is attributable to confounding by obesity is not clear.

Another situation in which to assess the genetic component in diabetes is to observe diabetes rates among the offspring of conjugal diabetics. Usually only 6 percent to 10 percent of the offspring are found to have overt diabetes (Ganda and Soeldner, 1977). Glucose tolerance testing shows that 25 percent to 40 percent of the offspring of conjugal diabetic parents have chemical or latent diabetes. Prevalence of diabetes in the offspring of 37 conjugal diabetic parents were investigated (Tattersall, 1975). Some families with no diabetic offspring were found, thus supporting heterogeneity. As reported, at most only 50 percent of offspring of two diabetic parents have been found to be affected (Rimoin, 1971). Obviously, these findings make the autosomal recessive theory most questionable; however, the proponents of the theory would argue that "lack of penetrance" may exist, and mutation may also account for the diverse patterns of inheritance.

Autoimmunity—Virus—HLA System

Within the past five years, the search for a genetic marker for diabetes has spawned new research avenues. Reports have shown a relationship of diabetes with alleles of the major histocompatibility system—human leukocyte antigen (HLA) locus of man. The HLA antigens are coded for by genes in the major histocompatibility complex on the sixth chromosome (see Figure 7-1). On a small part of this chromosome are located four loci: A, B, C, D. These loci control about 54 different HLA factors. An individual inherits two haplotypes; one maternal, one paternal, each of them with A, B, C, D specificities. A number of diseases (ankylosing spondylitis, psoriasis, celiac disease, and myasthenia) have been associated with increased frequencies of certain HLA antigens in patients with these diseases as compared with healthy controls. Mouse and guinea pig studies have shown that genes determining specific immune responses, and perhaps susceptibility to viral diseases, are present

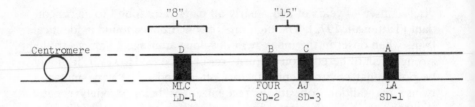

Figure 7-1. HLA region (major histocompatibility complex) on chromosome 6. Above the line are the current WHO Nomenclature Committee's designations for each locus; below the line are the previous designations.

"8" = Hypothesized approximate location of B8-associated diabetogenic gene; "15" = hypothesized approximate location of BW-15-associated diabetogenic gene.

From: Rotter, J. and Rimoin, D.: Heterogeneity in diabetes mellitus update. *Diabetes* 27:599–600, 1978. Reproduced with permission of the American Diabetes Association, Inc.

in the areas of the main histocompatibility locus (McDevitt and Benacerraf, 1969). There is evidence that the human HLA system is an important determinant of resistance or susceptibility to a variety of autoimmune and neoplastic disorders (McDevitt and Bodmer, 1974). The finding of specific HLA antigens in juvenile diabetics may suggest that viral susceptibility or autoimmune phenomena may be involved in the disease's causation.

The concept of autoimmunity in diabetes is not a new theory, but one that has aroused considerable renewed interest. Vulnerability of endocrine glands to autoimmune disease has been recognized for some time. The first pathological observations suggesting autoimmune components in diabetes mellitus were reported early in this century. The literature contains descriptions of mononuclear cell infiltration in and around the islets of Langerhans in the pancreas of patients afflicted with diabetes (Warren and Root, 1925; Stansfield and Warren, 1928). These early studies were not given much attention as the findings were thought to be rare. Pathological investigations of the pancreas of recent juvenile diabetics provided interesting data (LeCompte, 1958). LeCompte found that all four cases exhibited lymphocytic infiltration of the islets of Langerhans and suggested that these findings were not uncommon. He felt that the phenomenon was not recognized because it was not sought frequently enough. LeCompte's comparatively small study was supported by a similar large study (Gepts, 1965) that reviewed pathological findings from 54 pancreases of juvenile diabetics. Gepts concluded that mononuclear cell infiltration, mainly lymphocytes, could be found in and around the islets of Langerhans in 68 percent of the cases examined. He labeled this phenomenon as "insulitis." The pancreatic histopathological findings in recent onset JOD cases are indistinguishable from pathological findings in other organs of patients suffering from autoimmune disorders, such as Addison's disease (Nerup and Bendixen, 1969).

Indirect evidence to support the autoimmune hypothesis comes from the repeatedly documented clinical association of diabetes and known autoimmune diseases. Thyrotoxicosis (Perlman, 1961), Hashimoto's disease (Crome, Erdohaze, and Rivers, 1967), primary hypothyroidism (Ganz and Kozak, 1974), idiopathic hypoparathyroidism (Blizzard, 1969), Addison's disease (Irvine, et al., 1970), Schmidt syndrome (Carpenter, Solomon, and Silverberg, 1964), pernicious anemia (Irvine, et al., 1970), and myasthenia gravis (Osserman, 1969) have all shown a tendency to be present in patients who concurrently have diabetes. This association prompted investigators to examine specific antibody levels in patients with diabetes. The incidence of serum antibodies to thyroid, gastric, and adrenal tissue in both JOD and MOD patients was determined (Goldstein, et al., 1970). Overall, the data showed a greater incidence of thyroid and gastric antibodies in JOD cases as compared with controls. The finding was not true for the MOD patients. An increased incidence of various organ-specific antibodies in young patients with insulin dependent diabetes, particularly directed against thyroid, adrenal, and gastric cells, has been repeatedly documented (Whittingham et al., 1971; Bottazzo, Florin-Christensen, and Doniach, 1974; Fialkow, Zovala, and Neilsen, 1975). Antibody levels to thyroglobulin, thyroid cytoplasm, and gastric parietal-cell cytoplasm for diabetics and controls have been investigated (Irvine et al., 1970). Both JOD and MOD diabetics were analyzed. Among insulin dependent diabetics aged 10 to 39 years, the increased incidence of antibodies to thyroid cytoplasm and to gastric parietal-cell cytoplasm was highly significant compared to controls. Interestingly, patients aged 40 to 69 years and of insulin dependent classification also exhibited significant levels of antibodies. The antibody levels examined for those with MOD were found not to be different from levels obtained for controls.

Two thoughts are suggested by these findings. First, immunologically, JOD appears to manifest itself similarly in the young and the old. Second, the immunologic markers of autoimmune disease are more frequent in insulin-dependent diabetics than in insulin-independent diabetics. This illustrates, again, the heterogeneity existing in diabetes.

Within the last few years, other evidence in support of an autoimmune hypothesis has come from in vitro studies of cellular immunity in diabetes. The use of the leukocyte migration test (LMT) (Soborg and Bendixen, 1967) to detect cellular-type hypersensitivity has been instrumental in this work. Using the LMT (Nerup et al., 1971; MacCuish et al., 1974), the occurrence of autoimmune phenomena in insulin-dependent diabetics was reported. Insulin-induced lymphocyte transformation in six of ten newly diagnosed juvenile diabetics was also measured, four of whom never received insulin therapy (MacCuish et al., 1975). This implied that these patients had an insulin-sensitized lymphocyte population before exogenous insulin was given. Thus, cell-mediated autoimmunity to insulin may coexist with early-onset juvenile diabetes.

Viral Diseases

The search for the cause of diabetes has also included investigations of viral etiologies. Remembering the early pathological studies by Le-Compte and Gepts, the identification of a cellular infiltrate in the islets of Langerhans could be explained as a result of direct invasion of the islets by some infectious agent. An association between viral infection and diabetes has been known at least since 1899. A case of diabetes with onset shortly after mumps was perhaps the first recorded occurrence of viral-associated diabetes (Harris, 1899). There have been sporadic reports of diabetes following mumps infections documented in the literature (Hindin, 1962; Kremer, 1947). Severe juvenile-onset diabetes has also been reported in association with infectious mononucleosis (Burgess, Kirkpatrick, and Menser, 1974) and infectious hepatitis (Adi, 1974). In the past decade, much work has been undertaken of specific potential viral agents (Bloom, 1971; Craighead, 1975).

Animal models have helped to strengthen the suspected association between viral disease and induced diabetes mellitus. In the late 1960s, researchers observed hyperglycemia and pancreatic lesions of cattle infected with foot and mouth disease (Barbonic, 1966). Reports of mice infected with an M variant of the encephalomyocarditis (EMC) virus developing a diabetes-like syndrome with associated insulitis was observed (Craighead and McLane, 1968). A contagious form of diabetes mellitus has been described in a colony of guinea pigs; 50–60 percent of normal guinea pigs introduced to the colony developed diabetes within six weeks to three months (Lang, Munger, and Rapp, 1977). A search for the etiologic agent proved fruitless. The authors concluded that if diabetes was induced by a virus, the infection was probably short-lived and had been eliminated from the host sometime before clinical manifestation of the disease.

Mumps virus and members of the Coxsackie B group have been most often implicated as possible causes of juvenile diabetes. Recently, it has been shown that in vitro, human beta cells can be infected and destroyed by mumps virus (Prince et al., 1978) and Coxsackie virus B3 (Yoon and Onodera, 1978). Another recent report has investigated reovirus type 3 (Onodera et al., 1978). Infants and young children are prone to infection with this agent. The disease, however, is thought to be mild and often asymptomatic. Yet reovirus type 3 has been found to infect mouse beta cells, altering host capacity to metabolize glucose. Coxsackie-virus related work in humans further examined a suspected viral role (Craighead, 1974). Examining pancreatic tissue from infants dying with Coxsackie B4 infection, Craighead found lesions which were pathologically very similar to those reported by Gepts.

Many infectious diseases show seasonal variation. Regarding JOD, a seasonal trend in occurrence has been reported. An increase in the incidence of new JOD cases in the fall and winter with the nadir taking place in the summer has been observed (Adams, 1926; Gamble and Taylor, 1969). Seasonal variation was determined for insulin-dependent juvenile diabetics in Pittsburgh, Gainesville, Galveston, and Melbourne (Fleegler et al, 1979). The U.S. cities showed a decrease in new cases during the summer with a peak incidence in January through April. Observations of peak incidence in Melbourne were also found during the winter months. However, work by researchers in Boston (Gleason et al., 1977) suggests that this trend is slight or absent. More studies are needed to investigate this apparent trend before conclusive statements are made. Another study examined the relationship of Coxsackie virus prevalence and annual diabetes incidence (Gamble, Kinsley, and Fitzgerald, 1969). Correlations between the incidence of Coxsackie B4 infections and the incidence of JOD cases were found to be statistically significant. In another similar study, JOD patients of recent onset were examined for neutralizing antibody to Coxsackie virus types B1, B2, B3, B4, B5, and B6 (Gamble, Taylor, and Cumming, 1973). The results show that JOD cases had high neutralizing antibody titers only to Coxsackie B4 virus. Furthermore, these high titers were found to be present within three months of disease onset. Controls had a lower frequency of such antibodies. It is worthy of mention that not all studies have found an association between Coxsackie B4 virus and juvenile-onset diabetes. In some studies a negative association was found (Gamble, Taylor, and Cumming, 1973; Huff et al., 1974). Future studies inspecting Coxsackie virus infections and the occurrence of juvenile diabetes should help to clarify this relationship.

Epidemics of mumps followed by increases in deaths from diabetes have been observed (Gundersen, 1927). Interestingly, these deaths were noted only after three or four years had passed. Other data report that the incidence of diabetes parallels the incidence of mumps disease given a four-year time-lag (Sultz, 1975). Recently offspring of women who had rubella during the first trimester of pregnancy have been identified as having classical insulin-deficiency diabetes (Menser, Forrest, and Bransby, 1978). Several investigators have now confirmed the original observations, and it appears that up to 50 percent of such individuals eventually become diabetic. However, the identification of diabetes has generally not occurred prior to late adolescence or early adult life. The "lag phase" between viral exposure and clinical symptomatology of diabetes is surprisingly long and suggests the possibility of a "slow virus conversion" or delayed autoimmunity.

The degenerative changes observed in the diabetic individual could hypothetically be the result of an autoimmune response to a "slow" virus which would take from two to four years to institute damage in the pancreas. The possibility of diabetes being the result of a "slow" virus infection is intriguing. However, the hypothesis, although appealing, is as yet still conjecture. The lesions describing an "insulitis" were reported to be found in diabetics of recent onset; this would weigh against slow virus or delayed autoimmune phenomenon (Craighead, 1971; Gepts, 1965).

Possible Pathophysiologic Explanations

Assuming a viral role in the etiology of diabetes, the theoretical chain of causation could be as follows. If an individual were genetically predisposed to diabetes, a viral infection could cause irreversible change in the islets of Langerhans resulting in beta cell failure. For a normal individual (not predisposed to diabetes), infection by a virus might cause reversible damage to the beta cells followed by total regeneration. Those predisposed to diabetes may be perhaps identified by specific HLA antigens. Frequency of HLA in MOD and JOD patients provides further clues in the pattern of diabetes inheritance.

HLA antigens in MOD and JOD cases compared to normal controls found antigen BW15 significantly higher in the insulin-dependent group (Singal and Blajchman, 1973). In a similar study, increased antigens HLA B8 and BW15 in diabetics were found (Nerup et al., 1974). The results showed that most of the increase in HLA B8 originated from the JOD cases. Antigen BW15 was increased in both diabetic types with no apparent preference. In general, juvenile-onset diabetes has been associated with the findings of HLA B8 and BW15 antigens, both in the SD-2 series (B locus). A new locus (D), responsible for the mixed lymphocyte response (MLR), has been found to lie very close to the SD-2 locus on the sixth chromosome (Carpenter, 1976). A strong association of two other antigens within this series, DW3 and DW4, has been shown to exist for juvenile diabetics compared to controls (Creutzfeldt, Kobberling, and Neel, 1976; Thomsen et al., 1975). Not every study has produced a positive association between HLA types and juvenile diabetes. One study failed to find any relationship between HLA antigens and the presence of diabetes (Finkelstein et al., 1972). Interestingly, one HLA antigen, namely B7, has been associated with a reduced risk for juvenile-onset diabetes (Ludwig, Schernthaner, and Mayr, 1976). The literature reveals that this decrease in B7 occurs only in the presence of the B8 form of the disease.

Thus, for typical JOD there seem to be at least two distinct inherited forms of the disease (Rotter and Rimoin, 1978). One form is characterized by HLA B8 with increased prevalence of the DW3 allele at the D locus and a decreased frequency of B7. The second form is related to the presence of HLA BW15. The specifics of this characterization are presently being investigated. Implications suggest an association with the CW3 allele of the C locus.

One hypothesis suggests that all JOD results from a single recessive inheritance with 50 percent penetrance of the gene (Rubenstein, Suciu-Foca, and Nicholson, 1977). This hypothesis requires that two diabetogenic genes are necessary for diabetes onset. Most studies have suggested that only one HLA-associated gene is required for JOD susceptibility. Diabetes can occur if an individual has one or two B8 genes or one or two BW15 genes (Svejgaard, and Ryder, 1977). Following this trend further, an almost equal prevalence of HLA identity where both haplotypes are shared and HLA haplo-identity where only one haplotype was shared among affected siblings of JOD diabetics has been reported (Cudworth and Woodrow, 1975; Barboza et al., 1977). Clearly, these data imply that only one HLA gene in common is needed for predisposition to diabetes onset. Future HLA work investigating multiple siblings will help to unravel these inconsistencies.

An HLA role in predisposing to diabetes is likely. Specific HLA antigens seem to increase the risk for diabetes development. Pancreatic pathologic "insulitis" strongly suggests autoimmune phenomena may be operative. Antibodies to specific organs involved in proper glucose metabolism have been demonstrated. A temporal association between viral disease and diabetes onset has been intimated. Particular antibody titers seem to be higher among diabetics compared to controls. Viral agents, some capable of pancreatic destruction, may act to trigger irreversible beta cell failure and elicit diabetes.

The precise etiology of insulin-deficiency diabetes remains obscure (Drash, 1979), but evidence from a variety of sources suggests that the basic genetic alteration is a defect in immunological integrity in some way associated with the HLA system located on chromosome six. This immunological defect results in an increased likelihood of viremia and virus localization in the islet cells of the pancreas. It appears quite clear now that some cases may be a direct result of islet cell destruction secondary to virus multiplication and inflammation (Yoon et al., 1979). What percentage of new cases of insulin-deficiency diabetes are a direct result of virus infection is not clear but probably is relatively small. It is theorized that most cases result from autoimmune destruction of the beta cells either directly or as a consequence of initial viral inflammation. This indicates that major new insights into the causation and natural history of this disease should result from research activities presently underway in several centers. It is entirely clear that indiscriminate screening for diabetes mellitus in childhood in the general population is a futile and inappropriate approach if it exclusively utilizes fasting glucose, two-hour postprandial glucose, or the standard oral glucose-tolerance test. However, by selectively screening families with known insulin-dependent diabetics, valid and important observations can be made. Glucose-tolerance testing combined with HLA typing and detection of islet cell antibodies will allow for a classification of parents and siblings into various "at-risk groups." Careful observation of this population of subjects over time should allow for the dissection out of those factors that increase the likelihood of development of overt diabetes and those factors that may be in some way protective. With this information it is conceivable that intervention techniques may be possible. Theoretically, the development of a virus vaccine such as against Coxsackie B4 might prevent the development of diabetes in certain susceptible individuals. However, until much more is known about the frequency of virus-induced diabetes and its relationship to specific virus agents, the development and application of a virus vaccine is clearly premature.

Insulin-deficiency diabetes mellitus and maturity-onset diabetes are two distinctly different diseases, having different etiologies, course, and outcomes. Studies on diabetes mellitus must differentiate between the two disorders and utilize appropriate research methodology and design in order to clarify the differences and similarities.

REFERENCES

Adams, S.F.: Seasonal variation in the onset of acute diabetes. *Arch. Intern. Med.* 37:861–864, 1926.

Adi, F.: Diabetes mellitus associated with epidemic of infectious hepatitis in Nigeria. *Br. Med. J.* 1:183–185, 1974.

Allan, W.: Heredity in diabetes. *Ann. Intern. Med.* 6:1272–1274, 1933.

Barboni, E.: Observations on diabetes mellitus associated with experimental foot and mouth disease in cattle. *Arch. Vet. Ital.* 17:362–369, 1966.

Barboza, J., King, R., Noreen, H., and Yunis, E.J.: The histocompatibility (HLA) system in juvenile insulin dependent diabetic multiplex kindreds. *J. Clin. Invest.* 60:989–998, 1977.

Barrai, I., and Cann, H.: Segregation analysis of juvenile diabetes mellitus. *J. Med. Genet.* 2:8–11, 1965.

Blizzard, R.M.: Idopathic hypoparathyroidism: A probably autoimmune disease, in P.A. Miescher, and H.J. Mueller-Eberhard, editors, *Textbook of Immunopathology*, Vol. 2. New York: Grune and Stratton, 1969, pp.547–550.

Bloom, B.: Mechanism of cell-mediated immune reactions. *Adv. Immunol.* 13:104–110, 1971.

Bottazzo, G.F., Florin-Christensen, A., and Doniach, D.: Islet-cell antibodies in diabetes mellitus with auto immune polyendocrine deficiencies. *Lancet* 2:1279–1283, 1974.

Burgess, J., Kirkpatrick, K., and Menser, M.: Fulminent onset of diabetes mellitus during an attack of infectious mononucleosis. *Med. J. Aust.* 2:706–707, 1974.

Carpenter, C., Solomon, N., and Silverberg, S.: Schmidt's Syndrome (thyroid and adrenal insufficiency): A review of the literature and a report of 15 new cases including ten instances of coexistent diabetes mellitus. *Medicine* 43:153–180, 1964.

Carpenter, C.: The new HLA nomenclature. *N. Engl. J. Med.* 294:1005–1006, 1976.

Cornblath, M., and Schwartz, R.: *Disorders of Carbohydrate Metabolism in Infancy*. Philadelphia: Saunders, 1976, p. 218.

Craighead, J.E.: The role of viruses in the pathogenesis of pancreatic disease and diabetes mellitus. *Prog. Med. Virol.* 19:161–214, 1975.

Craighead, J.E., Insulitis associated with viral infection, in P.A. Basterie and W. Gepts, editors, *Immunity and Autoimmunity in Diabetes Mellitus*. New York: Elsevier North Holland Inc., 1974.

Craighead, J.E., and McLane, M.F.: Diabetes mellitus: Induction in mice by encephalomyocarditis virus. *Science* 162:913–914, 1968.

Creutzfeldt, W., Kobberling, J., and Neel, J.V., editors: *The Genetics of Diabetes Mellitus.* New York: Springer Verlag, 1976.

Crome, L., Erdohaze, M., and Rivers, R.: Fulminating diabetes with lymphocytic thyroiditis. *Arch. Dis. Child.* 42:677–681, 1967.

Cudworth, A., and Woodrow, J.: Evidence for HLA linked genes in juvenile diabetes mellitus. *Br. Med. J.* 3:133–135, 1975.

Drash, A.L. et al: A Registry for JODs. 1965–1977. In preparation.

Drash, A.L. The etiology of diabetes mellitus. *N. Engl. J. Med.* 300:1211–1213, 1979.

Drash, A.L.: Chemical diabetes mellitus in the child. *Metabolism* 22:255–267, 1973a.

Drash, A.L.: Relationship between diabetes mellitus and obesity in the child. *Metabolism* 22:337–344, 1973b.

Fialkow, P.J., Zovala, C., and Neilsen, R.: Thyroid auto-immunity: Increased frequency in relatives of insulin-dependent diabetic patients. *Ann. Intern. Med.* 83:170–176, 1975.

Finkelstein, S., et al.: No relations between HLA and juvenile diabetes. *Tissue Antigens* 2:74, 1972.

Fishbein, H., Faich, G., and Belloni, J.: Statewide Diabetes Control Project, Rhode Island Department of Health, Division of Epidemiology. *R. I. Med. J.* 62(6):229–231, 1979.

Fleegler, F., Rogers, K., Drash, A., et al: Age, sex and season of onset of juvenile diabetes in different geographic areas. *Pediatrics* 63:(3), 1979.

Gamble, D.R., Kinsley, M.L., Fitzgerald, M.G., et al.: Viral antibodies in diabetes mellitus. *Br. Med. J.* 3:627–630, 1969.

Gamble, D.R., and Taylor, K.W.: Seasonal incidence of diabetes mellitus. *Br. Med. J.* 3:631–633, 1969.

Gamble, D.R., Taylor, K.W., and Cumming, H.: Coxsackie viruses and diabetes mellitus. *Br. Med. J.* 4:260–262, 1973.

Ganda, O.P., and Soeldner, S.: Genetic, acquired, and related factors in the etiology of diabetes mellitus. *Arch. Intern. Med.* 137:461–469, 1977.

Ganz, K., and Kozak, G.P.: Diabetes mellitus and primary hypothyroidism. *Arch. Intern. Med.* 134:430–432, 1974.

Gepts, W.: Pathologic anatomy of the pancreas in juvenile diabetes mellitus. *Diabetes* 14:619–633, 1965.

Gleason, R.E., Kahn, C.B., Funk, I.B., et al.: Seasonal distribution of juvenile diabetes (JD) onset in Massachusetts, 1964–1973, Boston, MA. *Diabetes* 26:abstract H 183, 399, 1977.

Goldstein, D., Drash, A., Gibbs, J., et al.: Diabetes mellitus: The incidence of circulating antibodies against thyroid, gastric and adrenal tissue. *J. Pediatr.* 77:304–306, 1970.

Gorwitz, K., Howen, G., and Thompson, T.: Prevalence of diabetes in Michigan school-age children. *Diabetes* 25:122–127, 1976.

Gottlieb, M., and Root, H.: Diabetes mellitus in twins. *Diabetes 17:693–704, 1968.*

Gunderson, E.: Is diabetes of infectious origin? *J. Infec. Dis.* 41:197–202, 1927.

Handwerger, S., and Roth, J.: Glucose intolerance in cystic fibrosis of the pancreas. *Mod. Prob. Paediatr.* 12:172, 1975.

Harris, H.F.: A case of diabetes mellitus quickly following mumps. *Boston Med. Surg. J.* 140:465–469, 1899.

Hindin, E.: Mumps followed by diabetes. *Lancet* 1:1381, 1962.

Huff, J.C., Hierholzen, J., Farris, W., et al.: An "outbreak" of juvenile diabetes mellitus: Considerations of a viral etiology. *Am. J. Epidemiol.* 100(4):277–287, 1974.

Irvine, W.J., Clarke, B.F., Scarth, L. et al.: Thyroid and gastric autoimmunity in patients with diabetes mellitus. *Lancet* 2:163–168, 1970.

Kremer, H.: Juvenile diabetes as a sequel to mumps. *Am. J. Med.* 3:257, 1947.

Lang, C.M., Munger, B.L., and Rapp, F.: The guinea pig as an animal model of diabetes mellitus. *Laboratory Animal Science* 27(5), Part 2:789–805, 1977.

LeCompte, P.: Insulitis in early juvenile diabetes. *Arch. Pathol.* 66:450–457, 1958.

Lippe, B., Sperling, M., and Dooley, R.: Pancreatic alpha and beta cell function in cystic fibrosis. *J. Pediatr.* 90:751, 1977.

Ludwig, H., Schernthaner, G., and Mayr, W.: Is HLA-B7 a marker associated with a protective gene in juvenile onset diabetes mellitus? *N. Engl. J. Med.* 294:1006, 1976.

MacCuish, A., Jordan, J., Campbell, C.J., et al: Cell-mediated immunity in diabetes mellitus. *Diabetes* 24:36–43, 1975.

MacCuish, A., Jordan, J., Campbell, C.J., et al: Cell-mediated immunity to human pancreas in diabetes mellitus. *Diabetes* 23:693–697, 1974.

McDevitt, H.O., and Benacerraf, B.: Genetic control of specific immune responses. *Adv. Immunol.* 11:31–74, 1969.

McDevitt, H., and Bodmer, W.: HLA immune-response genes and disease. *Lancet* 1:1269–1275, 1974.

Menser, M.A., Forrest, J.M., and Bransby, R.D. Rubella infection and diabetes mellitus. *Lancet* 1:57–60, 1978.

Murthy, D.Y.N., Guthrie, R.A., and Womack, W.N.: Chemical and early overt diabetes mellitus in children. *Diabetes* 18:686, 1969.

Nerup, J., and Bendixen, G.: Anti-andrenal cellular hypersensitivity in Addison's disease. *Clin. Exp. Immun.* 5:341–353, 1969.

Nerup, J., Andersen, O., Bendixen, G., et al: Antipancreatic cellular hypersensitivity in diabetes mellitus. *Diabetes* 20:424–427, 1971.

Nerup, J., Platz, P., Andersen, O., et al: HLA antigens and diabetes mellitus. *Lancet* 2:864–866, 1974.

North, F., Gorwitz, K., and Sultz, H.: A secular increase in the incidence of juvenile diabetes mellitus. *J. Pediatr.* 91(5):706–710, 1977.

Onodera, T., Jenson, A., Yoon, J.W., et al: Virus-induced diabetes mellitus: Reovirus infection of pancreatic B cells in mice. *Science* 201:529–531, 1978.

Osserman, K.E.: Muscles, in P.A. Miescher, and M. Mueller-Eberhard, editors, *Textbook of Immunopathology,* Vol. 2. New York: Grune and Stratton, 1969, pp. 605–623.

Perlman, L.V.: Familial incidence of diabetes in hyperthyroidism. *Ann. Intern. Med.* 55:796–799, 1961.

Pildes, R.: Adult-onset diabetes mellitus in childhood. *Metabolism* 22:307–315, 1973.

Pimstone, B., Becker, D., Weinkove, C., and Mann, M.: Glucose intolerance and insulin in protein calorie malnutrition. *Mod. Prob. Paediatr.* 12:154, 1975.

Pincus, G., and White, P.: On the inheritance of diabetes mellitus. 1. An analysis of 675 family histories. *Am. J. Med. Sci.* 186(1):1933.

Post, R.H.: An approach to the question—Does all diabetes depend upon a single genetic locus? *Diabetes* 11:56–65, 1962.

Prince, G.A., Jenson, A.B., Billups, L.C., et al: Infection of human pancreatic beta cell cultures with mumps virus. *Nature* 271:158–161, 1978.

Rimoin, D.: Inheritance in diabetes mellitus. *Med. Clinic. North Am.* 55(4):807–819, 1971.

Rippy, E.L.: Juvenile diabetes: Early observations of 181 cases. *Texas Med.* 60:226, 1964.

Rosenbaum, P.: Juvenile diabetes mellitus at Charity Hospital. *St. Louis Med. Soc.* 119(10):89, 1967.

Rosenbloom, A.L.: Insulin responses of children with chemical diabetes mellitus. *N. Engl. J. Med.* 282:1228, 1970.

Rosenbloom, A.L. editor: *Metabolism* 22 (February):209–421, 1973.

Rosenbloom, A.L., Drash, A.L., and Guthrie, R.: Chemical diabetes in childhood. *Metabolism* 22:413–419, 1973.

Rotter, J., and Rimoin, D.: Heterogeneity in diabetes mellitus update, 1978. *Diabetes* 27:599–608, 1978.

Rubenstein, D., Suciu-Foca, N., and Nicholson, J.F.: Genetics of juvenile diabetes mellitus: A recessive gene closely linked to HLA D and with 50% penetrance. *N. Engl. J. Med.* 297:1036–1040, 1977.

Seltzer, C.: Physiopathology of adipose tissue. Proc. 3rd Int. Meeting of Endocrinology. J. Vague, and R. Denton, editors, *Genetics and Obesity.* Marseilles, 1968, pp. 324–344.

Seltzer, H.S.: Diagnosis of diabetes, in M. Ellenbert, and H. Rifkin, editors, *Diabetes Mellitus: Theory and Practice.* New York: McGraw-Hill, 1970, p. 437.

Simpson, N.E.: The genetics of diabetes: A study of 233 families of juvenile diabetics. *Ann. Hum. Genet.* London, 26:1–21, 1962.

Singal, D., and Blajchman, M.A.: HLA antigens, lymphocytotoxic antibodies and tissue antibodies in patients with diabetes mellitus. *Diabetes* 22:429–432, 1973.

Soborg, M., and Bendixen, G.: Human lymphocyte migration as a parameter of hypersensitivity. *Acta Med. Scand.* 181:247–256, 1967.

Stansfield, O., and Warren, S.: Inflammation involving the Islets of Langerhans in diabetes. *N. Engl. J. Med.* 198:686, 1928.

Steinberg, A.: Heredity in diabetes mellitus. *Diabetes* 10:269–274, 1961.

Sultz, H.A., Schlesinger, E., and Mosher, W.: The Erie County Survey of Long-Term Childhood Illnesses: II. Incidence and Prevalence. *Am. J. Public Health* 58:491–498, 1968.

Sultz, H.A.: Epidemiologic Evidence for Mumps Virus Etiology of Childhood Diabetes. Presented at the American Diabetes Association, 1975.

Svejgaard, A., and Ryder, L.: Associations between HLA and disease: Notes on methodology and a report from the HLA and Disease Registry, in J. Dausset, and A. Svejgaard, editors, *HLA and Disease* Copenhagen, 1977, pp. 46–71.

Tattersall, R., and Pyke, D.A.: Diabetes in identical twins. *Lancet 2:1120–1125, 1972.*

Tattersall, R., Fajans, S., and Arbor, A.: Prevalence of diabetes and glucose intolerance in 199 offspring of thirty-seven conjugal diabetic parents. *Diabetes* 24:452–462, 1975.

Thomsen, M., Platz, P., Andersen, O., et al: MLC typing in juvenile diabetes mellitus and idiopathic Addison's Disease. *Transplant Rev.* 22:125–147, 1975.

U.S. Department HEW: Report of the National Commission on Diabetes to the Congress of the U.S. Vol. III, Part 1, 19, 1975.

Warren, S., and Root, H.: The pathology of diabetes with special reference to pancreatic regeneration. *Am. J. Pathol.* 1:415, 1925.

West, K.: *The Epidemiology of Diabetes and Its Vascular Lesions,* Chapter 8, New York: Elsevier North-Holland, 1978.

West, K., editor: Symposium on epidemiology of diabetes and its macrovascular complications. *Diabetes Care* 2:63–215, 1979.

White, P.: Natural course and prognosis of juvenile diabetes. *Diabetes* 5:445–450, 1956.

Whittingham, S., Mathews, J.D., Mackay, I.R., et al: Diabetes mellitus, autoimmunity and aging. *Lancet* 1:763–767, 1971.

Yoon, J.W., and Onodera, T.: Virus-induced diabetes mellitus. *Diabetes* 27(7):778–781, 1978.

Yoon, J.W., Austin, M., Onodera, T., and Notkins, A.: Virus-induced diabetes mellitus: Isolation of a virus from the pancreas of a child with diabetic ketoacidosis. *N. Engl. J. Med.* 300:1173–1179, 1979.

CHAPTER 8

Environmental and Occupational Health

WALTER ROGAN, M.D.

In principle, all diseases caused by exposure to noxious agents in the environment are preventable. Exposure can be limited to "safe" levels, or abolished completely. In practice, there are many obstacles to achieving a totally safe environment, for either the population or the worker. Foremost is the sheer number of agents; there are at present at least 30,000 synthetic chemicals in the environment, and an additional 1,000 are introduced each year. Other agents, like asbestos, radiation, vibration, and noise, add to the total. To choose which to act on and which to tolerate involves balancing many considerations, but one aspect that is always key is the toxicity of an agent to human beings exposed to it, and the dose at which such toxicity occurs.

The identification of the toxicity of workplace or environmental exposures has historically been a clinical role; the alert practitioner has provided the first warning for most of the well-documented environmental hazards. Examples range from scrotal cancer among chimney sweeps generations ago to angiosarcoma of the liver among vinyl chloride workers in modern times. The establishment of dose-response relationships has been the job of the epidemiologist and toxicologist, and public health or regulatory action then results. In order for the practitioner to exploit his or her unique position—at the bedside—in the recognition of known or new environmentally related diseases, two principles must be kept in mind. The first is that a high "index of suspicion" for etiology must be present. This leads logically to a complete occupational history, as well as inquiry into residence, and jobs of other household members who may have brought contaminants into the home. The second is the concept of latency period. Diseases that result from environmental exposures can take up to 50 years to appear;

This chapter was prepared by Walter Rogan as an employee of the Public Health Service, U.S. Department of Health and Human Services.

therefore exposures that took place early in a patient's career or even during childhood may be important.

In this chapter, three kinds of environmental exposures and the clinical results of them will be examined. This seems more useful than a catalogue of agents and their accompanying diseases. The three agents are asbestos, lead, and the polyhalogenated hydrocarbons. Asbestos is the paradigmatic occupational hazard and has been under suspicion as a hazard outside the workplace as well. Lead is known to clinicians as a cause of encephalophathy in children and colic in painters. It too is a very widespread polutant and may be toxic at levels previously thought to be benign. The polyhalogenated hydrocarbons are a disparate group of chemicals that include certain pesticides and industrial chemicals. Some of them, such as DDT and the polychlorinated biphenyls (PCBs), have become widespread environmental pollutants, and the consequences for human health are as yet unknown.

ASBESTOS

Asbestos has been known for its fire-resistant properties for hundreds of years. Its uses as a fire retardant, insulator, and acoustical material increased rapidly over the last century, and millions of persons are alive today who were occupationally exposed to asbestos. There are now about 3,000 articles in the literature dealing with the health hazards of asbestos exposure. Two reviews have appeared in the last three years, both by experienced investigators—a book by Selikoff and Lee (1978), and a short, quite clinical article by Margaret Becklake (1976). The interested clinician is referred to these for more detailed information. In accord with current thinking, four manifestations of asbestos exposure—pulmonary parenchymal asbestosis, pleural asbestosis, asbestos-related cancer (particularly lung cancer), and diffuse malignant mesothelioma—will be treated somewhat separately. It should, of course, be borne in mind that these processes are not mutually exclusive, and more than one can and often does occur in the same person.

Epidemiology

Mr. H. Montague Murray, a British physician, performed an autopsy on an asbestos textile worker in 1900. He found extensive pulmonary fibrosis, presumably related to the patient's occupation. Although he never published the case, he did report it to the Departmental Committee on Industrial Disease of the British Parliament (Cooke, 1929). Case reports of asbestosis accumulated (Auribault, 1906; Scarpa, 1907; Pancoast, Miller, and Landis, 1918; Fahr, 1914), companies that insured asbestos workers noted increased mortality (Hoffman, 1918), and by 1924 there was recognition of asbestos as a potentially lethal hazard to those occupationally exposed (Cooke, 1924). The first epidemiologic study was begun by an insurance company in 1929; by 1930 the British Medical Inspector of Factories could report that the incidence of fibrosis was directly related to the duration of dust exposure. Haslam's *Recent Advances in Preventive Medicine* noted asbestosis in 1930; thus, potential for prevention was noted even then.

Pleural disease runs a more indolent course, in general, than does parenchymal fibrosis. Selikoff (1965) suggests that those with high exposure may die before the formation of plaques and their subsequent calcification can occur. Nevertheless, the radiographic and pathologic appearance of plaques is sufficiently striking, and their prevalence among workers sufficiently high, that the association with asbestos exposure was reported by 1943 (Siegal, Smith, and Greenburg, 1943). Because of the unusual radiographic appearance and the high prevalence among workers, calcified plaques without other obvious cause should raise a strong suspicion of previous asbestos exposure.

The occurrence of bronchogenic carcinoma in a worker with asbestosis was first noted in a 1935 case report (Lynch and Smith, 1935). The reason for publication might well have been no more than the fact that two rare diseases had occurred in one patient; lung cancer was uncommon in the 1930s. Many case reports were published over the next 20 years (e.g., Homburger, 1943; Wyers, 1949), but a causal relationship was doubted by many. In 1955, Sir Richard Doll reported on the results of a study of all coroner's autopsies among British asbestos workers (Doll, 1955). He showed that asbestos workers with 20 or more years of exposure carried approximately tenfold higher risk for lung cancer than the general population. The Mount Sinai experience with long-term surveillance of 632 asbestos workers was reported in 1964, and confirmed the elevated risk (Selikoff, Hammond, and Churg, 1968). In 1968, the Mt. Sinai group reported that cigarette smoking and asbestos exposure were more than additive in their effect on risk for lung cancer (Selikoff, Churg, and Hammond, 1964). The role of asbestos as a factor in the development of lung cancer in heavily exposed workers is now accepted as fact; controversy remains, however, about the existence of a "safe" dose and, if it exists, what it might be.

Diffuse malignant mesothelioma is another disease which, like lung cancer, has increased remarkably in incidence in this century. The first report of its occurrence in association with asbestos exposure came from south Africa in 1960 (Wagner, Sleggs, and Marchand, 1960). A most unusual aspect of this report was that mesothelioma was seen not only among workers, but also among people who lived or worked in areas near asbestos mines. The idea that asbestos represented an "environmental" hazard as well as an "occupational" one was rather startling, since asbestos is present in the environment of huge numbers of people, albeit at very low doses. Confirmatory reports of mesothelioma in workers appeared in the United States in 1963 (Mancuso and Coulter, 1963). By the late 1960s, sufficient experience in surveillance of occupationally exposed cohorts had accrued that mesothelioma was recognizable as an occupational hazard (Selikoff, 1976). In addition, case reports continued of mesothelioma in wives and offspring of workers, and in adults who, as children, had played in mine tailings (Anderson et al., 1976). In 1977, Hasan, Nash, and Kazemi reviewed the Massachusetts General Hospital experience with mesothelioma, and found that 17 of 36 cases gave a clear history of occupational exposures, half of those exposures had been for less than five years, and the latent period from termination of exposure ranged from 18 to 42 years. All but one of the "asbestos" cases were clearly mesothelioma at autopsy; few of the "non-asbestos" cases could be so confirmed.

The clinical spectrum of asbestos related disease has been outlined by Selikoff from the more than 30 years of his experience at Mt. Sinai. High exposures to susceptible people result in pulmonary fibrosis and early death from pulmonary or right heart failure. The risk of fibrosis increases with duration of exposure. Pleural calcification occurs later in the natural history, perhaps only in those somewhat resistant to the fibrotic effects. The combined effects of smoking and exposure to asbestos results in an increased risk of lung cancers that is greater than the additive effect of each agent alone. Such cancers occur in a younger age group than usual, and are distributed more toward the lower lung fields. Cancer emerges also in those somewhat resistant to fibrosis, or to those insufficiently exposed to die of it. Mesothelioma can occur with even less exposure; it seems unrelated to cigarette smoking, and the time from exposure until development of disease is very long. All of these conditions have long latency periods, and it is likely that, on the average, the lower the dose, the longer the time until disease becomes clinically apparent.

Mechanisms of Asbestos-Induced Disease

The prototype of fibrogenic dusts in the pulmonary parenchyma is silica, and the similarity of asbestosis to silicosis lead many investigators to suppose that the mechanism of fibrosis would be the same. However, not all asbestos fibers are cytotoxic to a sufficient degree to exert their effect in this way. Basically, asbestos fibers of sufficient size are unsuccessfully phagocytized by one or more macrophages. This leads to the dissolution of the cell and subsequent release of substances that recruit fibroblasts. The resulting fibrosis takes longer and is less exuberant than that produced by silica. Despite the differences between silica and asbestos, it is fibrogenic in lung tissue, and eventually fibers are captured and walled off (Selikoff and Lee, 1978, 413). Such fibers, however, continue to have carcinogenic potential (Selikoff and Lee, 1978, p. 417).

The mechanism by which asbestos produces adenocarcinoma or mesodermal tumors is not known. Asbestos fibers can and do have, absorbed to their surfaces, traces of metals and halogenated hydrocarbons. Asbestos fibers treated to remove organic residues remain able to induce neoplasia, however, and the metals fail to produce cancer in instillation experiments where asbestos is successful. It is known that various inert agents, such as fibrous glass, can produce tumors when implanted subcutaneously in animals (Pott, Huth, and Friedrichs, 1974). Fibers of different kinds of asbestos, as well as fibrous glass, or aluminum oxide whiskers, can produce pleural tumors. Coupled with epidemiologic observation, it seems that asbestos is a physical carcinogen, at least for mesothelioma. The basis of its interactive role with cigarette smoke in carcinogenesis may be through a physical action. Alternatively, absorbed chemicals, general stimulation of cell proliferation, or some other factor may be key. Long fibers are likely more fibrogenic; however, shorter fibers have not been proven to be free of tumorigenic activity (Selikoff and Lee, 1978, pp. 413–430).

Research Issues and Open Questions

The most pressing question concerning asbestos-related disease is the same for many known industrial hazards: How low an exposure is low enough? In previous years, very dusty workplace situations led to fibrosis, sometimes at an early age. As exposures have lessened and workers live longer, diseases with longer latency periods, such as lung cancer and mesothelioma, have emerged as hazards. Abolition of asbestos exposure, either in the workplace or the ambient environment, would be a task of enormous proportions if possible at all, and the benefits that accrue to society from the use of asbestos are considerable.

Open questions that remain clinically are mostly in the realm of intervention. There is some evidence that limiting exposure when restrictive disease first appears might halt progression. Whether or not cancer risk declines is not known. The cessation of cigarette smoking reduces cancer risk among those unexposed to asbestos and should do so among those exposed, but again this is not clear. Finally, the role of early detection of cancer by screening, and therapy once the diagnosis is established, need a great deal more investigation in terms of outcome before we can confidently state that they are of major benefit.

Preventive Care and Management

History. In many cases, history of exposure to asbestos is either volunteered by the patient or readily obtained through even superficial inquiry into occupations. Those who mixed or milled the fiber may even know the type of asbestos to which they were exposed. Shipbuilders and refitters and insulation workers are usually aware of exposure. Automobile repair or assembly personnel who work with gaskets, undercoatings, or brake linings may not be so aware. A more exhaustive list of potentially exposed occupations can be found in Becklake (1976). Environmental exposure, from dusty work clothes or discharge from a mine or mill, has been associated with mesothelioma.

The patient with asbestosis usually presents with dyspnea of varying degree. Morning cough is reported usually in association with cigarette smoking. Chest pain or tightness is less common (Murphy and Ferris, 1967). The patient with lung cancer, unfortunately, needs no introduction to the modern clinician. However, in the presence of a history of cigarette smoking and asbestos exposure, the diagnosis should be considered in younger patients (even the late 30s) (Selikoff and Lee, 1978, p. 270). Mesothelioma may present only after ascites or large pleural effusions have appeared. If the tumor involves a sensory nerve, it may give rise to chest pain, or it may interfere with the thoracic duct by impingement. Eventually the tumor usually causes persistent nonpleuritic chest pain (Selikoff and Lee, 1978, p. 135). Of note is that the pleural effusions seen with asbestos exposure have not been clearly shown to be harbingers of mesothelioma. Effusions may come and go and mesothelioma never develop. An effusion accompanied by pain, or by symptoms of any mass effect, however, should raise the suspicion of tumor (Eisenstadt, 1974).

Physical Examination. Basilar crepitations, or fine dry rales are a distinctive physical finding in parenchymal asbestosis. They are not cleared by cough and usually do not occur at the apices. The patient who smokes may have additional findings, such as coarse rales or rhonchi. Wheezing is not a feature. The asbestotic lung is not emphysematous, and thus no increased A-P diameter nor signs of hyperinflation should be expected. Breath sounds may be diminished, and if functional capacity of gas exchange is sufficiently comprised, hyperpnea or tachypnea may be present. Clubbing and cyanosis are present commonly in long-standing or severe disease (Murphy and Ferris, 1967).

There are no specific markers of asbestos-related lung cancer on physical examination. There seems to be a predilection for the lower lobes, perhaps for more distal locations, and for younger than usual age groups.

Pleural effusion related to mesothelioma or occurring by itself has no particular features. In the presence of mesothelioma, there may be rib retraction or restriction of movement on the affected side. Tenderness is not very common, but sometimes pain is elicited by movement of the side.

X-Ray and Laboratory Findings. The X-ray findings of asbestosis are those of fine fibrosis. Reticulation appears in the lower lobes first, and Kerley B lines may be present. The upper lobes are generally spared early in disease. More specific changes take place in the pleura: thickening, adhesions, and calcified plaques. Pleural effusion may be present in the asymptomatic patient and resolve spontaneously or be accompanied by mesothelioma. The mesothelioma itself may appear only as irregular pleural thickening or may be a shadow that appears to lie within the lung substance rather than in the pleura. As with any neoplastic intrapleural process, draining the effusion may make radiography more interpretable. Again, lung cancer in those exposed to asbestos has no specific radiographic appearance. However, the lower lobe predisposition and the younger age group should be borne in mind; in addition, some investigators note more sites of tumor more distal in the lung than usual. Almost any combination of the above findings may be present in the individual patient; the presence of one manifestation of asbestos-related disease should increase suspicion that others may be there (Preger, 1978).

Pulmonary Function Tests. Early asbestosis does not appear radiographically; changes in pulmonary function or symptoms present first. Asbestosis per se produces mostly a "restrictive" pattern of abnormalities on pulmonary function testing, although some "obstructive" elements may be present due to peribronchiolar fibrosis and the effects of cigarette smoke (Becklake, 1973). Thus, most authors report decreases in total lung volume and vital capacity, variable effects on FEV, and reduction of CO diffusing capacity. This last finding, indicating the effect of fibrosis at the alveolar capillary interface, is the earliest abnormality detectable. Its occurrence in the patient without significant other lung disease should raise suspicion of asbestos exposure.

Management and Prevention. Prevention of asbestos-related diseases rests on prevention of exposure to asbestos and elimination of cigarette smoking. The occupationally exposed person removed from a dusty environment at the stage before radiographic changes appear may suffer no progression of disease. Eliminating or reducing exposure after radiographic changes are present probably does not alter the progression of fibrosis. For lung cancer, cessation of the cigarette habit, if present, should be strongly advised, although such advice may not be taken. Alternatives, such as not allowing those who smoke to work with asbestos, and/or screening before employment for existing lung disease, have been proposed (Preger, 1978). The physician with a number of patients engaged in this type of work should seek the more detailed treatments of this subject that are available.

Prevention of exposure is not limited to workers. In the past, family members of workers and those living near mines have developed mesothelioma years later. Close attention to work practices should prevent this route.

The problem of the worker exposed long in the past and requiring care now is a vexing one (DHEW, 1978). Screening for lung cancer among such patients is without documented benefit thus far; even screening populations known to have had long-term high-dose exposure does not seem to have affected mortality. The treatment of mesothelioma is a current area of investigation at some centers (Aisner and Wiernik, 1978), but no regimen has yet emerged as effective. Another problem is in response to the occasional "accidental" exposures, from ceilings in school sprayed with asbestos and now deteriorating or from demolition (EPA, 1978). In general, chest X-ray or pulmonary function tests are not useful as measures of acute morbidity. The latency period for all asbestos-related disease is very long, and abnormalities discovered in those with very recent exposure are almost certainly due to other causes.

LEAD

Despite years of intense hazard-abatement activity, lead exposure absorption, and intoxication remains a source of morbidity. Center for Disease Control (CDC) screening programs still find 2–3 percent of screened children to be in need of chelation therapy (CDC, Environmental Health Services Division, 1978). Both scientific and regulatory interest in this long-recognized toxin continue: Ambient exposure through air and occupational exposure have been the subject of recent regulation (EPA, 1978; Department of Labor, 1978), and a rather emotional debate on so-called low-dose effects on CNS function enlivens the 1979 pediatric clinical literature. Exposure of human beings to lead elicits a wide range of toxic responses. With the exception of acute encephalopathy of childhood, however, lead is more important as a cause of morbidity than of mortality. Because effective treatment is available, the diagnosis of lead intoxication should be considered even when obvious sources for exposure are not present. When such sources are present, screening of children is clinically justified, even in the absence of symptoms.

Epidemiologic Aspects

Lead in Paint. Numerous studies have shown that older houses, painted on interior surfaces with lead-based paint, afford children the opportunity to ingest and absorb toxic amounts of lead (CDC, 1978). If enough lead is ingested, such children will eventually show both laboratory and clinical evidence of lead poisoning. The most severe form is acute lead encephalopathy, which presents as convulsions and/or coma, anemia, and vomiting. The case fatality rate varies in different series. Even with effective therapy, however, about 25–50 percent of children will be left with some neurologic residual; this is a comparable figure to long-term sequelae in any severe encephalitis of childhood. Despite the fact that etiology, epidemiology, preventive tactics, and therapy are known, about 50 children per year die of this disease in the U.S. About 15,000 children per year are hospitalized for chelation (Wessel and Dominski, 1977); they are either symptomatic or have such high levels that they are thought to be in imminent danger of becoming so.

The relationship between lead in paint and lead encephalopathy is not in doubt. The contribution of non-paint sources to body burden of lead, other morbidity that might occur due to lead, and the levels at which such morbidity occurs are all somewhat controversial.

Other Sources of Lead. The studies of CDC and others (Landrigan et al., 1976; Baker et al., 1977b) around lead smelters have shown that children's blood lead is increased in the vicinity of lead smelters and that the increase is roughly proportional to the proximity to the emission source. Decrease in the amount of lead emitted resulted in a decrease in the mean level of blood lead in children (Rosenblum et al., 1978). Air lead is absorbed at least partly through dustfall and subsequent ingestion. However, lead can also be absorbed through the respiratory tract, if particle sizes are appropriate. The "fouling the nest" (Chisholm 1978a) syndrome also contributes to children's exposure. Both male and female lead workers have been shown to carry dust home on work clothes (Baker et al., 1977a; Dolcourt et al., 1978). This dust contaminates the house, and children subsequently show increased absorption. In one case, the diagnosis of lead intoxication in a female battery worker was made only after her son was found to have elevated levels on screening (O'Tauma, Rogers, and Rogan, 1979).

Soft, acidic water can leach lead from plumbing (old plumbing [Fr. *plumbus* (lead)] was done mostly with lead pipe, thus the name) and is thought to be responsible for elevated levels occurring in part of Scotland (Beevers et al., 1976) and in older parts of Boston, Massachusetts (Greathouse, Craun, and Worth, 1976). Lead is not used in newer pipes in this country, although solder contains lead. Lead occurs as a contaminant in many foodstuffs; the exact source is unknown (Kehoe, 1960, pp. 1–17). While low-level contaminations occur, high levels are now sporadic and rare.

It is also likely that lead in ambient air contributes to lead body burden. EPA based its recent standard of 1.5 µg/l on relationship of about 2 µg/dl blood lead per 1 µg/l of air lead, when air lead is in the 1–2 µg/l range (EPA, 1978). Most airborne lead is related to automobiles: of the 268,000 metric tones emitted into the atmosphere in 1968, about 98 percent came from cars burning leaded gas (National Academy of Sciences, 1972).

Improperly glazed pottery occasionally leads to outbreaks of lead absorption. With increased awareness of the hazard, however, there will likely be fewer of these incidents. Burning batteries for home heating has resulted in increased absorption and in the transplacental intoxication of at least one child (Angle and McIntire, 1964). Moonshine whiskey is usually heavily lead contaminated, both because it is distilled in automobile radiators and leaches the solder and because it is often flocculated with lead acetate (Palmisano, Sneed, and Cassady, 1969).

Occupational exposure occurs through smelting, mining, ship breaking, and so on. A comprehensive list can be found in Chisholm (1978c).

Metabolic Studies

Intake and Output. Kehoe's (1960) extensive studies show that about 10 percent of orally administered lead is absorbed; the remainder is excreted in the feces. Iron-deficient children may absorb more. Some absorbed lead is excreted in the urine, in proportion to the amount in the blood. Some is retained and stored in both soft tissue and bone; a body burden of lead gradually accretes over years. Lead can also be absorbed from the respiratory tract.

Hematologic Toxicity. Lead produces anemia both by interference with heme production and by shortening the life span of the red cell. The effects of lead on heme production may be demonstrated biochemically at quite low levels (Chisholm, 1978b). The enzyme amino levulenate dehydratase condenses two moles of amino levulenic acid to produce porphobilinogen. Lead inhibits this step, with a resulting increase in the production of ALA, through a feedback derepression mechanism. ALA can be found in excess in the urine at blood lead levels of 20–30 μg%. Inhibition of ALA-D is the most sensitive index of lead absorption and biochemical effect; however, it is not known to have clinical significance when it occurs in isolation. The next step in heme synthesis affected by lead is the incorporation of iron into the closing ring by ferrochelatase. Inhibition leads to an accumulation of free erythrocyte protoporphyrin and then zinc protoporphyrin. This effect is detectable at lead levels of about 30 μg%, on the average, although some children show this abnormality at lead levels of 15 μg%. Elevation of ZPP need not be accompanied by anemia. Its measurement is part of the clinical evaluation of the lead-exposed child.

Lead inhibits at least one other red cell enzyme that is not part of the heme pathway: 5′ nucleotidase (Valentine et al., 1976). This enzyme varies genetically in its susceptibility to lead. The intriguing hypothesis has been made that its inhibition results in incomplete degradation of the red cell's nucleic acids, producing the basophilic stippling of the cells seen in lead poisoning.

Lead increases the fragility of red cell membranes and is also directly hemolytic, although the mechanisms of these effects are not clear (Goyer and Rhyne, 1973).

Renal Toxicity. During episodes of acute lead intoxication, there is an acute tubular dysfunction similar to Fanconi's syndrome: amino aciduria, glycosuria, and hyperphosphaturia. In those dying of lead poisoning, relatively nonspecific changes—degeneration, cloudy swelling—of proximal tubular cells occur. The glomerulus is spared. The biochemical abnormalities reverse on successful treatment, but there is not yet evidence that the morphologic lesions do so (Goyer and Rhyne, 1973). The evidence for a chronic form of renal toxicity is not clear. Although a cohort of Queensland children who were lead poisoned in childhood showed evidence of renal failure on follow-up (Goyer and Rhyne, 1973), these findings have not been confirmed in U.S. studies. Similar studies in occupationally exposed groups and in consumers of moonshine whiskey have raised suspicion of both lead-related renal disease and hypertension, but these have not been consistent. So-called saturnine gout [Latin *saturn* (lead)], described by no less an authority than Garrod, has also not yielded consistently to study. However, abnormalities of urate secretion have been described in lead intoxication, and the clinical presentation (more women, no family history, absence of associated lipid abnormalities) may differ (Goyer and Rhyne, 1973). The reasons for these many inconsistencies is probably differences in dose. The very heavy exposures that occurred early in this century have been largely eliminated, and those who accrue a heavy burden are treated. Thus patients with long-term high levels do not appear so frequently now.

Nervous System. Despite extensive study, the mechanism of the acute encephalopathy of lead remains an enigma. The most consistent findings are those of cerebral edema, and sometimes diffuse astrocytic proliferation, but even these relatively nonspecific findings are not universal. Lead is known to produce a peripheral motor neuropathy, commonly presenting as wrist drop, and perhaps a motor neuron disease, but again the mechanism is not clear. Animal studies have shown a segmental demyelinization and axonal degeneration, but this has not been well demonstrated in humans (Goyer and Rhyne, 1973).

Clinical Studies

Current clinical study of lead is focusing on the effects of low-level, environmental exposure. In children, the nervous system is thought to be most sensitive to such levels, and various manifestations of CNS or peripheral nervous system toxicity have been sought in association with lead. David, Clark, and Voeller (1972) showed that children with so-called pure hyperactivity had slightly higher lead levels than either normal children or hyperactive children whose disorder was thought to be secondary to some other cause. They then treated a group of hyperactive children with chelating agents, and found improvement, most marked in children without any obvious etiology (David et al., 1976). Landrigan and colleagues (1976) described a negative correlation between nerve conduction velocity and relatively low lead levels. However, all of the nerve conduction velocities were normal. Needleman has shown that lead body burden, as measured by dentine levels, correlates inversely with performance on various intelligence scales (Needleman et al., 1979), and Landrigan has shown a relationship between finger-tapping tests of motor performance and blood lead (Landrigan et al., 1975). None of these studies has been universally regarded as conclusive; however, responsible investigators and editorialists shy away from discounting completely the possibility that low levels of lead may have some effect on cognitive or higher cortical functioning (Lin-Fu, 1979; Anonymous, 1978). There have also been studies of blood pressure and lead levels in children, but these also have been conflicting (Rogan et al., 1978; Jhaveri et al., 1979).

"Low level" effects have also been sought in adults. Lancranjan and associates (1975) studied 150 male lead workers and found abnormalities of sperm morphology and hypospermia that was dose related. The group with the lowest levels among the exposed workers (mean level 23 μg%) still showed slight increases in abnormalities compared with controls (mean level 13 μg%). There was no evidence of pituitary dysfunction.

In females, lead has long been regarded as an abortifacient. Nogaki's (1958) study of Japanese lead workers showed about a doubling of the frequency of miscarriages after beginning work. Other studies have shown higher rates of low birth weight babies among women exposed to lead. Although there is no clear evidence of human teratogenesis for lead, various birth defects have been reported in children born to mothers with high lead levels. In addition, lead is known to cross the placenta and perhaps intoxicate the unborn child (Rom, 1976). Pregnancy is a time of relative iron deficiency and calcium deficiency, both of which increase absorption of lead; bone is also mobilized, releasing stored lead into the circulation.

Research Issues

The mechanism by which lead produces its most devastating consequences—lead encephalopathy and death—is primary; yet the difficult questions arising from low-dose exposures have great public health significance. The central question of environmental toxicology—how low is low enough?—is nowhere more vexing than when asked about lead. Intelligence, cognition, motor performance, reproduction, blood pressure are all "continuous" sorts of attributes, in the sense that an alteration in any one of them would affect (at least potentially) the whole population. Factors that affect susceptibility—genetic, nutritional, physical—have shown intriguing hints that need exploration. Although cadmium is synergistic with lead in toxicity, zinc seems antagonistic: lead toxicity may be reduced in the presence of zinc. Screening programs find higher levels in the summer months, perhaps related to sunlight-induced alterations in divalencation metabolism. Genetic variability in susceptibility probably exists (Sassa, Granick, and Kappas, 1975), but has not yet been described well.

Preventive Care and Management

History. A history of exposure to lead, from occupation, pica, moonshine, or other sources varies widely in the ease with which it is obtained. In children, it is up to the physician to expect lead exposure in the Eastern metropolitan areas. Chisholm (1978b) suggests that lists of high-risk addresses be posted in clinics where inner-city children are cared for.

Symptoms of lead intoxication are protean and nonspecific. Colic and peripheral weakness occur with high levels of exposure, but disturbances of memory, muscle pain, or anxiety may be the only symptoms present. Hyperactivity in children and disturbances in reproduction have been noted in association with lead, but the specificity of these complaints for lead exposure is probably quite low. Thus there are no pathognomonic historical syndromes of lead intoxication, except perhaps at the highest levels of exposure. Diagnosis depends on a high index of suspicion and the laboratory.

Physical Findings. There are no obvious findings specific for lead intoxication except at high levels of exposure. In adults, there are some well-described classic findings of lead poisoning. Lead lines are bluish-gray discolorations just at the gingival edge. They occur usually in association with poor dental hygiene. Wrist drop or, less commonly, peroneal nerve palsy, are not specific for lead poisoning but are consistent with that diagnosis. In children with acute lead encephalopathy, the findings are those of raised intracranial pressure as well as dehydration from associated vomiting. There are no specific findings at lower levels.

X-ray and Laboratory Findings. X-rays of the long bones in children may show "lead lines"—fine deposition at the metaphyseal plates. In children with pica, flecks of the radiodense paint chips may be seen in the GI tract. Neither of these findings is present in adults.

The diagnosis of increased lead absorption and lead poisoning, however, depends for the most part on two tests: blood lead level, and erythrocyte protoporphyrin.

Prior to the development of the hematofluorimeter, screening programs used finger stick blood leads. That test, however, is subject to contamination from finger dirt or even from paper towels used to dry the hands, and thus resulted in a high number of false positives. The hematofluorimeter measures fluorescence of zinc protoporphyrin in a monolayer of cells and is not subject to contamination. It is a micro method, and thus can be done in finger stick samples. It is specific for three conditions: erthryopoetic protoporphyria, iron deficiency, and increased lead absorption. The first is a rare hereditary condition marked by severe photosensitivity and is unlikely to pose diagnostic problems. Iron deficiency is common, but is of interest to detect. It also results in generally moderate elevations of ZPP. Elevation of ZPP due to lead begins at a lead level of about 15–30 μg% in children and continues to go up logarithmically as lead levels increase. CDC (1978) has constructed a flow chart for evaluation of children using a combination of blood lead and ZPP. Since these guidelines change, those responsible for treatment are encouraged to consult the latest CDC publication. Basically, diagnostic guidelines are based on departures from a "normal" blood lead of less than 30 μg% and a normal ZPP of less than 49 μg%.

There are other biochemical disturbances detectable in those with increased lead absorption; they are, in general, not available at most institutions and unnecessary for making the diagnosis. In particular, the presence of basophilic stippling is not a reliable indicator of increased lead absorption and should not be used either as a screening test or as a treatment criterion.

Management and Treatment. The primary therapeutic intervention in increased lead absorption is the separation of the patient from the source of lead. Chelation should be thought of as an adjunct measure when prevention has failed. Detailed guidelines for treatment of both children and adults can be found in Chisholm (1978b) and are periodically updated by CDC. In nonemergency cases, "chelatable" lead can be first estimated by a test dose of Ca EDTA, followed by a therapeutic course of Ca EDTA, BAL, or pencillamine, depending on the severity of lead absorption and the clinical presentation. In the case of children, social services and local health department personnel should be involved early, so that no child is returned from the hospital to a leaded home. For occupationally exposed adults, consultation with the responsible physician at the workplace or with management will be necessary. Nonoccupational sources must be identified so that reintoxication does not occur. Even in the absence of continued exposure, lead may be mobilized from depot tissues, so careful follow-up is necessary.

POLYHALOGENATED HYDROCARBONS

The polyhalogenated aromatic hydrocarbons of environmental importance are a diverse group of compounds that include both pesticides and industrial chemicals. The importance of this group of chemicals to environmental medicine comes not so much from their great toxicity (although some are very toxic) as from their extremely widespread occurrence and long persistence in the environment and in human tissue. The consequences for human health of the body burden of these environmental chemicals is, for the most part, unknown.

The so-called chemical age began in the middle of this century; diseases with long latencies may not yet have emerged as the result of chemical exposures. This part of the chapter will be considerably less clinical than the preceding, since clinical diseases known to result from these chemicals are generally not seen or are poorly characterized. The potential for the clinician to encounter those exposed is increasing, however, and some familiarity with the problem is becoming necessary.

Epidemiologic Studies

The epidemiologic approach to these chemicals has proceeded along many lines: the establishment of exposure, through food, water, air, and other special routes; the establishment of storage or body burden by chemical examination of blood, fat, or other body tissues; the description of toxicity in exposed persons; and the relationship of the occurrence of toxicity to dose. Chemicals are chosen for some or all of this attention because they have potential for widespread occurrence, because they are peculiarly toxic in animal systems, or because they have been associated with some disease in humans.

DDT is probably the best known of these chemicals. It was used widely for 30 years as a pesticide, but was banned in 1972, because, among other reasons, it was shown to be a carcinogen that accumulated in human tissue (Ruckelshaus, 1972). DDT resists ultimate degradation both in the environment and in tissue; it was this stability, in fact, that made repeated applications unnecessary and made it desirable as a pesticide. However, traces of DDT were transported from sites of application, remained as residues on food, and contaminated open oceans and estuaries. Since the compound has not metabolized completely, and since it is fat soluble and thus is unavailable for renal excretion, it can concentrate in a food chain. Small organisms may come to steady state with the low ambient levels, but predators absorb and store such contaminants over a lifetime (Bevenue, 1976). Man lives very high on the food chain and is long lived, and human fat has been shown to be contaminated by DDT at levels much higher than are found in the general environment. The levels of DDT found in the general population, perhaps 6–7 ppm in adipose tissue (Sobelman, 1976), are not associated with any known disease. Indeed DDT is a remarkably nontoxic substance for adult human beings, as shown both by the studies of workers and by dosed volunteers (Hayes, Dale, and Perkle, 1971; Laws, Curley, and Biros, 1967). Nevertheless, the idea that these residues are present virtually universally is disquieting, and it is difficult to believe that they convey any benefit to the population.

A second widespread group of polyhalogenated hydrocarbons is the industrial chemicals that were introduced in the 1930s. Their principal application was as an insulating fluid in large electrical transformers, where they replaced flammable mineral oil (Durfee, 1976). PCBs are essentially nonflammable, nonconductive oils that resist degradation. They were also used in capacitors and ballasts, were part of microscope immersion oil, and were the oily suspending fluid for the pigment in carbonless copy paper. No thought was given to the environmental impact of PCBs, since it was not forseen that they could or would get into the environment. However, transformers wear out and are discarded, carbonless copy paper is discarded or recycled, and PCBs gradually found their way into the environment, the food supply, and the tissues of man. PCBs are now present in trace quantities in the adipose tissue of the general population, one-third of which may have quantifiable levels (Kutz and Strassman, 1976). Again, no specific diseases have been identified that are produced by the presence of PCBs at these levels.

Other halogenated pesticides, such as oxychlordane, lindane, and benzene hexachloride, occur in trace amounts in the general population. In addition to the "background" chemicals, specific "epidemic" exposures can occur, such as the town of Hopewell, Virginia, experienced with Kepone (Cannon et al., 1978), or the entire state of Michigan with PBB (Kay, 1977). Since these chemicals are usually manufactured, formulated, applied, or otherwise handled in such a way that workers are exposed to much higher doses than the general population, it would seem to be straightforward to investigate toxicity among such groups. Sometimes this can be done, as happened in the Kepone exposure. Usually, however, large stable groups of workers who are exposed to specific chemicals are not available, and short-term study of small groups may not be informative: a relatively small increment of risk for a specific condition might well be undetectable in such a study, yet important when the actual population at risk is very large. For diseases with long latency periods, exposures may not have been present long enough for the consequences to have emerged.

Although most of the halogenated hydrocarbons to which human beings are exposed have not been extensively studied in human populations, there are data available on a few, and the findings will be reviewed here briefly.

Kepone. An illness characterized by nervousness and tremor occurring in a Kepone production worker prompted a Hopewell, Virginia, internist to submit a serum sample to the Center for Disease Control (CDC) for analysis. Kepone was identified in serum, and subsequent investigation showed that the production facility practiced poor industrial hygiene. The toxicity of Kepone, known as the "Kepone shakes" among workers, was characterized as nervousness, tremor, ataxia, and opsoclonus. Seventy-six of 133 workers experienced some or all of those signs and symptoms; in addition, many had hepatomegaly and abnormal liver function tests. Two family members also became ill, presumably from dust carried home on worker clothes (Cannon et al., 1978). Fortunately, Kepone is rather more acidic than most halogenated hydrocarbons, a property that led to successful treatment of exposed symptomatic patients with cholestyramine (Cohn et al., 1978).

Polychlorinated Biphenyls (PCBs). In 1968, an epidemic of an acnelike eruption, nausea, vomiting, and myalgias occurred in Kyushu, Japan. Investigation showed that many of those affected were heavy eaters of tempura—a Japanese dish of batter-fried fish or vegetables. In addition, many belonged to a food buying cooperative that had purchased a large lot of rice oil for cooking. Analysis of the oil at that time showed that it contained 2,000–3,000 ppm PCBs. The oil had been produced in one lot at the Krice Oil Company, where examination of the final heating vat showed leaks in the heat transfer rods. These were filled with Kanechlor 400, a Japanese PCB mixture. Eventually, cases diagnosed as having Yusho disease (oil disease) numbered over 1,100. A number of affected women were pregnant or lactating at the time of the exposure or soon afterward; an investigation of 13 such pregnancies showed one stillborn, as well as jaundice, skin pigmentation (cola color), conjunctivitis, and low birth weight (Kuratsune et al., 1972). Because of the fat soluble nature of the chemicals, they were found in the fat of breast milk; breastfed babies had somewhat higher serum values than those bottle fed. Growth of these children was retarded somewhat to age four or so, but they have subsequently returned to normal (Yoshimura and Ikeda, 1978). There is some doubt, however, as to their neurological and developmental status (Harada, 1976). The severe skin rashes present in adult cases have faded somewhat over the years, and no striking mortality pattern has yet emerged from this cohort (Urabe, Koda, and Asahi, 1978).

Polybrominated Biphenyls (PBBs). Chemical analysis of dairy cow food from a farm where the cows had sickened identified PBB as a contaminant. In 1973, Firemaster BP-6, a flame retardant, had been mixed up in shipment with Nutrimaster, a MgO_2 supplement for dairy cows. Thousands of cows, swine, and other livestock either sickened and died or were destroyed because of contamination. However, food chain contamination had already occurred; by 1976, it was estimated that 90 percent of adult Michigan residents had measurable amounts of PBB in body fat (Brilliant et al., 1978). Symptoms reported in conjunction with PBB exposure included joint pain, fatigue with secondary hypersomnia, headache, paresthesias, and insomnia. Laboratory abnormalities included elevated liver enzyme values and depression of circulating T cells. None of the signs, symptoms, or laboratory values reported, however, have shown a consistent relationship to level of the chemical in blood or in fat when fat was measured. Investigations of the long-term consequences of PBB body burden are continuing; few of the over 4,000 persons under surveillance thus far have died, and it will be years before any clear picture of morbidity and/or mortality emerges (Landrigan et al., 1978). PBBs were also found in breast milk in Michigan (Brilliant et al., 1978); although no morbidity was recognized in association with such exposure, women were offered testing and were advised not to breast feed if levels were high.

DDT. DDT appears to be a remarkably nontoxic chemical for human beings, or at least for adult males. Studies of occupationally exposed groups as well as prisoner volunteers have not demonstrated measurable toxicity even with long-term dosing. It is possible to poison a human being with DDT, but the dose required is in grams. Although probably safe in adults, the toxicity of DDT for very young children, fetuses, or pregnant women has not been investigated extensively, and again, DDT appears in breast milk (Hayes et al., 1971).

Metabolic Studies

Distribution. These compounds are readily absorbed from the GI tract, and the PCBs can be absorbed through the skin (Crow, 1970). Once absorbed, they associate with the lipid portion of the blood or are bound to plasma proteins. They distribute into fat and reach a steady state that is related to their very high lipid/water solubility coefficient; they are virtually insoluble in water. The more persistent compounds—those with higher levels of halogenation among the PCBs and PBB, and DDE, the primary metabolite of DDT—resist the attachment of the glucuronide moiety or other mechanisms for rendering them water soluble. Thus, they persist in fat and other tissues for long periods of time and can have half-lives (LD_{50}) of years to decades once they are in the fat. They do not appear in urine or feces in large amounts (Matthews et al., 1977).

Toxicity. The LD_{50} varies widely among these compounds, depending on whether the commercial mixture or specific congeners and isomers are used. The PCBs are inducers of hepatic microsomal enzymes (Alvares et al., 1977), are carcinogenic in rats (Kimbrough et al., 1975), and are known to cross the placenta. In a series of experiments on the transplacental toxicity of PCBs, James Allen at the University of Wisconsin fed female Rhesus monkeys 2.5 and 5 ppm in the total diet. The animals fed the higher doses failed to reproduce; those on the lower regimen were subfertile and produced low-birth-weight infants. On breast feeding, the infant monkeys developed chloracne and suffered increased early mortality (Barsotti, Marlar, and Allen, 1976).

PBBs have not been subjected to testing as extensively as have PCBs, but their toxicity seems broadly similar. Kepone has not been tested extensively, but it does produce excitability, increased liver to body weight ratios, and skin lesions in rodents that are comparable to the syndrome found in workers.

DDT is a hepatic enzyme inducer (Welch, Levin, and Conney, 1967) and is carcinogenic in mice (EPA, 1975). The human syndrome of excitability, tremor, and convulsions has been reproduced in animals. Other animal studies have shown such effects as adrenal atrophy (in dogs) and estrous abnormalities. These have not been investigated in detail in humans.

Clinically Related Studies

Cohn and co-workers (1978) reported on the successful treatment of Kepone poisoning with cholestyramine; he followed levels of the pesticide in abdominal fat tissue and was able to show reduction as well as symptomatic improvement.

No specific therapy has emerged from the Yusho incident for PCB poisoning, although the skin lesions, at least, have tended to decrease in severity over time (Urabe et al., 1978). PCB workers have been shown to have shortened antipyrine clearance (Alvares et al., 1977), but the levels of the chemical at which this effect occurred was not reported.

Bekesi and colleagues (1978) reported on immune function abnormalities associated with PBB exposure in Michigan farmers; the effects were mostly on levels of circulating T cells and bore no obvious relationship to level in blood or fat. There are reports of DDT intoxication in the clinical literature, but no toxicity in association with occupational or ambient exposure has been reported.

Research Issues and Open Questions. The significance of the "body burden" phenomenon of fat soluble chemicals for human health or disease is essentially unknown. Such population-based exposures are very difficult to study adequately, since there is little variability of levels in tissue in the general population. Population in very underdeveloped nations may have lower body burdens, but they also differ in many other ways from industrialized groups. A number of occupationally exposed groups are or have been under surveillance, but marked toxicity has thus far not been a feature. The fact that levels are detectable in the parts per million or even part per billion range is certainly a triumph of analytical capability, but the usefulness of these measurements in terms of disease prevention is still obscure.

Preventive Care and Management

Chloracne is the only established occupational hazard from the PCBs, but it can be caused by other halogenated hydrocarbons as well. The distribution of the lesions tends to be malar, and at the outer canthi or on areas of direct exposure. Pigmented comedones with cyst formation are the hallmarks of the disease, with somewhat less inflammation than seen in acne vulgaris (Crow, 1970). Abnormalities of liver function have been reported in the older literature in association with PCBs, but this has not been a feature of current studies. Treatment of chloracne has not been evaluated extensively, and newer methods such as the use of retinoic acid or the tetracyclines have not been reported on. Management of the person occupationally exposed to PCBs consists of recommending good work practices and the avoidance of exposure. Chloracne due to PCBs should not occur if current OSHA guidelines are respected; the physician who diagnoses chloracne should examine carefully the occupational history of the patients, seeking evidence of exposure to the PCBs, chlorinated naphthalenes, or furans or dioxins.

Kepone toxicity should no longer occur; there are no newly occupationally exposed workers. The potential for new incidents similar to the Kepone one, however, is very real, and the physician confronted with an unusual illness should keep in mind the possibility of an acute or subacute industrial intoxication.

With rare exceptions, there is no DDT available, and thus the possibility of either exposed workers or accidentally poisoned children is minimal. The significance of the body burden for adults or for exposure transplacentally is not known. The clinical sequelae of PBB absorption among Michigan residents is not known and will be under investigation for many years. Reports of altered T-cell function have not yet been confirmed, although efforts are underway.

Perhaps the most troublesome aspects of exposure to these chemicals is defining an appropriate approach to deal with the "worried exposed." Public consciousness of the real, supposed, or unknown dangers of environmental chemicals is increasing. The list of instances in which exposures to chemicals of poorly understood human toxicity increases constantly. At the Love Canal area in upstate New York, families had a black sludge of chemical waste seep into their basements from an abandoned chemical dump on which their houses were built. Residents of central North Carolina living on a 200-mile strip were exposed to PCBs that had been intentionally spilled along the roadside. Although public health officials are often involved quickly, the clinician is usually the first to see those exposed. Guidelines that apply in all instances have not been formulated. However, the physician seeing such patients early might make a significant contribution by gathering data that may later be clouded or unavailable. A careful history, taken from the viewpoint that unusual or nonspecific complaints might be due to environmental exposures, is the first step. Such a history should include detailed attention to dates of exposure as well as onset of symptoms. Any physical findings should be recorded carefully, and evanescent findings like skin rashes might be photographed. If blood or tissue is obtained for other purposes, portions might be stored for later analysis. If some effect on reproduction is suspected, then aliquots of placenta, cord or cord blood, or breast milk should be saved. The availability of these specimens might later prove invaluable in the investigation of "epidemic" exposures. Unfortunately, uncontrolled specimens are not as useful for the more widespread chemicals: PCBs, for example, are now expected contaminants of human tissue and demonstrating their presence would not be revealing.

CONCLUSIONS

Exposure to environmental toxins is now virtually ubiquitous, and accidental exposures to unusual chemicals can be expected to continue. Although increasing legislative activity has limited exposure to many agents, potential toxins are proliferating even more rapidly. The clinician may have a unique opportunity to help identify the hazards associated with the more widespread ones. Such familiarity may lead only to reassurance for the "worried exposed," but this is an appropriate function that can be enormously helpful for the individual patient.

REFERENCES

Aisner, J., and Wiernik, P.H.: Malignant mesothelioma. *Chest* 74(4): 438–444, 1978.

Alvares, A.P., Fischbein, A., Anderson, K.E., and Kappas, A.: Alternations in drug metabolism in workers exposed to polychlorinated biphenyls. *Clin. Pharmacol. Ther.* 22(2):143, 1977.

Anderson, H.A., Lilis, R., Daum, S.M., Fischbein, A.S., and Selikoff, I.J.: Household-contact asbestos neoplastic risk. *Ann. N.Y. Acad. Sci.* 271:311, 1976.

Angle, C.R., and McIntire, M.S.: Lead poisoning during pregnancy. *Am. J. Dis. Child.* 108:431, 1964.

Anonymous: Lead and mental handicap. *Lancet,* February 18:365–369, 1978.

Auribault, M.: Note sur l'hygiene et la securite des ouvriers dans les filateurs et tissages d'amiante. *Bull. Insp. Trav.* Paris 14:120, 1906.

Baker, E.L., Folland, D.S., Taylor, T.A., Frank, M., Peterson, W., Lovejoy, G., Cox, D., Houseworth, J., and Landrigan, P.J.: Lead poisoning in children of lead workers. *N. Engl. J. Med.* 296:260, 1977a.

Baker, E.L., Hayes, C.G., Landrigan, P.J., Handke, J.L., Leger, R.T., Houseworth, W.J., and Harrington, J.M.: A nationwide survey of heavy metal absorption in children living near primary copper, lead and zinc smelters. *Am. J. Epidemiol.* 106(4):261, 1977b.

Barsotti, D.A., Marlar, R.J., and Allen, J.R.: Reproductive dysfunction in Rhesus monkeys exposed to low levels of PBCB's. *Fed. Cosmet. Toxicol.* 14:99–103, 1976.

Becklake, M.R.: Asbestos-related diseases of the lung and other organs: Their epidemiology and implications for clinical practice. *Am. Rev. Respir. Dis.* 114:187–227, 1976.

Becklake, M.: Lung function, in P. Bogovski et al., editors, *Biological Effects of Asbestos. IARC Sci. Publ* 8:31, IARC, Lyon.

Beevers, D.G., Erskine, E., Robertson, M., Beattie, A.D., Campbell, B.C., Goldberg, A., and Moore, M.R.: Blood-lead and hypertension. *Lancet,* 7965:1–3, 1976.

Bekesi, J.G., Holland, J.F., Anderson, H.A., Fischbein, A.S., Rom, W., Wolff, M.S., and Selikoff, I.J.: Lymphocyte function of Michigan dairy farmers exposed to polybrominated biphenyls. *Science* 199:1207–1209, 1978.

Bevenue, A.: The "bioconcentration" aspects of DDT in the environment. *Residue Rev.* 61:37–112, 1976.

Brilliant, L.B., VanAmburg, G., Isbister, J., Humphrey, H., Wilcox, K., Eyster, J., Bloomer, A.W., and Price, H.: Breast-milk monitoring to measure Michigan's contamination with PBBs. *Lancet* 8091(2):643–646, 1978.

Cannon, S.B., Veazey, J.M., Jackson, R.S., Burse, V.W., Hayes, C., Straub, W.E., Landrigan, P.J., and Liddle, J.A.: Epidemic Kepone poisoning in chemical workers. *Am. J. Epidemiol.* 107(6):530, 1978.

CDC: Environmental evaluation and lead hazard abatement, *Preventing Lead Poisoning in Young Children,* 1978, pp. 11–12.

CDC, Environmental Health Services Division: Surveillance of childhood lead poisoning—United States. *Morbid. Mortal. Wkly. Rept.* 27(48):484–485, 1978.

Chisholm, J.J.: Fouling one's own nest. *Pediatrics* 62(4):614–617, 1978a.

Chisholm, J.J.: Treatment of lead poisoning. *Preventing Lead Poisoning in Young Children.* Atlanta: CDC, 1978b, pp. 22–40.

Cohn, W.J., Boylan, J.J., Blanke, R.V., Faris, M.W., Howell, J.R., and Philip, G.S.: Treatment of chlordecone (Kepone) toxicity with choles- tryramine: Results of a controlled clinical trial. *N. Engl. J. Med.* 298:243– 248, 1978.

Cooke, W.E., Fibrosis of the lungs due to the inhalation of asbestos dust. *Br. Med. J.* II:147, 1924.

Cooke, W.E.: Asbestos dust and the curious bodies found in pulmonary asbes- tosis. *Br. Med. J.* II: 578, 1929.

Crow, K.D.: Chloracne. *Trans. St. John's Dermatol. Soc.* 56:79–99, 1970.

David, O., Clark, J., and Voeller, K.: Lead and hyperactivity. *Lancet* 2:900– 903, 1972.

David, O., Hoffman, S.P., Sverd, J., Clark, J., and Voeller, K.: Lead and hyperactivity: Behavioral response to chelation: A pilot study. *Am. J. Psychiatry* 133(10):1155–1158, 1976.

DHEW: Statement of Secretary Joseph A. Califano, Jr., April 26, 1978.

Department of Labor, Occupational Safety and Health Administration: Occu- pational exposure to lead: Final standard. *Fed. Reg.* Part IV, November 14, 1978.

Dolcourt, J.L., Hamrick, H.J., O'Tauma, L.A., Wooten, J., and Barker, E.L.: Increased lead burden in children of battery workers: Asymptomatic exposure resulting from contaminated work clothing. *Pediatrics* 62(4): 563–566, 1978.

Doll, R.: Mortality from lung cancer in asbestos workers. *Br. J. Indust. Med.* 12:81–86, 1955.

Durfee, R.L.: Production and Usage of PCB's in the United States. Presented at the National Conference on Polychlorinated Biphenyls, November 19–21, 1975. EPA 560/6-75-004, pp. 103–107.

Eisenstadt, H.B.: Pleural effusions in asbestosis. *N. Engl. J. Med.* 290:1025, 1974.

EPA: Carcinogenicity of DDT in mice. *DDT—A Review of Scientific and Economic Aspects of the Decision to Ban its Use as a Pesticide*, 1975, pp. 83–85.

EPA: National ambient air quality standard for lead: Final rules and proposed rulemaking. *Fed. Reg.*, Part IV, October 5, 1978.

Fahr, T.: Demonstrationen: Preparate und mikrophotogrammes von einem falle von pneurumokoniose. *Muench. Med. Wochenschr.* 11:624, 1914.

Goyer, R.A., and Rhyne, B.C.: Pathological effects of lead. *Int. Rev. Exp. Pathol.* 12:30–44, 1973.

Greathouse, D.G., Craun, G.F., and Worth, D.: Epidemiologic study of the relationship between lead in drinking water and blood lead levels. *Trace Subst. Environ. Hlth.* X:9–24, 1976.

Harada, M.: Intrauterine poisoning: Clinical and epidemiologic studies and significance of the problem. *Bull. Instit. Constit. Med., Kumamoto University* XXV(Supplement):38, March 25, 1976.

Hasan, F.M., Nash, G., and Kazemi, H.: The significance of asbestos exposure in the diagnosis of mesothelioma: A 28-year experience from a major urban hospital. *Am. Rev. Respir. Dis.* 115(5):761–768, 1977.

Hayes, W.S., Dale, W.E., and Perkle, C.I.: Evidence of safety of long-term, high, oral doses of DDT for man. *Arch. Environ. Hlth.* 22:119–135, 1971.

Hoffman, F.L.: Mortality from respiratory disease in dusty trades. Inorganic dusts. *Bull. U.S. Census Bur. Labor Statist.*, No. 231, Washington, D.C.: U.S. Bureau of Labor, 1918.

Homburger, F.: The co-incidence of primary carcinoma of the lungs and pulmonary asbestosis. *Am. J. Pathol.* 19:749, 1943.

Jhaveri, R.C., Lavorgna, L., Dube, S.K., Glass, L., Khan F., and Evans, H.E.: Relationship of blood pressure to blood lead concentrations in small children. *Pediatrics* 63(4):674–676, 1979.

Kay, K.: Polybrominated biphenyls (PBB) environmental contamination in Michigan, 1973–1976. *Environ. Res.* 13(1): 74–93, 1977.

Kehoe, R.A., The Harben Lectures, 1960: The Metabolism of Lead in Man in Health and Disease. *J. Roy. Instit. Pub. Hlth. Hygiene*, pp. 1–81.

Kimbrough, R., Squire, R.A., Linder, R.E., Strandberg, J.D., Montali, F.J., and Burse, V.W.: Induction of liver tumors in Sherman strain female rats by polychlorinated biphenyl Aroclor 1260. *J. Natl. Cancer Inst.* 55:1453–1459, 1975.

Kotin, P.: The industrial medical officer and corporate responsibility, in L. Preger, editor, *Asbestos-Related Disease*. New York: Grune and Stratton, 1978, pp. 239–245.

Kuratsune, M., Yoshimura, T., Matsuzaka, J., and Yamaguchi, A.: Epidemiologic study of Yusho, a poisoning caused by ingestion of rice oil con-taminated with a commercial brand of polychlorinated biphenyls. *Envi-ron. Hlth. Perspec.* 1:125, 1972.

Kutz, F.W., and Strassman, S.C.: Residues of polychlorinated biphenyls in the general population of the United States. Presented at the National Con-ference on Polychlorinated Biphenyls. EPA, 1976, pp. 139–143.

Lancranjan, I., Popescu, H.I., Havenescu, O., Klepsch, I., and Serbanescu, M. Reproductive ability of workmen occupationally exposed to lead. *Arch. Environ. Hlth.* 30:395–401, 1975.

Landrigan, P.J., Baker, E.L., Feldman, R.G., Cox, D.H., Eden, K.V., Oren-stein, W.A., Mather, J.A., Yankel, A.J., and von Lindern, I.H.: In-creased lead absorption with anemia and slowed nerve conduction in chil-dren near a lead smelter. *J. Pediatr.* 89(6):904–910, 1976.

Landrigan, P.J., Whitworth, R., Balough, R.D., Staehling, N.D., Barthel, W.F., and Rosenblum, B.F.: Neuropsychological dysfunction in children with chronic low level lead absorption. *Lancet* 1:708–712, 1975.

Landrigan, P.J., Wilcox, K.R., Silva, J., Humphrey, H.E.B., Kaufman, C., and Heath, C.W.: Cohort Study of MI Residents Exposed to Polybromi-nated Biphenyls: Epidemiological and Immunological Findings. Presented at the New York Academy of Sciences, June, 1978.

Laws, E.R., Curley, A., and Biros, F.J.: Men with intensive occupational exposure to DDT. *Arch. Environ. Hlth.* 15:766–775, 1967.

Lin-Fu, J.S.: Lead exposure among children—a reassessment. *N. Engl. J. Med.* 300(13):731–732, 1979.

Lynch, K.M., and Smith, W.A.: Pulmonary asbestosis. III. Carcinoma of lung in asbesto-silicosis. *Am. J. Cancer* 24:56, 1935.

Mancuso, T.F., and Coulter, E.J.: Methodology in industrial health studies—the cohort approach, with special reference to an asbestos company. *Arch. Environ. Hlth.* 6:210, 1963.

Matthews, H.B., Kato, S., Morales, N.M., and Tuey, D.B.: Distribution and excretion of 2,4,5,2',4',5'-hexabromobiphenyl, the major components of Firemaster BP-6. *J. Toxicol. Environ. Hlth.* 3:599–605, 1977.

Murphy, R.L.H., and Ferris, B.G.: Manifestations of asbestosis v. duration of exposure and age. Personal communication with I.J. Selikoff, 1967; cited in Selikoff and Lee.

National Academy of Sciences, Division of Medical Sciences, National Re-search Council, Committee on Biologic Effects of Atmospheric Pollutants: Airborne Lead in Perspective, 1972.

Needleman, H.L., Gunnoe, C., Leviton, A., Reed, R., Peresie, H., Maher, C., and Barrett, P.: Psychological performance of children with elevated lead levels. *N. Engl. J. Med.* 300(13):689–695, 1979.

Nogaki, K.: On action of lead on body of lead refinery workers: Particularly conception, pregnancy and paturition in case of females and on vitality of their newborn. *Excerpta Med.* XVII 4:2176, 1958.

O'Tauma, L.A., Rogers, J.F., and Rogan, W.: Lead absorption by children of battery workers. Letter to the Editor. *JAMA* 241(18):1893, 1979.

Palmisano, P.A., Sneed, R.C., and Cassady, G.: Untaxed whiskey and fetal lead exposure. *J. Pediatr.* 75(5):869–871, 1969.

Pancoast, H.K., Miller, T.G., and Landis, H.R.M.: A roentgenologic study of the effects of dust inhalation upon the lungs. *Am. J. Roentgenol.* 5:129, 1918.

Pott, F., Huth, F., and Friedrichs, K.H.: Tumorigenic effect of fibrous dusts in experimental animals. *Environ. Hlth. Perspec.* 9:313–315, 1974.

Preger, L.: ILO U/C International Classification of radiographs of the pneumoconioses, in L. Preger, editor, *Asbestos-Related Disease.* New York: Grune and Stratton, pp. 227–238.

Rogan, W.J., Hogan, M.D., Chi, P.Y., and Cowan, D.: Blood pressure and lead levels in children. *J. Environ. Pathol. Toxicol.* 2:517–518, 1978.

Rom, W.N.: Effects of lead on the female and reproduction: A review. *Mt. Sinai J. Med.* 43(5):542–552, 1976.

Rosenblum, B.F., Kretzschmar, R., Candelaris, F., Hubert, J., Bradley, J., and Webb, C.R.: Follow-up on lead poisoning—Texas. *Morbid. Mortal. Wkly. Rept.* 27(8):57, 1978.

Ruckelshaus, W.D.: Order banning general use of DDT. EPA. *Fed. Reg.* 37(131):13369–13376, 1972.

Sassa, S., Granick, S., and Kappas, A.: Effect of lead and genetic factors on heme biosynthesis in the human red cell. *Ann. N.Y. Acad. Sci.* 244:419–440, 1975.

Scarpa, L.: Industria dell'amianto e tuberculosi. *Proc. 18th Intnatl Med. Congr.,* 1908, p. 358.

Selikoff, I.J.: Lung cancer and mesothelioma during prospective surveillance of 1249 asbestos insulation workers, 1963–1974. *Ann. N.Y. Acad. Sci.* 271:448–456, 1976.

Selikoff, I.J.: The occurrence of pleural calcification among asbestos insulation workers. *Ann. N.Y. Acad. Sci.* 132:351, 1965.

Selikoff, I.J., Churg, J., and Hammond, E.C.: Asbestos exposure and neoplasia. *JAMA* 188:22, 1964.

Selikoff, I.J., Hammond, E.C., and Churg, J.: Asbestos exposure, smoking and neoplasia. *JAMA* 204(2):206–112, 1968.

Selikoff, I.J., and Lee, D.H.K.: *Asbestos and Disease.* New York: Academic Press, 1978.

Siegal, W., Smith, A.R., and Greenburg, L.: The dust hazard in tremolite talc mining, including roentgenologic findings in talc workers. *Am. J. Roentgenol. Radium Ther.* 49:11, 1943.

Sobelman, M.: Average DDT intake and storage for humans in U.S.: For the record. Letter to the Editor. *Clin. Toxicol.* 9(1):123, 1976.

Urabe, H., Koda, H. and Asahi, M.: Present state of Yusho patients. Presented at the New York Academy of Science, June, 1978.

Valentine, W.N., Paglia, D.E., Fink, K., and Madokoro, G.: Association with hemolytic anemia, basophilic stippling, erythrocyte pyrimidine 5'-nucleotidase deficiency, and intraerythrocytic accumulation of pyrimidines. *J. Clin. Invest.* 58:926, 1976.

Wagner, J.C., Sleggs, C.A., Marchand, P.: Diffuse pleural mesothelioma and asbestos exposure in the Northwestern cape province. *Br. J. Industr. Med.* 17:160, 1960.

Welch, R.M., Levin, W., and Conney, A.M.: Insecticide inhibition and stimulation of steroid hydroxylases in rat liver. *J. Pharmcol. Exp. Ther.* 155:167, 1967.

Wessel, M.A., and Dominski, A.: Our children's daily lead. *Am. Sci.* 65(3):294, 1977.

Wyers, H: Asbestosis. *Postgrad. Med. J.* 25:631, 1949.

Yoshimura, T., and Ikeda, M.: Growth of school children with polychlorinated biphenyl poisoning or Yusho. *Environ. Res.* 17:416–425, 1978.

Index